NOBEL PRIZES

and

Nature's Surprises

NOBEL PRIZES *and* *Nature's Surprises*

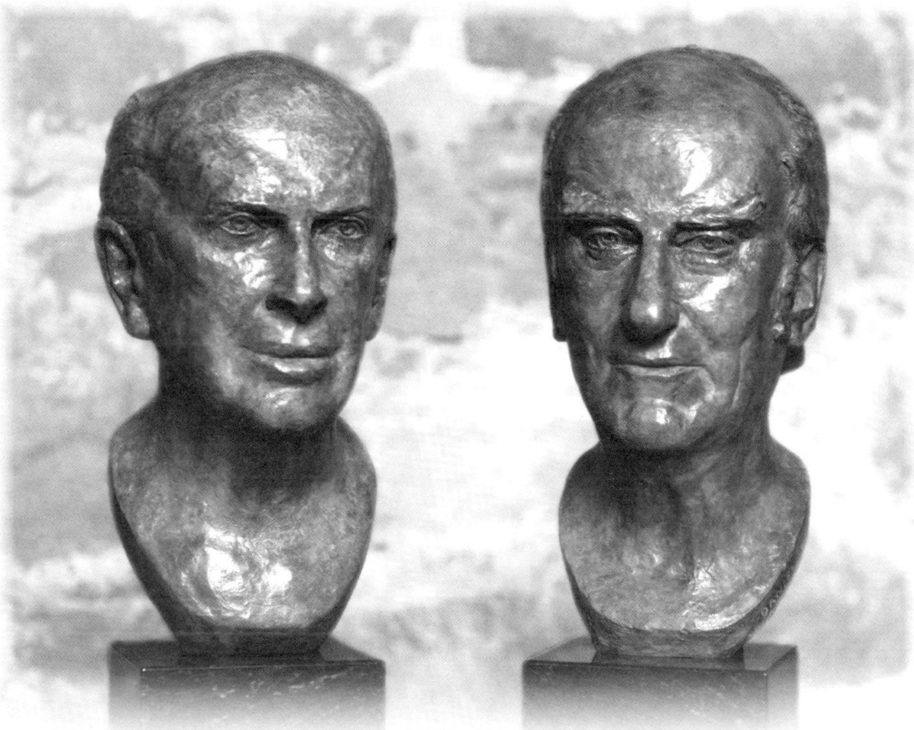

Erling Norrby

The Royal Swedish Academy of Sciences, Sweden

World Scientific

NEW JERSEY • LONDON • SINGAPORE • BEIJING • SHANGHAI • HONG KONG • TAIPEI • CHENNAI

Published by

World Scientific Publishing Co. Pte. Ltd.
5 Toh Tuck Link, Singapore 596224
USA office: 27 Warren Street, Suite 401-402, Hackensack, NJ 07601
UK office: 57 Shelton Street, Covent Garden, London WC2H 9HE

Library of Congress Cataloging-in-Publication Data
Norrby, Erling, author.
Nobel prizes and nature's surprises / by Erling Norrby.
p. ; cm.
Includes bibliographical references and index.
ISBN 978-9814520980 (hard cover : alk. paper) --
ISBN 978-9814520997 (pbk. : alk. paper)
I. Title.
[DNLM: 1. Allergy and Immunology--history. 2. Nobel Prize. 3. Biological Science Disciplines--history. 4. Biomedical Research--history. 5. History, 20th Century. QW 511.1]
QH315
570.79--dc23
2013036833

British Library Cataloguing-in-Publication Data
A catalogue record for this book is available from the British Library.

Printed in Singapore by Mainland Press Pte Ltd.

Preface

The more I have used the Nobel archives the more I have come to appreciate their unique value. It is unlikely that there is any matching historical material in any other part of the world. The invited obligatory nominations vary in comprehensibility and content, but can sometimes be very informative. The core material, however, is the reviews made by the members of the Nobel Committees, at the time the only referees used. The reviews are generally very thorough and provide the best possible evaluation to be expected from a particular Swedish scientist, who might benefit from his close interactions with other members of the committee. In order to fully interpret the proposed priorities one needs to be well familiarized with idiomatic Swedish and the traditional academic tuning of the time. Following the gradual shift and maturation of evaluations of a given candidate(s) it is possible to develop an insight into the progressive change in understanding — the gradual erosion of prevailing dogmas — with time. This is of particular interest during the sixth decade of the previous century when it was eventually appreciated that it was nucleic acids which played the critical role in information storage in biology and not the proteins. The latter instead provided structures, tools and messages for the diversified cellular functions. By use of the Nobel archives it is possible to examine this kind of revolution in real time. The relative stability of member representation in the committees during the 1950s and 1960s further substantiates the significance of the assessments in linear time.

This book is a sequel to my previous book *Nobel Prizes and Life Sciences*, but it has a different origin. The chapters have been written directly for the book, whereas in the earlier book several chapters were adaptations of review articles written for scientific journals. The time covered in the present book, with one exception, relates to the period 1960–1962, and the focus is mainly on Nobel Prizes in physiology or medicine. However the archives both at the Karolinska Institute and at the Center for the History of Science at the Royal Swedish Academy of Sciences, throughout these years have been reviewed in parallel, although among the prizes in chemistry only the one in 1962 is presented in detail. In addition, somewhat extended comments have also been given on the chemistry prizes in 1954 and 1964. It should be emphasized that as a consequence of the emergence of molecular biology in the 1950s, with time there has been an increasing overlap between candidates reviewed for a Nobel Prize in either chemistry or in physiology or medicine.

Chapter 5 presents a different time frame, since it concerns the Nobel Prize in chemistry of 1943, awarded in 1944 to Georg de Hevesy. There are several reasons for the inclusion of this chapter in the present book. It deals with the discovery of a new technique to label biological products by use of radioactive isotopes, which became an indispensable tool in the development of the field of molecular biology. In the presentation of Hevesy, a physicist, who received a Nobel Prize in chemistry, for the development of a technique with wide applications in biology, I have profited enormously from information provided by his son Georg Hevesy, Stockholm, and his son-in-law Gustaf Arrhenius, La Jolla, CA. I was also greatly helped by material from Siegfried Niese, who kindly shared with me his comprehensive biography in German of Hevesy. Additional material about Hevesy was provided by Anders Lundgren, Uppsala University. Jonas Frisén provided copies of articles to assist in describing the recent work by his research group.

The first chapter describes the Australian virologist Burnet to whom I was introduced by my predecessor in the chair of virology at the Karolinska Institute, Sven Gard. Although Gard argued very strongly throughout the 1950s for a prize in virology for Burnet, this never came about. The committee resolved the problem of acknowledging Burnet's entitlement to a prize by awarding him a shared prize in immunology in 1960. The process of writing about scientists who later receive Nobel Prizes leads to a varying degree of familiarization with each one of them.

Among the candidates discussed in this book Burnet was second in terms of such a familiarity, mostly because of his prolific writing, not only autobiographically but also about a wide range of existential problems. I am grateful to his Australian colleagues, his successor as Director of the Walter and Eliza Hall Institute, Gus Nossal, and his early student and later professorial colleague Derek Denton, for personal information about Burnet. Denton in collaboration with Suzanne Cory, kindly arranged for pictures of Burnet's

Nobel Prize gold medal and diploma, kept at the Institute. Another Australian colleague, the immunologist and Nobel Laureate Peter Doherty, kindly read some early versions of the first chapters on immunology and also generously provided some comments for the back cover of the book.

The second chapter presents Burnet's co-recipient of a Nobel Prize in 1960 for the discovery of immunological tolerance, Peter Medawar. Like Burnet he has presented himself and his thoughts on a wide range of topics on life in books. Additional comments on this prize and on these two statesmen of science have been provided by George Klein. He represents an exceptional source of information because he has been involved in the Nobel work at the Karolinska Institute since the late 1950s and in addition he has written a number of essays (mostly in Swedish) frequently involving his scientific colleagues. Also at the stage when full texts for the chapters of the book had been finalized I have continued to receive comments from colleagues with whom I have shared some texts. It is apparent that it was the Nobel Committee which took the initiative to combine Burnet and Medawar. Arthur Silverstein has pointed out to me that this initiative was taken at the time when immunological tolerance had not as yet become a scientific household word.

Thirty years had passed since the previous recognition of the discipline of immunology by a Nobel Prize when the 1960 prize to Burnet and Medawar was awarded. Since then the field has been repeatedly recognized, reflecting the major steps of advances that have been made. It was therefore decided to present these milestone advances in immunology and also to reflect on whether certain omissions might have been made. This is presented in Chapter 3. The field of immunology has indeed advanced into a very complex science and we still need to gain further understanding of the fundamentals of immune regulations to intervene rationally in the etiological process of, for example, autoimmune diseases.

The success story of managing a balanced immune suppression which has allowed successful transplantation of organs is dealt with in Chapter 4. It was discussed against the background of the widening understanding of persistent virus infections in our bodies. Doherty and Klas Kärre made some comments on both Chapters 3 and 4. Bodvar Vandvik, a neuroimmunologist, read Chapters 1 to 4 and provided some constructive criticism. He also recommended that some sections from the chapters might be taken out to form a separate concluding chapter, which finally was done. Jan Lindsten provided important information and also pictures from the work of the Nobel Committee at the Karolinska Institute during the 1970s and 1980s. He also shared important material for discussion of Georg von Békésy's interest in the arts in Chapter 6. Eva Myrdal, the director of research and documentation at the World Cultural Museums (a consortium of four museums; the World Cultural Museum in Gothenburg, and in Stockholm, the Ethnographic museum, the East Asiatic museum and the Mediterranean Museum) provided important information about the deposition at the three museums in Stockholm of the objects donated by Békésy to the Nobel Foundation. Additional information about the art at the office of the Nobel Committee at the Karolinska Institute was supplied by its secretary Göran Hansson. Bertil Hamberger provided a picture of his father, Carl-Axel Hamberger, a central figure in the developments that led to a prize to Békésy.

1962 was a particularly important year in the history of Nobel prizes in chemistry and in physiology or medicine. Two exceptionally critical advances were recognized, the principles of folding of large protein molecules and the structure of DNA. Two extensive chapters deal with these major events. Anders Liljas provided valuable information for the section on Lawrence Bragg and also shared two pictures. One of them had been taken by Ivar Olofsson, who also provided an additional picture from his own collection. Another private picture was provided by Carol Corillon. In Chapter 8 Per-Åke Albertsson provided information about Tiselius. Aaron Klug gave encouraging support to the text and kindly provided some comments for the back cover. Crick's son from his first marriage, Michael, kindly pointed out to me that in addition to the participation in the Nobel ceremonies of Crick's two daughters together with Odile Crick, he himself was also present at the Stockholm events. Wilhelm Engström provided some private archival material and also a picture of his father Arne Engström, which was eventually used in Chapter 6. Another picture of Crick and Rich was kindly made available by Shuguang Zhang. James Darnell gave perspectives on the gene concept and Istvan Hargittai provided valuable information both through his different books on Nobel Prizes and by personal exchange of information. Craig Venter generously provided comments on the composition of Chapter 8.

The person I felt that I got to know the best among all those investigated was Rosalind Franklin, although admittedly there are probably parts of her personality that might have remained hidden even to her closest friends and relatives. In the archives of the J. Craig Venter Institute there is rich material about Franklin, including several of her handwritten letters. Seeing the hand-writing of a person, although they have been dead for a long time, gives a feeling of a more immediate contact. After I had finished the writing of

Chapter 8 on the structure of DNA, I came upon one more book on Franklin, in addition to the valuable books by Anne Sayre and Brenda Maddox. It had been published in 2012 and was written by Jenifer Glynn. Its title is *My Sister Rosalind Franklin* and it is a charming book. Glynn kindly gave some comments to the text of Chapter 8, which resulted in some late minute changes. Finally, Jan Witkowsky at the Cold Spring Harbor Laboratory also gave very valuable comments on the final version of this chapter.

It is my hope that the present book will serve to further discussion about the conduct of science and about the personalities of those who pursue it. In this Preface I would like to quote from one letter, presented in Glynn's book, by Franklin to her father during her time in Paris. It provides a general illustration of the particular involvements of scientists:

> You enquire about the importance of my job. Perhaps it misleads you that it is called a job. The place where I work is purely a research establishment, and my particular work has no immediate industrial objective (some people would call it "pure research", while others argue that there is no such thing as "pure research", since all scientific advancement is ultimately useful). The position, therefore, is that I am paid and given facilities to work on my own ideas — and anybody else's I may be able to borrow. Its importance depends, of course, on what I make of it — what results I get, if any.

It is difficult to describe the position of a scientist better, and others did indeed borrow her ideas and findings!

My association with the J. Craig Venter Institute as the vice-chairman of its board of trustees has provided great benefits for the development of this book. It has been possible for me to get access to selected books of value for the work, requests kindly taken care of by Julie Adelson, and in particular to take advantage of the rich collection of archival material available at the Institute. The core of the assembled material is a part of the Jeremy Norman collection acquired by the Institute some years ago. Since the autumn of 2012 the collection has been skillfully managed by Crystal Carpenter. She has provided invaluable help in finding selected items and she has also kindly taken photographs of particular objects included in the picture material of the book.

I would also like to extend my thanks for the many pleasant contacts at World Scientific Publishing in Singapore. In particular I am grateful to its Chairman Professor Kok Khoo Phua for the confidence he has displayed in my writing about Nobel Prizes — the stories about individuals, environments and advancing frontiers of knowledge. My editor Kim Tan has provided a very efficient professional support and has arranged a pleasant working environment during my visits to Singapore. Colleagues at the Nanyang Technical University, Singapore, Bertil Andersson and Jan Vasbinder have given kind encouragement to my work.

Since English is not my native language I have had all texts read by Harry D. Watson. His insightful and expedient correcting of the texts is much appreciated. The fees for his assistance were covered by a grant from the Sven and Dagmar Salén Foundation

Many different organizations that are a part of the Nobel system have provided valuable assistance to my work. At the Nobel Foundation Jonna Petterson and her temporary substitute Siavash Pournouri kindly helped me to obtain pictures of Jim Watson taken during the Nobel Week Dialogue arranged in December 2012 and also transferred information about Nobel medals. At the Nobel Museum Olov (Olle) Amelin informed me about the busts of Watson and Crick donated to the museum in December 2012. In collaboration with him, Watson and in particular the artist Daniel Altschuler it was arranged to use pictures of the busts on the book cover. At the Karolinska Institute, the secretary of the Nobel committee for physiology or medicine, Göran Hansson, gave me permission to examine the archives that progressively became available for analysis. In the office of the committee Ann-Mari Dumanski and Tatiana Goriatcheva looked after me well during my January visits and on other occasions.

I have my office at the Center for the History of Science at the Royal Swedish Academy of Sciences. It is a very attractive working environment, not only because the Nobel Archives are 30 seconds away but in particular because of the people working at the Center. Its director Karl (Kalle) Grandin has arranged for all the support I need for my work and in particular he has spent many hours working on the table and picture materials for this book. He has always been generous with his time helping me out also when I had problems with my computer. Maria Asp, Anne Miche de Malleray, Jonas Häggblom, Åse Frid and not least my next door neighbor Bengt Jangfeldt — a great humanist, writer and intellectual sparring-partner — have all contributed to a working environment colored by happiness and engaged professional insights. An unrestricted number of diverse subjects have been discussed during coffee and lunch breaks.

My final thanks go to my family. My wife Margareta's unfailing support and endurance of my writing obsessions has made it possible to bring the project of producing this book to a conclusion. My first Nobel book was dedicated to her, but this second book I would like to dedicate to our three children Jacob, Lars (Lasse) and Christina (Titti). Their importance for the richness and joy of our life cannot be overestimated.

Contents

Chapter 8

Chapter 1

A Magician of Virology from Australia

Packages of Genes
Evolution Always at Work
Clever parasites

Nobel Prizes are rarely predictable. This is illustrated well by the 1960 prize in physiology or medicine. It recognized Frank Macfarlane Burnet and Peter Brian Medawar, two relative newcomers to the field of immunology. There was *no* nomination proposing that these candidates should receive a joint prize for their studies of immunological tolerance. The recommendation to recognize this discovery was made on a proposal by a narrow majority of the Nobel committee. This initiative made it possible to resolve a recurring problem that haunted it.

It had become apparent that Burnet should be awarded a Nobel Prize, but the problem was the richness of his different discoveries. He was clearly *the* leading virologist of his generation and he had been nominated for a prize in physiology or medicine repeatedly since 1948. Even in this first year of nomination he had been declared worthy of a prize, a pattern that continued through the following years. The many nominations focused on his various important contributions to the field of virus diseases. It was not until 1960 that, for the first time, there was a serious proposal that his theories on fundamental immunology could also serve as a basis for a prize. By way of contrast, Medawar was nominated for the first time in 1958 and again in 1960, both times for his contributions to the field of immunological tolerance.

The Shaping of a Biologist

There are excellent sources providing an insight into Burnet's rich life as a scientist. He himself wrote a book about his life called *Changing Patterns*[1] with a particular subtitle *An atypical autobiography*. He focused on his life as a visionary scientist and left out most of the different personal influences that are normally considered so decisive in the shaping of a life. He justified this approach by saying that "Like in any significant segment of biology the story of an individual is too complex, too multi-faceted to be presented satisfactorily in a smooth linear continuum of narrative." Overall Burnet was a very skilled writer and throughout his life he was to produce a very large number of scientific publications as well as several books and monographs. Many of the latter were published towards the end of his long life. It seems that writing for him was a way of sorting out his many thoughts and testing the validity of the numerous ideas that evolved in his highly efficient and capacious brain. When writing for the general public, in particular during later years, he did not mind provoking his audience. With time he did indeed build up a considerable confidence in his own intellectual capacity. In fact it seems that even during the early phase of his life he took comfort in his exceptional capacity to integrate facts and identify relationships that others had not understood. It is said that he wrote effortlessly, and that the first draft often became the final text. To someone who, like most authors, has to struggle with words and formulations to convey the proper meaning, it can only be hoped that this statement is partly a myth. Towards the later part of his life, he agreed to be interviewed by Christopher Sexton, who succeeded in establishing an informative relationship with this naturally shy and introspective scientist. Burnet was a man of paradoxes. At the same time that he was a deeply private man he was also a public figure, perhaps the best-known Australian of his generation. The insights that Sexton eventually gained materialized in a biography, originally called *The Seeds of Time*, with reference to a quote from Shakespeare's *Macbeth*, and later simply *Burnet. A Life*[2].

Burnet was born three months short of the new 20th century. On his paternal side the family originated from Scotland. His father, Frank Burnet, immigrated to Australia as a young banker in 1880. After holding various positions in different branches of the Colonial Bank of Victoria he became manager at Koroit, a minor town in the Western District of Victoria. There he met and married Hadassah Mackay who was fourteen years his junior, the daughter of an influential teacher of the town. The family moved to Traralgon, where their first child Doris was born in 1896. Sadly the delivery was attended with complications and the child was severely handicapped, something the family tried to keep secret. This had major consequences, since the mother had to spend most of her time with Doris and much less with the six children that later arrived in the family. Frank Macfarlane, the second child, was a precocious boy, who at an early stage showed a particular interest in the variety of life forms in nature. He loved to explore the valley, clearing and creek at the back of the family's home where he could catch butterflies, beetles and other creatures that stirred his interest in biology. As he grew up he became a serious collector of certain insects and enjoyed referring to the fact the he — like Darwin — was an avid coleopterist, a beetle collector. This interest became more sophisticated with time and stayed with him until age 30 or so.

During his first school years it was already apparent that Macfarlane, later in life generally referred to as Mac, was an exceptional student, quick in learning and with an impressive memory. He was a prodigious reader and devoured the older edition of *Chambers's Encyclopaedia* available in the sparse library of his home. Although his relationship with both his father and his mother has been said to be rather awkward, they did recognize his cleverness and stimulated him by subscribing to the fortnightly parts of the *Harmsworth Natural History*. The family was, in good Scottish tradition, Presbyterian and the Reverend of the community to which it belonged, Samuel Frazer, quickly recognized the talented young boy. He gave him the book *Ants and Their Ways* and also said to Macfarlane's father "Burnet, you must educate that boy." So Macfarlane got a scholarship and, in 1913, he started at Geelong College as the only full time boarder. He compensated for his natural timidity by excelling at school. Of course he also wanted to do well in sports, but except for some temporary success in becoming a member of the rowing team during the college years, that was not for him. Still he was well-built and good-looking. In 1916 he graduated as number one of his class — the Scottish term is "dux" — and it was clear that he should go on to university. The three obvious main options were theology, law or medicine. The contrasting influences of his growing religious scepticism and evolving interest in biology made medicine a natural choice. The move to Ormond College, one of the oldest residential colleges on the campus of the University of Melbourne and operated by the Presbyterian Church, opened new degrees of freedom for Macfarlane. The impressive developments of his faculties can be illustrated by a citation from Sexton's book:

> At the start of his second year, Burnet had already developed a commanding power of abstract thought, coupled with an unbridled desire to enquire into a broad range of philosophical and social issues. With his sharp wit and lucid intelligence, he had acquired a prose style of unobtrusive elegance which, though occasionally bordering on the esoteric or sentimental, equipped him to state profound things with a remarkable simplicity. His were the powers of cool, inexorable logic and serene observation and, as intellect united with sensibility, their harnessing in tandem prefigured the writer and thinker that he was destined to become.

Yet he was still the boy, now young man, who loved to get close to nature, as illustrated by another citation from the same book.

> Armed with a big, black umbrella, he would while away the afternoon collecting beetles, shaking the more easily reached eucalyptus branches whereupon an assortment of bugs and other insects would hopefully fall on to the open inverted umbrella. Out in the hot sun and open air, he relished the seclusion and permanence of the local bush; soothed by its familiar sounds and smells, almost a kindred soul. As if under some glorious, hypnotic power, all his self-doubts and fears of the future suddenly evaporated as he aimlessly wandered through the underwood.

He managed his studies without effort and the time came to decide on his future course. Patient-oriented bedside medicine did not seem suited to his shy personality. In addition, at an early stage, he developed an ambitious goal to improve the human condition at large and, as a consequence, he confided to his diary in 1921 that his major goal was "to become a member of a medical institute and make good therein". However, he first had to finish his internship. He did well in surgery and became intrigued by neurology and even contemplated for a while whether he should engage in that clinical discipline. In fact towards the end of his residency, he applied for a position as medical registrar. This was the only position he applied for in his life, and he was rejected. A wise supervisor reflecting on Burnet's unique qualities suggested that, if he agreed to withdraw his application, a position opening up in pathology a few months later would be reserved for him. The supervisor understood that Burnet fitted the laboratory and that his inclination was towards generating new knowledge in a research setting. In Burnet's own words, he took to laboratory work like "a duck to water". In March 1923 Burnet entered, for the first time, the portals of the Walter and Eliza Hall Institute of Medical Research, where during the coming four decades he would develop his unique capabilities. This is the second oldest (1915) institute for medical research in Australia and it is located close to the Royal Melbourne Hospital. The crest selected for the institute bears the insignia *Fiat lux* — the beginning of the Old Testament meaning "let there be light". As Burnet began his laboratory work there were a number of routine procedures to learn, but his brain was already ticking, searching for problems to solve. Within a few months he confided to his diary:

> On one such occasion, I clearly remember observing a culture from urine on an agar slope of uniform lawn of B coli with four large bacteriophage plaques. This was only a month or so after I had produced typhoid phage. D'Herelle's book (*The Bacteriophage; Its Role in Immunity*, 1922) was new then and I wondered whether, if I had seen those plaques before reading d'Herelle, I would have realized there was something worth studying before me.

Viruses that infect bacteria, the bacteriophages, from Greek *phagus* "to eat", were a hot topic at the time. Growing in a bacterial layer on a disc with agar, they form local clearings, the plaques mentioned in the citation. Each plaque originated in the infection by a single virus particle. The discovery of bacteriophages also caught the attention of the Nobel Committee at the Karolinska Institute and, in 1926, it recommended that d'Herelle should get the reserved 1925 Prize in physiology or medicine. This never came to be. In 1925–26 the Institute kept the money and no prizes were awarded[3]. Bacteriophages came to be Burnet's first *tour de force* into virology, but his initial work in microbial science had a different orientation.

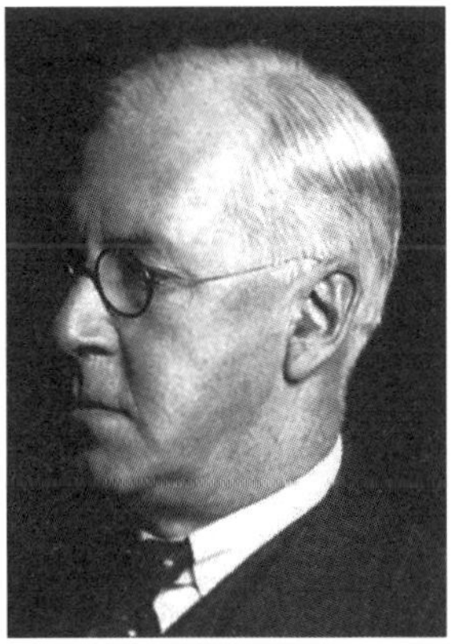

Henry H. Dale (1875–1968), recipient of a shared Nobel Prize in physiology or medicine 1936. [From *Les Prix Nobel en 1936*.]

In September 1923 there was an important change in directorship of the Hall Institute. Dr Charles Kellaway had arrived from England, where he had trained on a scholarship from the Royal Society. He was a first rate physiologist and one of his sponsors in England was Henry Hallett Dale, later Sir Henry and the forthcoming recipient of the 1936 Nobel Prize in physiology or medicine.

He became an active nominator of candidates for Nobel Prizes as we shall see. Kellaway very soon set about making plans for Burnet. He was first encouraged to conclude his examination for an M.D., focussing on the agglutinins in sera from patients with typhoid fever. After this, it was time to deepen his training. Burnet received a scholarship allowing a two years study as a Beit Medical Research Fellow at the Lister Institute in London. He was intrigued by phages and made these viruses the topic of his PhD thesis, which he finished in 1928. It might be noted that Burnet did not have a mentor in the field he decided to embark on. In many cases, Nobel Prize recipients have had experiences of working under an influential and experienced researcher, frequently of a quality qualifying him for the prize, but Burnet ploughed his own fields.

Burnet also developed his taste for travelling during his time in England. He made two bicycle tours of the European continent. His British colleagues noticed the talent of the young Australian researcher and it was made obvious that, if he stayed in London he could get a professorship in bacteriology. However, he had two reasons for returning to his home country. The first was the solidarity he felt with Australia. He knew, of course, that the career possibilities were much better in England or in the United States, but he had such a confidence in his own capacity that he felt he wanted to prove he could be successful within the more isolated Australian research enterprise. He had no doubt that this would be beneficial to science in that country. As his career evolved there were many temptations to leave Australia, but he never succumbed. The only exception was two more years of advanced training and research in England in 1932–34. It may in fact have been fortunate that Burnet stayed in Australia. It is not certain that his shy personality would have been as productive in a more competitive large international university. The second reason for returning was that he wanted to start a family.

Burnet's contacts with the opposite sex were rather uncomfortable. However, at the age of 24 he was introduced to Edith Linda Marston Druce, who was two years his junior, by a good friend, Dr George Simpson. Simpson later came to have a distinguished career as one of the early famous flying doctors in Australia. The contact with Linda changed Burnet's life, but this is something he avoided reflecting on in his prolific writings. She managed to break the barrier of his reticence and shyness. During his time at the Lister Institute she visited England and they became engaged before she left in October 1927. Burnet gave her a copy of Sinclair Lewis' *Arrowsmith*[4], the story about the attempt to use bacteriophages to cure cancer, fictionalized using characters at the Rockefeller Institute in New York. This he thought was appropriate reading during her long travel back to Australia.

Some months later Burnet arrived home to take up the vice-directorship at the Hall Institute. He married Linda in July 1928. Throughout their long marriage she covered for her husband during many social gatherings. He used to refer to himself with formulations like "always been something of a social misfit". She was an out-going person and a pleasant and intelligent hostess. When Burnet withdrew within himself for reflection she effectively managed the socializing. She always respected his needs and the routine through many of the early years was that he worked in the laboratory during the day and did his writing at night. Overall it seems that Burnet had a very strict work ethic — sometimes referred to as (secularized) Calvinistic — and had a remarkable capacity to focus on the work at hand. In present-day terminology Burnet would have been referred to as a workaholic. Possibly Burnet even nursed his image as a social outcast for his own benefit. This is something which is not infrequently observed in the archetypes of science personality. As a young scientist I got the occasional advice from one internationally renowned scientist at the Karolinska Institute that one need not distinguish oneself in the first contacts with committee meetings and not necessarily open all brown envelopes — the official university mail. Possibly my career would have been even more dominated by science if I had followed such advice. Because of my upbringing I did not do this. Of course, Burnet also took time for his family which came to include three children born 1929, 1931 and 1937, but it was Linda's responsibility to manage the practical aspects of their upbringing. Among other things she shared Macfarlane's enthusiasm for travelling, which gave them a lot of pleasure and special shared time through the many years they came to have together.

In 1931 Kellaway was contacted by Dale, who had had become the director of the National Institute for Medical Research in London. This Institute had just initiated an extensive program for research on virus diseases, with economic support from the Rockefeller Foundation. In the letter Burnet was invited to come and join this program on a special fellowship. It was for two years. This offer was too good not to accept and the Burnet family with one newborn set out for his second working sojourn in London. His time in London came to be very productive and he also learned a lot from the other ongoing research activities at the institute. When his time as visiting scientist was coming to an end, he was again invited to stay in England, this time by Dale. He declined and instead, through the contacts he had established with the Rockefeller Foundation, managed to raise important support for his forthcoming research back home in Australia. As he returned to his native country with his family in 1934 he was made assistant director for the Walter and Eliza Hall Institute and ten years later he became its director, succeeding Kellaway.

Burnet never built any large research groups. For many years he worked on his own, often with just a single (female) technician. As the director of the Institute he, of course, came to inspire many local and visiting scientists and, progressively, this led to the establishment of an exceptional Australian research environment. We will meet many of the scientists who developed in his sphere of enlightenment. The main emphasis of the Institute for many years was on problems in the field of virology, but in the mid-1950s this was progressively changed to a focus on immunology, a discipline showing a rapid development not the least because of the introduction of new concepts by Burnet. His retirement speech, when he left the Directorship in 1965 after 21 years, is quite remarkable, as reflected in the following brief excerpt: "There may be men with sufficient intrinsic dominance and capacity to exert unquestioned authority and run their organization as they desire. At the other extreme are people like myself of considerable intellectual capacity but far down in the pecking order when it comes to matters of human interaction and conflict." Clearly Burnet had his own leadership style that might be described as reserved, polite and direct. As we shall see Burnet was very active during the 20 years allotted to him after his retirement. He did some experimental work, at least early on, and he wrote extensively and consistently.

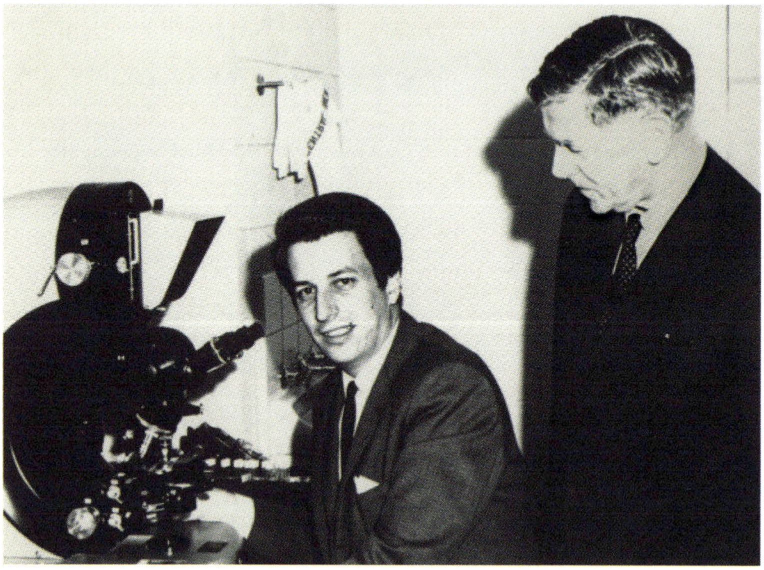

Gustav Nossal (*left*) and Burnet. [Photo kindly provided by Nossal.]

One of Burnet's junior immunology collaborators was Gustav (Gus) Nossal. Nossal is of Austrian origin, but when he was eight years old the family had to flee to Australia because of the Second World War. In his early research career, he did pioneering work supporting Burnet's revolutionary theory for antibody formation. When Burnet retired Nossal succeeded him as director of the Institute. Nossal carried this responsibility for more than 30 years nursing Burnet's legacy by maintaining the Institute as a first class research institution.

Virus as an Organism

Throughout Burnet's career he shifted his engagement between different kinds of viruses; bacteriophages, poliomyelitis virus, influenza viruses, viruses spread by insects, etc. In all these studies he retained a perspective as a general biologist with a deep understanding of the importance of evolutionary developments. He always considered both partners in an infectious process, the infectious agent and the host. As humans we have a tendency to overemphasize the significance of an agent from our own perspective or with consideration to the animals and plants that we exploit to sustain our living. Thus viruses may be seen as agents causing respiratory infections or enteric infections, but Burnet always wanted to give equal weight to the *anthropocentric* and *virocentric* perspectives. Many different viruses may infect the respiratory tract, and each one needs to be assessed from the perspective of the biology of the particular virus involved in that process. In order to make rational interventions, we always need to consider what is "in it for the virus". From an evolutionary perspective the virus, like us, strives to survive in nature. Causing a severe disease in man is a drawback for survival, as virus spread will be less efficient. The ideal situation should be a balance in the parasite-host relationship with moderate to no symptoms of the human host, but still efficient spread of virus. This insight shines through in all Burnet's work and is reflected in chapter or book titles like *Virus as Organism*[5] and *Viruses and Man*[6].

Burnet was also intrigued by the development and maintenance of immunity against infectious agents and this led him into deep speculations about the fundamental aspects of immunity. In these speculations he developed some of his most ingenious new concepts and towards the end of his career he shifted from virology to immunology. In fact he even stated that he had been through the most critical part of development of human and animal virology and that by the mid-1950s, all the major developments had occurred and the science of virus research was essentially over. Ten years later he also declared that the peak of immunological research had been reached. We will have reasons to come back to these very generalized and, today, obviously erroneous statements.

It is true that when Burnet started his career only very few viruses were known to cause disease in man, like yellow fever, polio, rabies and smallpox. The early studies of these viruses required infection of animals. With time, the developments of new techniques — embryonated hen's eggs and tissue culture — allowed the propagation of a large number of filterable agents. It was in the 1950s that particularly useful cell culture systems were developed. Their use was facilitated by the access to antibiotics, like penicillin and streptomycin, which had become available by that time. By use of these kinds of cultures many agents of importance for disease in man were identified. But the development of virology did not, as suggested by Burnet, stop there. It remained to identify large number of fastidious viruses, which were gradually understood to exist. These sorts of viruses can only replicate in the laboratory under very special conditions or, in a number of cases, not at all. The only way of identifying the latter category of viruses is by the use of molecular tools, developed during the later decades, for recognition of their genetic material in samples from diseased patients.

Burnet made a number of seminal contributions to the subject of virology throughout the 1930s to 1950s and became the dominant scientist in that field. His various contributions will be presented first from a general perspective and then, with a particular focus, using the rich Nobel archive materials and also his nomination for a foreign membership of the Royal Swedish Academy of Sciences. Interestingly, the nomination in June 1957 for such a membership exhaustively evaluated his contributions to understanding the dynamics of the biological equilibrium between infectious agents and their hosts but it did not mention his fundamental theorizing about mechanisms of antibody production. It is said that, when he was informed that he had been selected as a foreign member of the Academy in 1957, he took this as a consolation meaning that he would not receive a Nobel Prize. Apparently he had for many years been expecting to receive this prize. When it eventually happened, its timing and focus might have come as a surprise to him. Before we come to that in the next chapter, Burnet's deep engagement in many aspects of virology will first be discussed. They will be presented in the context of different kinds of viruses.

Phages and Receptors

The bacterial viruses stimulated Burnet's curiosity. He set out to study these agents in his PhD work and, more extensively, during his second research sojourn in England at the National Institute for Medical Research, London. The essence of his findings was summarized by Burnet himself in 1934[7] and the impact of his early research was also addressed in later books[8,9]. Burnet collected bacteriophages from many sources and characterized their growth characteristics on the appropriate host bacteria. According to his own words he was "by temperament an ecologist, a naturalist, a collector of beetles, a snapper-up of unconsidered trifles". This guided him in his approach to science. He simply pursued curiosity-driven research. From his own repository combined with various phages obtained from other researchers, he set out to divide them into groups. For this purpose he used their immunological properties and compared them by use of antisera prepared in experimental animals. He was able to sort the 50 different phages he was studying into 12 distinct groups. One of the larger groups was later shown to include the so called T-even phages. They came to play a particular role in future studies as expressed by Burnet's own words "Almost the whole of the modern structure (of phage genetic research) has been built on the standard strain of *Escherichia coli B* and two phages T2 and T4 … ."

Burnet also studied the growth curve characteristics under conditions when all bacteria in a culture were infected by phage. These experiments presaged the 1939 experiments by Emory Ellis and Max Delbrück which came to initiate the use of phages to study viral genetics. The pioneering contributions of the "phage school" came to be very influential for the development of genetics and led to a number of discoveries. A critical aspect of the studies of phages was that the effect of individual virus particles could be examined. When replicating in a layer of bacteria on an agar plate they gave focal lesions — so called *plaques*. Such plaques could display variable appearances. These advances were eventually recognized by a Nobel Prize in physiology or medicine in 1969 to Delbrück, Alfred Hershey and Salvador Luria, as discussed in my earlier book[3]. Burnet was also involved in determining the size of bacteriophages, together with Christopher Andrewes using Elford's fine filters with pores of graded calibrated sizes. He made further important observations concerning the capacity of phages to remain in a dormant form, a non-infectious *Anlage* (genetic rudiment). This state of virus-bacterium interaction later came to be referred to as *lysogeny* condition. Lysogeny was to be evaluated in depth by French researchers, in particular André Lwoff, leading to a shared Nobel Prize in physiology or medicine in 1964[3].

Still other important observations concerned the first step in the infectious cycle of bacteriophages. Burnet concluded that this occurred by adsorption of the virus to specific chemical groups at the surface of bacteria. These groups were called *receptors* and the introduction of this concept had wide importance and was further analysed in forthcoming studies of animal viruses, in particular influenza virus. Already at an early stage it was understood that blocking the receptors might be one way to prevent the infection of a cell by a virus. The membrane receptor concept with time developed to take on a major importance in studies of normal cellular functions. Signalling substances in the nervous and endocrine system were found to interact with specific receptors. These developments have led to the discovery of a number of pharmaceutically important drugs. About half of all drugs used in the early 21st century interact with receptors as evidenced by the 2012 Nobel Prize in chemistry to Robert J. Lefkowitz and Brian K. Kobilka "for studies of G-protein-coupled receptors".

Finally it can be added that, by the mid-1930s, the first chemical analyses of phages were made by the Hungarian scientist Martin Schlesinger. He started his studies in Frankfurt am Main, but moved to London after the Nazi takeover. The conclusion of his work was that the phage consisted of about half protein and half DNA[10]. These data, suggesting that phages were packages of genes and chromosomes were way ahead of their time. Due to his untimely death in 1936, further work on the chemistry of phages ceased. The huge importance of Schlesinger's original finding did not become apparent until the conceptual revolution some 20 years later showing that DNA represents the genetic material in all forms of life except certain groups of viruses, which instead use RNA (Ref. 3, Chapter 7). It was these early studies of bacteriophages that paved the way for the later explosive developments of molecular genetics, but Burnet did not follow up his phage work after 1940. Instead he came to focus on animal viruses. However by his own judgement he stated when looking back "... it had a major place in my enthusiasms and I believe that the phage work at Hampstead probably represents the peak of my scientific achievement." Still there was much to come and many more discoveries to make.

Poliovirus

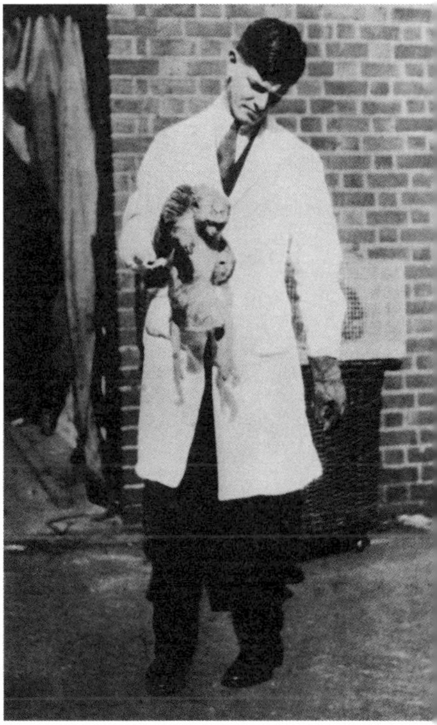

Burnet holding the first monkey paralyzed by an Australian poliovirus. Picture taken in 1929. [From Ref. 1.]

Burnet's involvements in studies of the virus causing poliomyelitis deserve to be discussed. Between 1928 and 1942, he was intermittently involved in experimental studies of the disease and, together with his collaborators, he made two rarely acknowledged original observations of considerable importance for our understanding of the infection and how to prevent it.

In connection with a relatively small epidemic in Melbourne in 1928, Burnet identified the virus by transfer to monkeys . Since, at the time, attempts were made to use serum from convalescent patients for early treatment — so called *passive immunization* — of acute polio cases, the effect of such a serum was tested in monkeys. It was then found, and published in 1931, that the serum protected against infection with the virus recovered from a case of the Melbourne epidemic but *not* against another strain of poliovirus obtained from the Rockefeller Institute in New York. This was the first indication of the existence of more than one strain of poliovirus. Later studies by others demonstrated that there were in fact three immunologically distinct types, named 1, 2 and 3. This explained how a single individual could have two attacks of the same kind of disease and also why epidemics unfold and return in repeated waves. It was also crucial knowledge for the proper design of vaccines when the time became ripe for this during the mid-1950s.

The second important observation was made in 1937–38, when Melbourne was hit by a major epidemic with some 1,900 cases. This was, by the way, the first time that Burnet exited his ivory tower and became a spokesman on public health matters. He became quietly comfortable with that and later he played the same role many times, progressively even extending outside his domain of infectious diseases. At the time the technique used to recover poliovirus was to inject material from patients into Indian *rhesus* monkeys. They were difficult to infect and had to be injected directly into the brain or some other part of the central nervous system like the spinal cord. An alternative procedure was to hold the monkey upside down and administer the virus via his nostrils onto the exposed olfactory nerves in the upper part of the nasal cavity. Via these nerves the virus could spread backwards — in a retrograde fashion — to the brain. These procedures were used by Burnet and his collaborators, but then there was a happy accident.

Temporarily no more monkeys were available from Calcutta and as an alternative Malay *cynomolgus* monkeys were obtained from Singapore. It was found that these animals were much more sensitive to infection than the previously used rhesus monkeys. The Malay monkey could be infected simply by swabbing the back of the throat with virus. This led to an ingenious, perhaps typical Burnet experiment. Two *cynomolgus* monkeys were anaesthetized and after a surgical incision virus was carefully delivered directly into the cavity of the intestine. Both animals became infected. This finding resurrected a theory proposed some decades earlier by the Swedish bacteriologist Carl Kling that polio spread as an intestinal infection. Burnet´s findings were soon confirmed by others examining the spread of poliovirus in the body during the infectious process. These observations eventually refuted the prevailing dogma at the time formulated by Simon Flexner and collaborators about 30 years earlier at the Rockefeller Institute. They had concluded that the olfactory epithelium is the single point of entry of poliovirus into the body, a misleading theory that eventually was proven wrong. Sadly this dominating concept led to many children having their olfactory epithelium destroyed by some caustic treatment as a presumed way of possibly preventing the terrifying polio disease. The only effect of such a treatment was a loss of the sense of smell.

The Embryonated Hen's Egg

Viruses can only replicate as parasites in live cells. Hence the traditional way of studying a virus was to have access to some suitable host cell in the laboratory. In the early 1930s Ernest W. Goodpasture introduced the embryonated hen's egg for studies of human and animal viruses. This was a major advance beyond the use of intact animals to demonstrate replication of viruses, and for preparation of stock materials for further studies. During his second stay in England Burnet expanded Goodpasture's method of using chick embryos to a much more diversified practical use. He found that the egg contained a number of very different, available sources of living cells useful for the replication of various viruses. Injections could be made into different compartments of the egg, allowing the replication of different kinds of human and animal viruses. For example, it was found that fresh strains of influenza viruses replicated more readily if the material was injected into the amniotic sac, which is in contact with the future respiratory tract of the embryo, than into the allantoic sac. Once the virus had adapted to grow in the amniotic compartment by repeated passages between eggs, it could also replicate in the more voluminous allantoic sac. These early developments made accessible a technique to prepare large quantities of human influenza viruses that could serve as a source of material to produce inactivated vaccines. In the early 1940s techniques to prepare such formalin inactivated products were developed and used in soldiers of the Second World War.

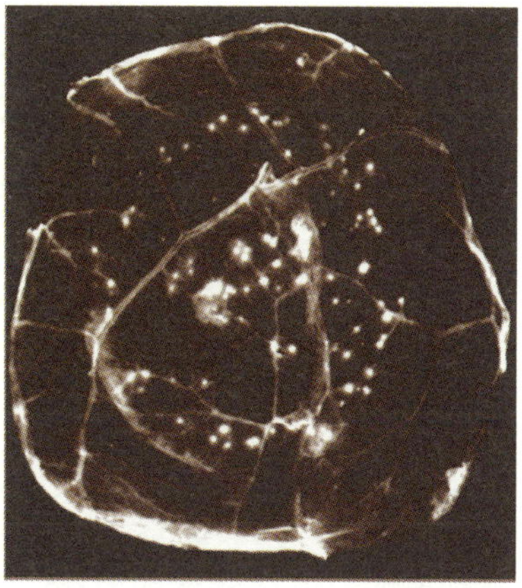

Local changes, pocks, caused by virus replicating in the chorioallantoic membrane of an embryonated hen's egg. [From Ref. 16.]

One other way of using the embryonated hen's egg was to grow virus on the chorioallantoic membrane. In order to make this accessible the egg was positioned in penetrating light and using a dentist's drill two holes were made through the egg shell, one on the top of the air sac and one on the side of the egg. Application of a negative pressure by suction at the former hole created an artificial air space, the bottom of which was not covered by the shell membrane as in the case of the normal air sac, but represented exposed chorioallantoic membrane. Inoculation of material into this artificial cavity allowed the virus to initiate infection in this membrane and, at a proper concentration, focal lesions, so called *pocks*, could be observed. Each such pock — like a plaque produced by a bacteriophage — originated from the infection with a single virus particle. The introduction of this technique allowed, for the first time, an exact quantification of the number of infectious particles in a particular sample from humans or from animals. However, in certain cases, it also allowed qualitative comparisons. It turned out that different strains of viruses could gave pocks that had varying characteristics. They might be of different sizes and the quality of the inflammatory process involving invasion of white blood cells and vascularization resulted in a range of appearances. The appreciation of the occurrence of such different qualitative behavior, of variants of one and the same kind of virus allowed the first genetic studies of an animal virus,

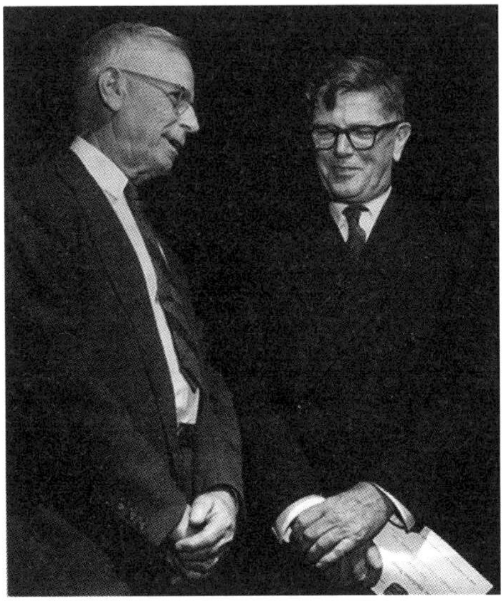

Ernest W. Goodpasture (1886–1960) and Burnet. [From Ref. 16.]

pioneering work that Burnet and colleagues developed using influenza virus during the 1940s.

Over the years Burnet and Goodpasture became good friends and it is with sadness that Burnet took note of their last encounter. This occurred in 1958 when Burnet was visiting Vanderbilt University in Nashville, Tennessee, where Goodpasture had spent almost his whole career. On this occasion Burnet gave one of his first lectures on his recently introduced theory on antibody production and clonal selection of cells. Goodpasture was nominated for a Nobel Prize but never received this recognition of his contribution, as we shall see.

Pioneering Studies of Influenza Virus

Burnet was present at the National Institute of Medical Research at Hampstead when influenza virus was first successfully made to grow in the laboratory. The story has already been told[3] how, in 1933, ferrets inoculated with material from patients with influenza developed symptoms and how the infection was transferred back to a scientist called Wilson Smith who was working with the animals. He developed symptoms of influenza and virus was recovered from his respiratory tract. This virus became the prototype WS strain of the dominating group of influenza viruses, the type A viruses. In the late 1950s a thorough investigation was made to determine if the identification of influenza virus was a discovery that should be recognized by a Nobel Prize. The conclusion was that this should not be the case since the leader of the group of scientists that successfully made the important demonstration of the virus, Patrick P. Laidlaw, was no longer alive. Burnet did not participate in these early pioneering studies at the National Institute of Medical Research in London. It was after he had returned to Australia that he initiated his groundbreaking studies of influenza virus. There are many facets to this work including both human and animal viruses. Two important ones based on the modified egg techniques were already alluded to, namely the introduction of a technique for isolating influenza viruses from man and also the possibility of preparing sufficient quantities of the virus to produce a vaccine. Two more examples of the Burnet's pioneering findings also deserve to be described.

Already in his early work with bacteriophages Burnet had postulated the occurrence of receptors on cells to which virus particles attached as the first step of their replication. He and his colleagues came to make detailed studies of such receptors for influenza virus. It all started with a discovery that Burnet according to his own words "should have made, but did not"[1]. He had made the occasional observation that red blood cells which had leaked into allantoic fluid containing influenza virus had a tendency to aggregate and form clumps. It was others, firstly George K. Hirst at the Rockefeller Institute, New York, who demonstrated that this agglutination of cells was a virus-specific phenomenon. The aggregate was formed by the linking together of red blood cells by virus particles. This *hemagglutination* phenomenon provided a very efficient means of measuring the amount of virus in a sample and also the amount of antibodies in a serum sample by quantifying its capacity to inhibit the hemagglutination by an adjusted limited amount of virus.

The hemagglutination phenomenon also conveniently allowed studies of the first step — the adsorption of virus particles to receptors — in the infectious process in a cell. It was found that the interaction between the influenza virus and the red blood cells had the characteristics of an enzyme-substrate reaction. After prolonged incubation at 37°C, but not at 4°C, the virus particles detached from the blood cells. One consequence of this interaction was that the red blood cells could not be agglutinated again if fresh virus was added, but the original virus that had detached from them could agglutinate fresh cells. The receptors on the cells had been stripped off by the original contact with virus. Based on his insight into microbiology and an intuitive deduction Burnet tested what effect a filtrate of the organism which causes cholera, the bacterium *Vibrio cholerae*, might have on the receptor for influenza virus on the red cells. They were destroyed! Burnet called his preparation the receptor destroying enzyme, RDE. By the aid of chemists in the laboratory, in particular Alfred Gottshalk, it was possible to further characterize the adsorption-elution process. The critical cell receptor was of a mucoid nature and included as a critical part neuraminic acid. The relevant enzyme therefore eventually was called neuraminidase. Later on the mucoid character of the identified receptor came to give a name to the group of different influenza viruses. They were called *orthomyxoviruses*. Another group of viruses which originally were thought to use a similar kind of receptors were called *paramyxoviruses*. The latter group of viruses includes members that have a major importance for diseases in humans, like measles virus, mumps virus and parainfluenza viruses. In 1960 it was discovered that also measles virus had a capacity to agglutinate red blood cells. Only such cells from grivet monkeys *(Cercopithecus aethiops)* could be used in the test. Since we had access to this kind of monkey — they were used for certain controls in the polio vaccine production — close to the laboratory where I had started to work, the capacity of the virus to hemagglutinate could be easily confirmed and hence there was a convenient test at hand to study the properties of the virus. These studies led to a number of interesting findings which came to be the core material of my PhD thesis presented four years later.

Later studies of these different viruses have revealed detailed information about the number of genes in their genome and the structure and function of their gene products. Particularly detailed studies have been performed with influenza virus and a modern schematic picture of the virus is shown below. The membranous structure surrounding the particle, the *envelope*, contains two protruding structures, the *hemagglutinin*, which dominates quantitatively, and the *neuraminidase*. These two components represent the main targets of our immune defence system. After each influenza infection we mount an efficient antibody response to these two components. The problem is only that in this particular virus the surface components continuously change their structure

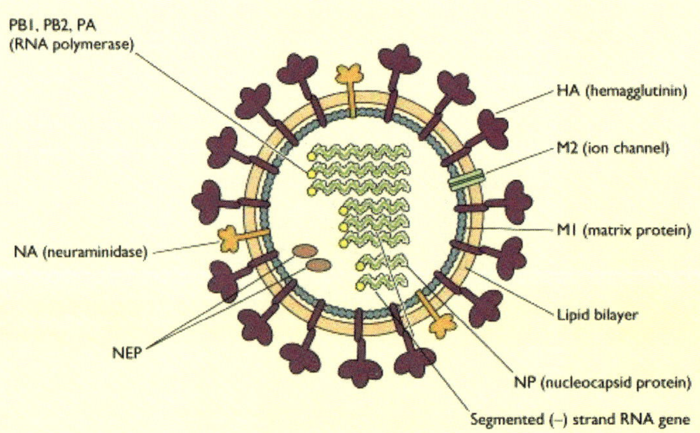

Schematic depiction of the components of influenza virus. The genome is composed of 8 individual pieces of RNA and the surface projections are the trimere hemagglutinin and the tetramere neuraminidase.

due to a high rate of mutations in the virus genome. It is because of these *antigenic drifts* that we repeatedly get infected by influenza viruses. The only way of preventing this is yearly immunizations with progressively modified vaccines. The virus strains to be included in the vaccine are selected to be as closely related as possible to the virus circulating at the time. However, the virus has one more trick up its sleeve. As illustrated in the figure the genome is divided into eight pieces. If two different influenza viruses — possibly one of human and one of animal origin — replicate in the same cell they can exchange equivalent pieces in a process called *genetic reassortment*. Such an exchange between viruses of different host origin — implying an *antigenic shift* — can lead to the emergence of a virus with completely new properties, potentially causing severe disease in man, like the 1918 swine flu epidemic.

The three-dimensional structure of both the trimere influenza hemagglutinin and the tetramere neuraminidase have been demonstrated in detail by X-ray crystallography and today we know a lot about the molecular mechanisms guiding the first steps of interaction between influenza viruses and cells, the attachment, and the fusion of the virus envelope and the cellular membrane. It is not obvious that Burnet would have applauded these advances. He generally referred to himself as a biologist and evolutionist and once the basic principles were clear he was not interested in the details. Not surprisingly later studies have proven the value of insights into molecular structures and functions of virus components. Still developments and applications of new knowledge take time and it is surprising that, in spite of all new knowledge, we are still today using influenza vaccines prepared in eggs by methods developed in the 1940s instead of using tissue cultures and avoiding the risks of egg allergy reactions. Furthermore although we have a deep insight into the molecular details of virus attachment to cells and the membrane fusion allowing the release of the genetic material into the interior of the cell, we have only had limited success in developing drugs that can block these early steps in virus replication.

The second example of a critical contribution to our understanding of influenza biology was Burnet's pioneering engagement in studies of the genetics of this animal virus. At the end of the 1940s it was known from studies of bacteriophages that the simultaneous infection of a bacterial culture with two distinct variants of phages could lead to the emergence of viruses with properties characteristic of both the parental strains, referred to as *recombinants*. By use of his egg technique Burnet could identify strains of influenza viruses with distinct different properties. These strains were used for concomitant infection of cells, which demonstrated that also in the case of animal viruses recombinant viruses could emerge. At this time it was not known that the virus genome is divided into pieces allowing the phenomenon of reassortment mentioned above. Burnet hoped to be able to use the technique of genetic recombination to produce useful live attenuated vaccine virus, but he and his collaborators were never successful in this and the attempts were given up in 1957.

During the more than 50 years that have passed since Burnet's early experiments to produce a live influenza virus vaccine several attempts have been made to develop such a product mostly by exploiting the mechanism of reassortment. Today such a live vaccine is available. It is given intranasally and the virus replicates in mucosal membranes giving a preferential stimulation of a local immunity. Although this may have some attractive features there are also some drawbacks and hence there is still a preference for using traditional inactivated vaccines injected parenterally. Whichever vaccine is used the critical factor, when it comes to efficacy of protection, is the degree of similarity between the antigenic make-up of the vaccine virus and of the circulating wild virus causing the epidemic at the time.

Viruses Can Persist in Man

Influenza viruses only give acute infections. Once the infection has been resolved all the virus has been cleared from the body. However, there are certain kinds of viruses in man and animals that like the dormant phages in bacteria can persist. One example is the virus causing the familiar cold sore on the lip, a disease known centuries ago. The agent responsible for this disease is called *herpes simplex virus*. Using a cohort of children, studied since they were toddlers in an orphanage, Burnet and his colleague Gray Anderson did some interesting investigations of infections with this virus. They could demonstrate that the children showed a resistance to infection by the virus during the major part of the first year of life because of antibodies transferred from the mother. Hereafter they became infected at a high rate and at the age of two years almost all of them had responded with an antibody production of their own. The frequency of early infections was lower in children from privileged homes reflecting the existence of higher hygiene standards, but infections were still quite common in the young age groups. In most individuals the virus remained hidden to the immune system throughout life. In some individuals it was repeatedly activated, mostly for unknown reasons. Sometimes fever or heavy exposure to sunlight could elicit a *recurrent infection*. Activated virus giving cold sores can serve as a source of infections in non-immune individuals.

Burnet discussed how herpes (simplex) virus has persisted way back into human history not only during our time of settled civilization, but also before that when we were hunters and gatherers. He concluded that in fact there is no reason why the virus spreading from one generation to the other — *vertically* — should not also have accompanied our ancestors at the time of our evolutionary separation from early hominids and the preceding primates/monkeys and possibly much further back in evolutionary time. Burnet also concluded that there must be a general rule that a virus that has evolved for a long time with its host has developed a tolerable association, acceptable to both partners. However, if this virus is spread to a completely different species, the outcome would be unpredictable. The importance of adaption to a host will be further discussed in Chapter 4.

Later studies have revealed that there exist two types of herpes simplex virus, type 1 and type 2. The virus studied by Burnet and colleagues was type 1. Type 2 virus infects the genital tract and is spread by sexual contacts. Studies of the age-dependent appearance of antibodies against type 2 — *seroepidemiology* — have revealed that they develop after infections during the teenage years, reflecting the time of the sexual debut. In general the first infection is harmless, but recurrent infections by activated latent virus, like the cold sores on the lips, can cause problems and serve as a source for further transmissions by sexual contacts.

The Sherlock Holmes of Epidemiology

Burnet thrived when he was confronted by a convoluted and enigmatic situation of epidemic spread of a previously unidentified disease. The situation of latent herpes simplex virus infections has just been discussed and in the following one additional selected example will be given. Other epidemics examined by Burnet could also have been discussed, like those of psittacosis and Q fever.

The epidemic to be discussed is Murray Valley Encephalitis (MVE), a severe disease caused by infection of the brain. As a background it is necessary to present a separate spread of a viral disease — an *epizootic* — among rabbits. This is the infectious disease *myxomatosis*, which was introduced into Australia in order to diminish the population of wild rabbits[11]. The person carrying the main responsibility for this initiative was Frank Fenner, an eminent virologist.

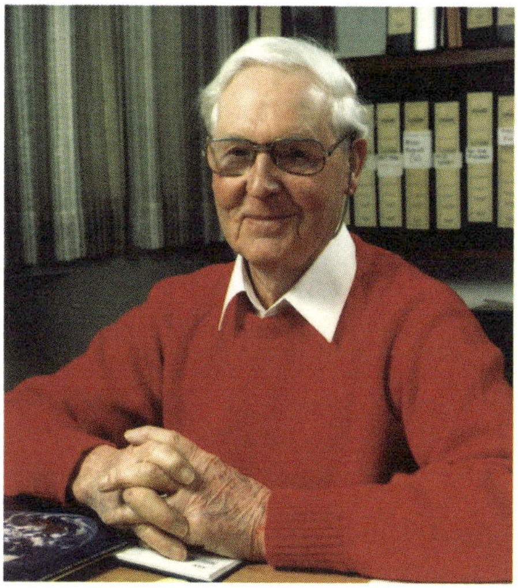

Frank Fenner (1914–2010). [Photo from Ref. 16.]

Besides Burnet he was the most respected virologist of Australian origin at the time. Fenner, who was 14 years younger than Burnet was recruited by him to work at the Walter and Eliza Hall Institute for Medical Research after the Second World War. He made exemplary and informative studies of the disease process — the pathogenesis — of poxviruses in mice and later became involved in studies of another poxvirus infecting rabbits, the *myxoma* agent. This virus was selected for use in an attempt to achieve a biological control of rabbits in Australia. Later in his professional life, Fenner made a very important contribution to the successful eradication of smallpox by the World Health Organization (WHO) in 1978 (Chapter 4). He was the chairman of the Global Commission for the Certification of Smallpox Eradication.

Rabbits have been a proverbial pest to Australian pastoralists since 1859. They were introduced by an enthusiastic "acclimatizer" Thomas Austin, who owned a large piece of land at Geelong in Victoria. He was successful in his initiative because he imported wild rabbits and not the inbred variants which had previously failed to survive. In the absence of natural enemies there was an intense replication and spread of rabbits and they came to occupy the major part of Australia south of the tropic. This was a heavy burden on the farmers since seven rabbits browse as much grass as one sheep. In an attempt to control the situation Fenner imported myxoma virus from North America and examined its properties. On that continent this virus and its rabbit host had established a balanced relationship, but the effect on the naturalized Australian rabbit, which represents a different genus, turned out to be dramatic. Laboratory experiments demonstrated that the infection essentially killed all the animals. When the virus after extensive deliberations was released into the natural Australian habitat the rabbit population was drastically reduced. The death rate initially was 99.7%. However with time a new balance between virus and animal established itself. The few surviving rabbits bred to give a stock of animals that were relatively more resistant to the virus. And the virus was also selected to give a less devastating disease and a longer time of survival of the animals. This prolonged time of survival had two consequences. One was the development of an additional method of spread of the virus. Originally the virus spread by direct contact between a diseased and a healthy animal. But the prolonged survival improved the opportunities for transfer of the infection also indirectly. Mosquitoes that had picked up the virus by biting the diseased animal could initiate an infection by biting a second animal, a *vector-borne transmission.*

After circulation of the virus for seven to eight years in Australia the mortality rate of rabbits had been reduced to about 50%. Among the animals that died, half succumbed directly from the infection and the rest, incapacitated by the disease, were killed by predators. Thus, in the end the introduction of the virus led to a reduced prevalence of rabbits and a relatively improved ecological balance. The release of myxoma virus had been made in 1950 and its initial spread occurred along the Murray River and its major tributaries. By the end of January 1951 it had spread to Mildura in the north-west corner of Victoria. Rabbits were dying in masses in the area but at the same time there happened to occur a dozen cases of severe encephalitis among children in the area. No such cases had been seen for a very long time. The question naturally was raised whether it possibly could be that the myxoma virus, released by the Federal authorities to kill the rabbits, had changed its character and also could infect man?

It did not take Burnet's collaborator Eric L. French long to determine that the virus giving the disease in the children was a different kind of agent than the one giving the rabbit epizootic initiated by man. The encephalitis in humans was caused by a virus related to a previously identified Japanese B encephalitis virus known to be transmitted from migratory birds by mosquitoes to man. The identification of the virus was made by the inoculation of material on chorioallantoic membranes in hen's eggs using Burnet's technique. It was the first time that the initial identification of a new virus had been made by this procedure. Burnet named the new virus Murray Valley encephalitis (MVE) virus. It still remained to convince the press and the public that the epidemic of encephalitis and the epizootic caused by myxoma virus were unrelated and at the same time to explain why they occurred simultaneously. This took some detective work. Before that Burnet and Fenner and the charismatic head of the CSIRO (a large government research organization) Ian Clunies-Ross, in order to calm the public, took the exceptional initiative to inoculate themselves with an amount of myxoma virus that would kill many rabbits. The outcome was, as expected, no disease — the researchers knew that many field investigators must have been bitten by mosquitoes carrying rabbit virus without any consequences — and its presentation (subjects being anonymous) in the Parliament had the expected calming effect on the public.

It remained to explain the MVE epidemic. It was recognized that back in 1917 and 1918 a large number of clustered cases of encephalitis had occurred in western New South Wales and northern Victoria. It had been possible to transmit an infectious agent to monkeys, but no further characterization of the nature of the agent had been possible at the time. The disease was referred to as Australian X-disease. To analyze a possible relationship of this disease to the MVE epidemic a search was made for antibodies against the newly isolated virus in different localities and in different age groups. Antibodies generally represent durable indicators of bygone infections. It was found that in certain areas where the impact of X-disease had been particularly heavy, people older than 35 years did in fact have antibodies against the MVE virus demonstrating a previous infection. The two outbreaks of diseases therefore were interpreted to be related.

In order to further understand the MVE epidemic and its origin extensive studies were performed over a long time looking for antibodies in humans and animals as a measure of previous infections. Entomologists and ornithologists were brought into the team to sample widely for the presence of virus. There were many negative results, but also a few critical findings of infected animals. Eventually a comprehensive picture emerged. It turned out that the MVE virus survived in a habitat of Indonesia, New Guinea and tropical Australia, being mostly a harmless parasite of birds and mosquitoes. It survived by being transmitted by the mosquitoes as a chain of infections in birds. After the mosquito had had a meal of infectious blood it took about ten days before the virus had replicated and spread to the salivary glands of the insect, the source of virus when a bird was infected by a mosquito bite.

It was deduced that the virus could spread to Mildura in southern Australia only under very exceptional weather conditions. Epidemics of encephalitis occurred in the years 1917, 1918 and 1951 with a smaller number of cases occurring also in 1925. The reason for this scattered occurrence of cases was deduced to be that in all cases there had been heavy and widespread rains over eastern Australia in the months of October and November during the year preceding the epidemic. By a random step by step alternating infection in birds and insects the virus managed to reach as far south as Mildura. When February of the following year was reached the repository of virus in the extensive colonies of different wild birds in the region had become so large that infections spilled over to domestic birds and from these to children.

It has been possible to identify many hundreds of virus infections in humans, which are transmitted from animals by different insects, like mosquitoes and ticks — usually referred to as *vectors*. In most cases vector-borne infections in man represent a point of no return for the virus. From a perspective of evolutionary survival the infection of man is of no value for the virus, but sadly it can be highly detrimental to the person attacked by the virus. There are special situations, like the urban form of yellow fever (Ref. 3, Chapter 4), when in fact humans can be the source of a virus infection in a mosquito, which then after some time can carry this infection to other humans. However, in almost all other vector-borne infections this is not the case and the persistent source of virus to infect the vector is some group of animals, not infrequently birds that sometimes may carry viruses over long distances. The spread of myxomatosis among rabbits in the latter phase of the epizootic was mainly from animal to animal via mosquitoes, like in the case of human urban yellow fever.

The Evaluations by Nobel Committees

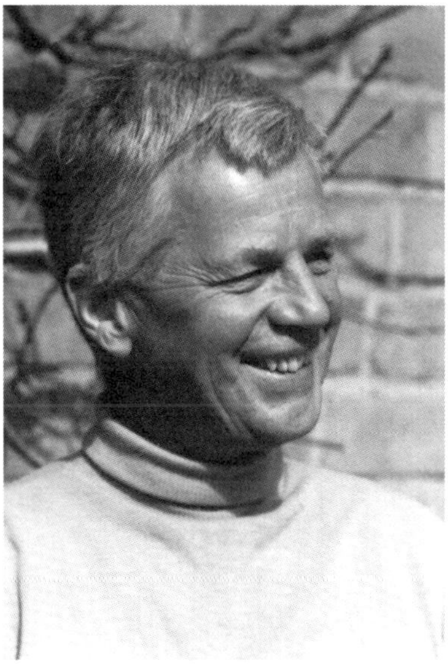

Berndt Malmgren (1906–1977). [Courtesy of Malmgren's daughter Marianne Liedström.]

Burnet was nominated for a Nobel Prize in physiology or medicine for the first time in 1948 and hereafter yearly until 1960, except in 1951, 1952 and 1957. In total there were 19 nominations and all except *one* (out of the three in 1960) were for his contributions to the field of virology. The exceptional nomination in 1960 highlighted his contributions to the field of immunology and this was in fact also mentioned in another of the three nominations that year. Sven Gard (p. 77) made repeated evaluations of Burnet. Gard was professor of virology at the Karolinska Institute, my mentor and predecessor as professor and chairman. He has been introduced in my previous book[3]. In addition to Gard's reviews, two evaluations were made by Berndt Malmgren, professor of bacteriology. Their impressions and the committee's evaluation of Burnet's work on viruses were as follows.

The first nomination of Burnet was by a professor of pathology in Adelaide, J. B. Cleland. In a five-page attachment he cited examples of Burnet's important contributions within all the different fields presented above. The committee asked Gard to make an in depth evaluation. He served as an adjunct member on the committee for the first time in 1948, the same year in which he had been appointed as professor and chairman for a department of virus research as a result of an initiative by the Swedish Parliament. Gard was kept busy by his engagement in the Nobel Prize work from the beginning and his first task on the committee became to make a preliminary investigation of Max Theiler nominated by Albert Sabin. This relatively thorough first investigation together with some supplementary comments formed the basis for the prize to Theiler three years later (Ref. 3, Chapter 4). However, Gard's main engagement during his first year was a 14 page investigation of Burnet submitted in early September.

Early Steps Towards Virus Chemoprophylaxis

There is no doubt that Gard has a considerable respect and admiration for Burnet's many important contributions to the development of the field of virology, but he had a problem. This was to select one particular discovery out of Burnet's many contributions to highlight to the Committee as *the* basis for a prize. He divided the material into three major fields; the formation of antibodies and the mechanisms of immune reactions; the nature and function of bacteriophages; and various questions regarding viruses infecting man. He decided to leave out Burnet's contribution in immunology, since he judged this at the time to be in a relatively preliminary state. During the 1950s Burnet progressively expanded and deepened his engagement in immunological problems, but it would take until 1960 before his contributions in this field were eventually reviewed in depth by Gard.

Concerning the phage studies Gard reviewed in particular Burnet's introduction of the receptor concept and the importance of such structures for the first step of a virus infection of a cell. Studies of receptors for phages were concluded to be important also for the understanding of how these bacterial viruses get into cells. Gard then turned his attention to the various studies of animal viruses. He discussed the visionary interpretations of the nature of herpes virus infections, including their propensity to establish a dormant latent stage from which they can be reactivated. He mentioned briefly the epidemiological studies of psittacosis and Q fever, none of which are caused by true viruses, but by more complex bacterial cellular parasites, collectively referred to as *Chlamydia* and *Rickettsia*, respectively.

Hereafter, Gard reviewed the development of the embryonated hen's egg techniques and its importance *inter alia* for studies of influenza virus. The main part of the review concerned the hemagglutinins of different viruses, especially influenza virus. Gard was intrigued by these groundbreaking studies and deduced that here was a possibility for the future development of a general way to treat virus infections. In fact there were some experiments in which Burnet and collaborators had treated the airways of animals with agents interfering with the function of receptors and hereafter tried to infect them. This led to a certain protection against disease. Gard wrote in an underlined text "The observation that eggs treated by RDE are completely resistant to infection.... This protective effect has been demonstrated also in mice." He concluded that Burnet was the driving force in all these epoch-making discoveries, but he briefly also mentioned Hirst as an interesting candidate. The concluding paragraphs in Gard's evaluation read:

> The importance of these observations need not be further discussed. From the theoretical point of view they represent the first step towards a deeper insight in the relations between a virus and a host cell. The practical consequences for human medicine in the form of an effective chemoprophylaxis against virus infections can already be seen as a possible reality.
>
> With reference to what I have presented above it is without hesitation my opinion to characterize Burnet's contributions as prize-worthy.

The committee agreed with Gard's conclusion and specified that it had found Burnet's method to make cells unsusceptible to certain virus infections prize-worthy. It recommended that the 1948 Prize should recognize Paul Müller's discovery of DDT as an effective insecticide, which also became the decision of the Faculty — the College of Professors (Ref. 3, Chapter 6).

Influenza Virus Grown in Eggs

Burnet was nominated again the following year, this time together with Goodpasture by two professors from Leiden, J. Mulder and J. D. Verlinde. There were also two nominations for Goodpasture alone. The nominations focussed on the development of different techniques for growing viruses in embryonated hen's eggs. Gard made two separate evaluations, one, of a preliminary nature, of Goodpasture and another, a full investigation, of Burnet. In the evaluation of Goodpasture he praised the introduction of the new techniques for growing viruses in eggs. However, this methodological advance was not by itself considered worthy of a Nobel Prize. It was not a discovery. The four page review of Burnet gave further support to his strength as a candidate for the prize. The committee concluded again that his discovery of a method to make cells unsusceptible to certain virus infections was prize-worthy, but it was of the opinion, following a supplementary note by Gard (an attachment A) that it should delay awarding a prize. The prize this year was split between Walter R. Hess "for his discovery of the functional organization of the diencephalon as a coordinator of the activities of the internal organs" and Antonio Egas Moniz "for his discovery of the therapeutic value of leucotomy in certain psychoses". This is a very much discussed prize; in particular the part that concerned the leucotomy procedure, which later came into disrepute[12].

Q Fever

In 1950 Burnet was nominated by Max S. Marshall, professor of bacteriology in San Francisco, on this occasion for his discovery of the etiology of Q fever. Back in 1934 an epidemic of fairly high fevers was observed in men working in abattoirs in Brisbane. The causative agent was recovered in guinea pigs by a Dr E. H. Derrick, but its nature was unravelled first when Burnet managed to transmit the infection to mice and performed careful light microscopy. Using the highest power he saw "herring-bone" like patterns. He concluded that it was a rickettsia, a cellular parasite larger and more complex than a virus. To honor its discoverer it later came to be called *Coxiella burnetii*, a fact which Burnet himself with amusement noted might give him a passport to immortality.

Gard made another full investigation and noted that the nomination identified another of Burnet's many seminal contributions. He commented that the range of "purposefulness, intuition and efficacy" were characteristics of Burnet's approach to science. However, Gard did not focus on the Q fever studies in his review, but made a follow-up analysis over some ten pages of Burnet's and colleagues work on the receptor for influenza virus. He noted again that treatment of mice with compounds that modify the cellular receptor for influenza virus could cause a delay, but not a blocking of an infection. Thus the goal to identify an effective prophylactic has not been reached. Still Gard argued strongly for a prize to Burnet and he concluded: "The theoretical and principal importance of these publications is, however, so large that I do not hesitate to characterize them as prize-worthy. In particular I would like to mention the discovery of RDE, the receptor destroying enzyme, with its capacity to change originally susceptible cells to cells insusceptible to infection." Gard's argumentations had an impact on the committee. In its recommendations to the Faculty Burnet remained on the list of prize-worthy candidates with the same motivation given in 1948, but in its final recommendations the committee was split, as described earlier (Ref. 3, Chapters 4 and 6). The majority of its 13 ordinary and adjunct members proposed that the Prize should be given to Philip S. Hench, Edward C. Kendall and Tadeous Reichstein for their discovery of hormones of the adrenal cortex and their clinical use, but four members including the chairman were of a different opinion. They recommended that the prize should be split between Max Theiler for his discovery of the yellow fever vaccine and Burnet for the discovery of methods that made cells resistant to certain virus infections. In the Faculty the majority opinion of the committee prevailed. Theiler received his Nobel Prize the following year but Burnet had to wait a good bit longer.

Nominations of Burnet were absent in 1951 and 1952 but in 1953 he was nominated again, now by two colleagues from Sydney, C. W. Stump and A. N. Burkitt. The Committee asked the bacteriologist Malmgren to make a supplementary review of Burnet. His five-page discussion of Burnet gave some supplementary information on recent experiments to be added to the information available in the previous reviews by Gard. The committee repeated its motivation for Burnet's prize-worthiness.

Hemagglutination

In 1954 Burnet was proposed by A. A. Moncrieff, London for his studies of virus hemagglutination and the significance of this phenomenon for the understanding of virus attachment to cells. He also emphasized Burnet's many additional contributions leading to a deeper understanding of the natural history of several virus diseases. In a separate nomination Hirst was proposed for his discovery of virus hemagglutination. Gard made another full evaluation of both of these two candidates together. He initially took note that the four previous evaluations of Burnet had concluded that he was considered highly worthy of a prize. Among his many different important contributions those made in his influenza studies were ranked the highest according to Gard's opinion.

Hirst started his work with influenza in 1940 when he was employed by the Rockefeller Foundation International Health Division. The Foundation ran a laboratory at Princeton University, supervised by Wendell M. Stanley, the recipient of a shared 1946 Nobel Prize in chemistry for his crystallization of tobacco mosaic virus (Ref. 3, Chapter 3). The main work of the laboratory concerned development of a vaccine against influenza. This was considered to have high priority at the beginning of the Second World War. A separate part of the research work concerning the vaccine was pursued at the Foundation's laboratories in New York. It was there that Hirst started his work after having received a scholarship from the Foundation. It did not take more than a year before he had made the important observation that the virus could agglutinate red blood cells. He characterized the mechanisms of interaction between virus and the cells — the adsorption and elution (release) — and the possibility of blocking this by antibodies. Hirst also managed to demonstrate that the cellular receptors appeared to be of mucopolysaccharide nature. However the chemical studies of the receptors in Burnet's laboratory were more detailed. After a further analyses of the detailed studies of the hemagglutination phenomenon Gard made the following summary statement:

> (The results of) Burnet's and Hirst's work appear to me without hesitation to be worthy of a prize. They supplement each other in a very fortunate way. Although there are many researchers who have contributed to the solving of the problem, it has not been possible for me to identify that any other contributions within this field can be compared to Burnet's and Hirst's. It therefore seems reasonable that a Nobel Prize for the work concerning the (virus) receptor mechanisms is divided equally between the two of them.

The committee agreed and declared both Burnet and Hirst prize-worthy. The prize in 1954 went to three other virologists John Enders, Thomas

Weller and Frederick Robbins for their growth of polio virus in non-nervous tissues, very much due to Gard's skilful and authoritative argumentation (Ref. 3, Chapter 5).

The Weakening Candidacy

In 1955 there were two more nominations of Burnet by J. I. Robertson, Adelaide and C. W. Jungeblut, New York. Malmgren made his second evaluation, but it was just a single page and did not contain any new information. The Committee retained Burnet as a strong candidate with the same motivation as before. There were three new nominations of Burnet in 1956, and in particular the one from Dale, the above-mentioned director of the National Institute for Medical Research in London and the 1936 Nobel laureate, was very comprehensive. It contained some very complimentary statements; the Institute in Melbourne that Burnet has developed as director "is second to none"; and that studies by the Committee of the documents he submitted should allow it to "recognize the brilliant and widely influential nature of the fundamental contributions which Sir Macfarlane Burnet has made, and is still making, to the special field of medical and biological knowledge with which they deal." The committee repeated its recognition of Burnet's prize-worthiness, but the impact of his candidacy was losing momentum because it added "but found that the future developments should be awaited". Thus there may have been some truth in Burnet's premonition that the strength of his candidacy for a prize had started to wane.

In the history of the work by the Nobel Committee at the Karolinska Institute one can find many examples of candidates who for a number of years are among the top candidates, but then gradually start to lag behind these. I have personally seen a number of cases of this kind during my involvement over two decades with the Nobel Prize in physiology or medicine. In a way it was fortunate that Burnet could make a comeback by his theoretical contributions to a completely different field, to immunology.

Nominations for Burnet's virus work continued. There were two more proposals in 1958 (F. Fenner, Canberra and J. Tornezik, Basel) and another two in 1959 (Dale and Banks, again). Finally in 1960, as already briefly mentioned, there were two more nominations of Burnet for his virus work by R. Lovell, London and J. Lederberg, Palo Alto, but the latter nomination also mentioned that "he has been instrumental in approaching the problems of immunology from a modern point of view". The third nomination by Jorgen M. Birkeland, Columbus, Ohio, only focused on Burnet's contributions to immunology. It proposed specifically to award his theory of antibody formation and referred to his very recent book *The Clonal Selection Theory of Acquired Immunity*[13]. The nomination mentioned Burnet's prediction that tolerance might evolve during the embryonic phase of life and it further stated "Billingham and Medawar tested this theory using skin homografts and found that it was true". The latter two scientists however were not included in this nomination. We will return to these nominations in the next chapter.

The Continued Studies of Virus Receptors

In the end it can be concluded that Burnet was never recognized by a Nobel Prize in physiology or medicine for his introduction of methods to make cells insusceptible to a virus infection, which Gard had selected to be the most outstanding discovery among his many prize-worthy contributions in virology. In a historical perspective this has turned out to be very fortunate since the conceptually attractive method of preventing virus infections by blocking the two first steps in the interaction between a virus particle and a cell — the adsorption (docking) and penetration — has not turned out, over the last 50 years, to be a particularly rewarding approach to the development of effective drugs against viruses — *anti-virals*. This is both surprising and disappointing considering the very impressive refined knowledge that in a number of cases has been gained in the understanding of the detailed molecular events of these early steps of virus replication.

Before describing the present state of affairs concerning development of new anti-virals some general comments should be made. The receptors on cells which make it possible for viruses to attack them are not present originally to serve this function but to have some other physiological role. During the course of evolution they have been hijacked by the virus for its own use. To this should be added that physiologically occurring structures at the surface of cells are continuously subjected to a turnover like all other structures in cells. Thus a cell from which structures used as receptors for a certain virus have been removed with (variable) time will regain susceptibility to the virus. This was what Burnet found when he tested receptor-destroying compounds in animals. The effect observed was moderate and transient.

In spite of this apparent limitation it would be very attractive to exploit any possibility to block, for example, the entry of common cold viruses into cells. There are some hundred different types of such viruses, which precludes any possibility of developing an effective vaccine. An alternative would be to attempt blocking the receptors used, since many members of groups of viruses causing the infection in the nasal mucosa use the same cell surface structure. In 1985 Michael Rossman and his colleagues at Purdue University, Indiana, managed, by use of X-ray crystallography, to define the fine structure of a type of common cold virus that looks like poliovirus. They were also successful in defining the groove at the virus surface which interacted with the receptor on cells. For many years they were searching, in collaboration with major pharmaceutical companies, for tailor-made chemical compounds that could block the critical function of the groove. Regrettably these extensive efforts have not as yet met with success.

Also in situations when the development of a vaccine has failed in spite of many efforts to produce one, as in the case of human immunodeficiency virus (HIV), there is an urgency to find effective anti-viral compounds. The latter case is in fact the best example of a highly successful development of a number of compounds which interfere effectively with different steps in virus replication, in fact also including both its adsorption and penetration. Thus there is one HIV anti-viral which blocks the CCR5 receptor of certain (M-tropic) type 1 strains and another that interferes with the fusion of virus and cell membranes, which is a prerequisite for the release of the virus genetic material into the cell. The highly successful development of antivirals controlling HIV infections can serve to illustrate another principally very important issue. This concerns the emergence of drug-resistant virus strains.

There is a major difference in the fidelity of replication of nucleic acids in a virus and in the cells constituting our bodies. The DNA in our cells replicates with a remarkably high precision, making a mistake in the insertion of only one in a million of the nucleotide bases used in the coded genetic message. By way of contrast the number of mistakes in the replication of a virus nucleic acid is about 100 times higher. One result of this fact is that it is relatively easy for a virus to spurn a mutant that escapes the inhibition by a certain compound. The only way of managing this problem is to use several — at least three — drugs which interfere with different steps in the virus replication cycle. The possibility for an escape of a resistant virus mutant is the multiple of the risks with each individual compound. If three different compounds are used simultaneously the possibility for emergence of a drug-resistant virus is one in ten thousand multiplied by itself twice. This gives a very low number meaning that essentially it is impossible for the virus to generate a triple mutant capable of replicating in the presence of all three drugs.

Many attempts have been made to develop anti-virals with an effect on influenza viruses. An access to drugs effectively blocking this virus would circumvent the limits of available vaccines, which have to be updated every year because of the antigenic drift and occasionally also shift that occurs. Drugs with some capacity to block virus replication have been developed and have come into a certain use. One kind of drugs is amantadine compounds which have an effect on one of the minor virus proteins, which form special channels for the transmission of ions into the infected cell, conjectured to influence the membrane fusion phenomenon. The second kind of compound has a blocking effect on the minor surface component of the virus (p.18), the neuraminidase. Interestingly, the effect of this compound is not on virus penetration but instead a blocking of the release of particles. During the final phase of virus replication particles are formed by being progressively budded off from the cytoplasmic membrane. It should be noted that it is important that the released particles are not adsorbed back onto receptors which have remained at the surface of the cell from which they were produced. This can be secured by some mechanism of removal of the receptors during the concluding phase of virus release from the infected cell. The neuraminidase component seems to serve this function.

Burnet came to advance the field of virology in many different ways due to his fundamental discoveries over more than three decades. In 1959 the complete knowledge in the field of virology at the time was summarized in three volumes: *The Viruses: Biochemical, Biological and Biophysical Properties*, Volumes 1, 2 and 3. They provided an encyclopedic presentation of a field of research that I had just entered. The editors of these volumes were Burnet and the Nobel laureate in chemistry, Stanley.

The Golden Age of Virology and the Changing Science

In his writings Burnet made frequent reference to how privileged he had been to have been active during the golden age of virology. It was first in 1958 that it became possible to give a resilient definition of a virus (Ref. 3, Chapter 3). From the 1930s through to the 1950s many of the medically important viruses were discovered and similar advances were made in studies of viruses infecting animals and plants exploited for the progress of human civilization. These impressive advances, which allowed the early development of a number of effective vaccines, like the ones against polio, measles, mumps, rubella, etc. led Burnet to conclude that the most important discoveries in the field of virology had been made – an end of science perspective.

It is also of interest to note that Burnet was relatively sceptical about the new technologies developed from the 1950s and onwards. He did not believe that the progressively introduced advanced techniques of molecular biology could provide results that would be of practical use in preventing infectious disease. Historical developments have shown that this sceptical attitude was unjustified. Just to give two examples, the viruses causing AIDS and severe acute respiratory syndrome (SARS) would not have been recognized at the time without access to molecular tools and the drugs we have access to today to successfully treat the former disease have been possible to develop only because we have a deep insight into the molecular mechanisms of replication of HIV.

My own engagement in virological research and teaching of this discipline started when Burnet argued that all was over. Not surprisingly my interpretation of developments in the field differs from the one expressed by Burnet. There have been impressive advances, many of which have allowed us to markedly improve our capacity to control virus infections. I was privileged to be a part of the process, which transformed virology from a discipline amenable to relatively crude biological examination to one employing sophisticated biochemical techniques. However in my teaching of medical students I evolved into a Burnetian. During the 1960s the subject was presented starting with the structure of the different kinds of virus particles, progressing to the replication of these viruses in cells and onwards to their interaction with the multicellular organism during the disease process. In the end the features of epidemics were reviewed. It was a bottom-up approach. After having used this outline for my lectures for a decade I completely reversed the sequence of presentation of the discipline. Initially the particular features of virus epidemics were reviewed and then it was described how these had their origin in the features of the unique interactions between viruses and man in the infectious process. Equal weight was given to the role of the two actors. The process was then further dissected until the importance of the genetic make-up of the different viruses had come into focus. This approach, which was appreciated by my students, reflected Burnet's attitude to his science. He started with the wide perspective and then worked his way towards finer and finer details.

It was a characteristic of Burnet that he was bold in formulating hypotheses. Georg Klein has written about Burnet in one of his books[14] and he cited a story about him that has been widely circulated. It runs as follows:

> It takes Sir Mac five days and five hen's eggs to make an experiment from which he can derive a new theory, which is often published rapidly and in the form of a book. Hereafter it takes 500 virologists about five years of work and the use of half a million hen's eggs before the theory has been proven wrong. However, all this work has led to the development of a new branch of science. In the meantime Burnet has lost interest in this field and has moved on to another one.

And it is true that Burnet was unique in his capacity to spurn new theories. Nossal has made a remark about Burnet's approach to science that is quite illuminating:

> Burnet believed totally that nature was always trying to tell him something. So he would take the unexpected, uninterpretable results and turn them this way and that, add and subtract figures in various simple ways, *play* with the data until they were forced into some kind of order. Somewhat mischievously he would say, "Nossal, I never repeat an experiment". He didn't mean it literally, of course. What he meant was that each experiment, no matter how small, would suggest some extra step, an extra control, an extra slight experimental variation, making the confirmatory experiment always into an elaboration, a broadening learning experience.

This citation brings to mind a statement ascribed to Francis Crick — "Do not let a good hypothesis be destroyed by a lousy experiment." We should also let Burnet use his own words to describe his approach to science. He said "I believe that scholarly work in science must aim at generalization and that research lacks meaning if it is not at every stage guided and stimulated by hypotheses, including major ones, devised on the best available data and analogies and put in such a form that in principle an experimental discussion, proof, disproof or modification, should eventually be possible." Thus it would seem that a critical aspect of the mind of a scientist is its capacity to exaggerate the relevant and to simplify or ignore the irrelevant aspects of reality. This problem will be discussed more extensively in Chapter 9. To further elaborate on Burnet's views one more citation from his autobiography could be given. "Great discoveries are usually made by the recognition of some wholly unexpected finding and just because the new phenomenon is outside of the design of their experimental programme it must be studied at first by the use of what for their time are amateurish techniques." This statement makes it clear that Burnet was aware of the limitations that techniques available at the time gave. He would certainly have agreed with Medawar's view, reflected in the title of one of his essays that science is *The art of the soluble*[15]. This was formulated to be antithetical to statements of the 1860s by the German iron chancellor Otto von Bismarck. He said that politics is not an exact science, but instead it is the *art of the possible*.

Since Burnet was aware of the limitations of available techniques in a certain situation one would have expected that he would have been curious about new techniques, but he was not. In fact he was openly critical of the introduction of new techniques in the rapidly emerging field of molecular biology in the early 1960s. Still one may ask if there might be a grain of truth in Burnet's statement that biological sciences changed their characteristics in the early 1960s when a range of molecular techniques were progressively introduced? Could it be that it became more difficult to make new dramatic hypotheses as time progressed and the work came to focus on finer and finer details? The answer to this question is probably both yes and no. We will return to this question in the last chapter, which will further consider the concept genius and its application to successful scientists.

It is now time to turn our attention to Medawar. He will be one of the two lead characters in the next chapter. By his versatile mind and intellect he was well aware of the value of words, including the etymological meaning of the word genius. Against this background it is interesting to note the following statement that he made about his fellow Nobel Prize recipient:

> *Genius* is not a word used lightly by scientists in referring to each other's work, but I have repeatedly said of Mac Burnet that he is a bit of a genius, not merely for the insight that anticipated the discovery of tolerance but for that even deeper insight that enabled him to interpret immunological reactions in terms of the population dynamics of lymphoid cells.

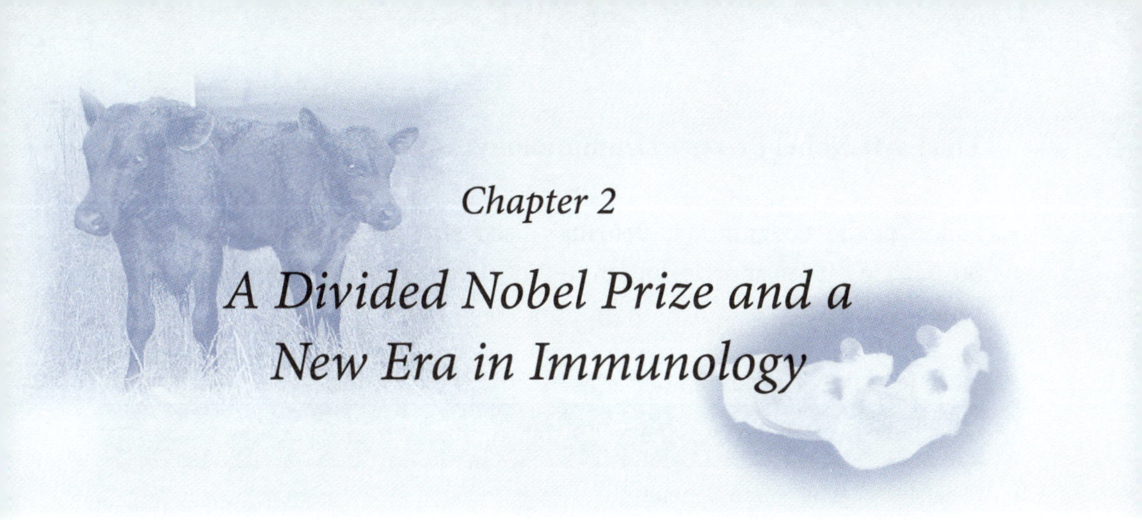

Chapter 2

A Divided Nobel Prize and a New Era in Immunology

THE SELF OR NON-SELF
A CREDO OF BIOLOGY
CLONAL SELECTION

It has been known since ancient times that individuals who have survived an attack by a well-recognized infectious disease may show resistance when exposed on the occasion of a new epidemic wave of the same disease. This insensitivity to a specific disease was referred to as immunity, from Latin *immunitas* meaning a temporary exemption from taxation for returned soldiers of the Roman Empire. The first Nobel Prize in physiology or medicine in 1901 was given to Emil A. von Behring for his discovery that an "anti"-serum generated by immunization of horses with bacterial products could prevent diphtheria[1,2]. The active substance came to be called *antibodies* — originally anti-toxin, because they inhibited the activity of the poisonous part of the bacterium which was the cause of the disease. These antibodies were demonstrated to be specific in their reaction with the substance used to stimulate their production. It was further recognized that the production of antibodies was facilitated by multiple injections over time of the selected substance, later called *antigen* (from *anti*body *gen*erator). There was some kind of memory in the immune system of multicellular organisms and after repeated injections there was an accelerated — a *boosted* — and more powerful immune response. During the later part of his professional life Behring was involved in developing procedures for stimulating production of antibodies by direct immunization of humans with inactivated toxins from the bacterium causing diphtheria and also the one causing tetanus.

The Early Nobel Prizes in Immunology

Following the recognition of Behring's discovery there were, prior to the 1960 Burnet and Medawar prize, four more Nobel Prizes in physiology or medicine, which focussed on advances in immunology (Table 2.1).

Table 2.1. Nobel Prizes in Physiology or Medicine (1901–1959) recognizing advances in immunology.

Year	Awardee(s)	Motivation
1901	Emil A. von Behring	for his work on serum therapy, especially application against diphtheria...
1908	Paul Ehrlich Ilya Ilyich Mechnicov	in recognition of their work on immunity
1913	Charles R. Richet	in recognition of his work on anaphylaxis
1919	Jules Bordet	for his discoveries relating to immunity
1930	Karl Landsteiner	for his discovery of human blood groups

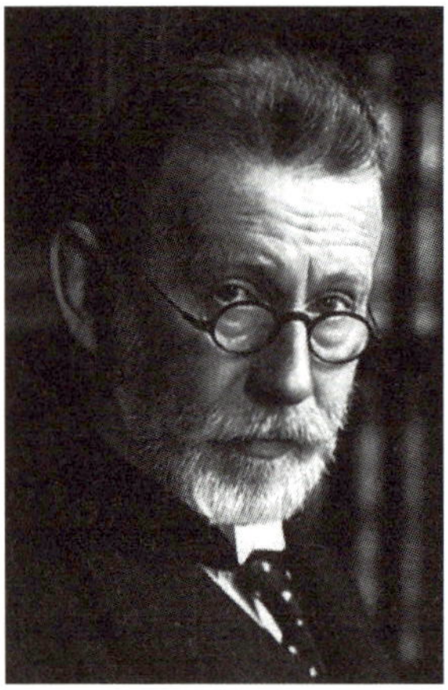

Paul Ehrlich (1854–1915), recipient of the shared 1908 Nobel Prize in physiology or medicine. [From *Les Prix Nobel en 1908.*]

The reaction between antigen and antibodies was studied in more detail by Paul Ehrlich, who like Behring got his initial training in Robert Koch's laboratory. Koch was one of the founding fathers of the field of bacteriology[1], but did not receive his Nobel Prize until 1905 "for his investigations and discoveries in relation to tuberculosis". Like Koch, Ehrlich can be named a father of a new discipline, immunology. Both of them had to wait for their Nobel Prizes and Ehrlich was not recognized until 1908. He was the first scientist to distinguish between the use of preformed antibodies in the treatment of infectious diseases — *passive immunization* — as compared to the use of a selected antigen for generation of immunity in an individual to prevent future disease. The latter procedure is called *active immunization* or today more generally referred to as *vaccination*. He was also the first to formulate ideas about the reaction between antigen and antibody. These were vague speculations since at this time the chemical nature of the interacting components was unknown.

Ehrlich also came to make pioneering contributions to developments in the field of chemotherapeutics leading to the introduction of a "magic bullet" against syphilis — Salvarsan — and very appropriately one of the two most important German prizes in biomedicine is the *Paul Ehrlich und Ludwig Darmstaedter Prize*. The other important prize in this field, not surprisingly, is the *Robert Koch Prize*. No prizes of the former kind were awarded for a long time in connection with the Second World War because Ehrlich had a Jewish ethnic background. For 18 years I was involved in the committee that selected the yearly recipients of the Paul Ehrlich und Ludwig Darmstaedter Prize and we were able to recognize many discoveries by front line immunologists. We also recognized other advances in biomedicine and one year we gave the prize to two crystallographers, one of whom was Michael Rossman, mentioned in the previous chapter. At the prize ceremony in the Frauenkirche (a deconsecrated building) in Frankfurt I learnt that Rossman, who like Ehrlich had a Jewish ethnic background, had had to flee the city together with his mother when he was 11 years old. It was a major emotional experience for him to now return to the city where he had been born, to receive his prize.

The 1908 Nobel Prize in physiology or medicine did not only recognize Ehrlich but also Ilya Mechnikov. A joint prize motivation — "for their work on immunity" — was used, but their contributions were very different. Ehrlich's work focused on antibodies circulating in serum — the *humoral* (from umor, *Lat.* moist, liquid) *immunity* — the way they can be induced and their specificity. By way of contrast Mechnikov's work focused on the importance of cells in the immune defence. This was a field of research he came to pioneer, but it was one that would take a long time to mature. He was primarily interested in macrophages — a word meaning large eaters — which could ingest foreign material like bacteria and potentially disarm them. The process of engulfing foreign material was called *phagocytosis*. This is a general mechanism that cannot be educated to specifically distinguish one microorganism from the other. Much later it has been found to be a part of a very complex system with different mechanisms acting as a first line of defence. These non-specific mechanisms are collectively referred to as *innate immunity*. Many important discoveries concerning different qualities

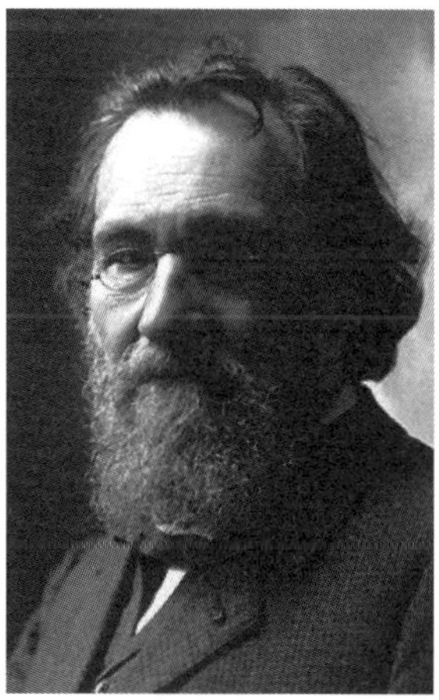

Ilya I. Mechnikov (1845–1916), recipient of the shared 1908 Nobel Prize in physiology or medicine. [From *Les Prix Nobel en 1908*.]

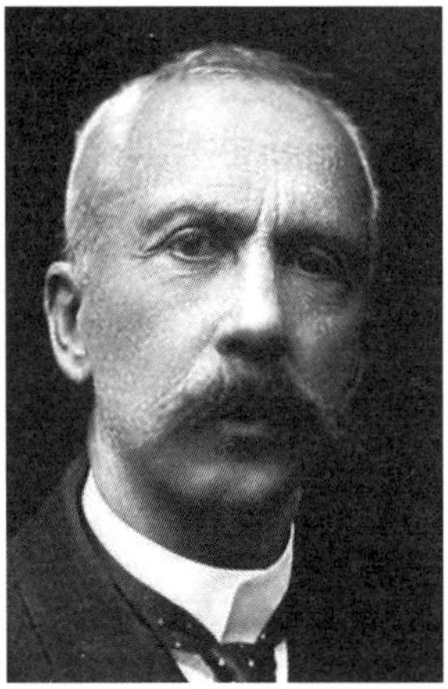

Charles R. Richet (1850–1935), recipient of the 1913 Nobel Prize in physiology or medicine. [From *Les Prix Nobel en 1913*.]

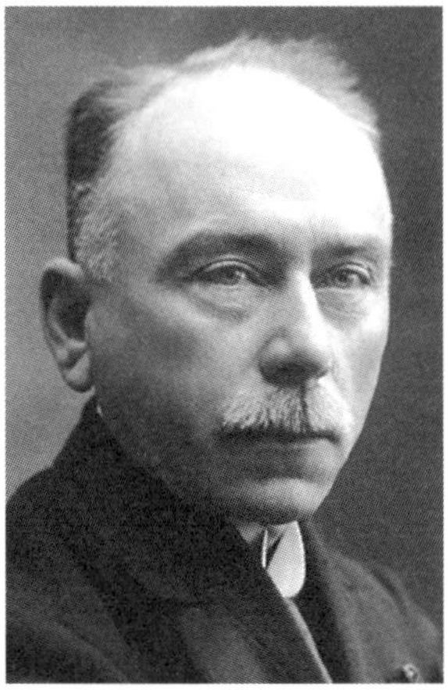

Jules Bordet (1870–1961), recipient of the 1919 Nobel Prize in physiology or medicine, awarded in 1920. [From *Les Prix Nobel en 1919*.]

of the innate immune defence have been made in our time, but it would take until 2011 before another Nobel Prize was awarded to recognize these advances as described in the next chapter. All other — specific and adjustable — mechanisms, targeted against a foreign intruder, be it a virus, bacterium, parasite or a helminth, are brought together under the term *adaptive immunity*. As this term indicates it is possible to adjust both the specificity and intensity of this kind of immunological reaction. For many decades the field concerned with adaptable immunity was dominated by "humoralists" — scientists focussing on the role of antibodies — and it was not until the 1940s that certain white blood cells — the *lymphocytes* — involved in immune responses began to become the focus of interest. Later on it turned out that the *cell-mediated immunity* was a very diversified and complex field.

In 1913 the Nobel Prize in physiology or medicine recognized studies by Charles Richet of the phenomenon of anaphylaxis, the potentially life-threatening allergic reactions to particular antigens. This was the first demonstration that the immune system not only can provide protection against invading infectious agents, but also under certain unfortunate circumstances be harmful to its host. Richet was a scientist with many different engagements, a renaissance man with deep cultural interests and at the same time a pioneer in aviation. His interests in extrasensory perception and hypnosis were particularly exotic. In hypnotic séances with the famous medium Eusapia Palladino he saw mist-like formations looking like fuzzy extremities, to which he gave the name teleplasma.

The 1919 Nobel Prize in physiology or medicine was awarded in 1920 to a Belgium microbiologist and immunologist Jules Bordet "for his discoveries relating to immunity". In parenthesis it can be mentioned that this is the first time that the word "discovery" has been used in a Prize motivation. Bordet's studies showed that the interaction between antibodies and bacteria can be more complex than previously found in studies of diphtheria and tetanus, in which case the critical effect was blocking the action of toxins. In other cases the antibodies acted directly on the bacterial cell, which under certain conditions may become destroyed — lysed — by the attack. In order to study immune reactions against foreign cells, like bacteria, Bordet used red blood cells from a different species as a model system. The disintegration of such cells could be readily measured by the release of the red pigment, haemoglobin, a phenomenon referred to as *hemolysis*. This experimental system allowed the analysis of the importance of various components in serum for the destruction of cells. Some of these, like the so-called *complement system*, later on turned out to be very complex and involve many different proteins normally present in serum. It was Bordet's original discovery of complement that made it possible to develop the Wassermann reaction, an antibody-dependent — *serological* — test that for the first time allowed a specific demonstration of syphilis. What Bordet recognized was that there is a difference between the normal cells of a body and foreign cells, be they bacteria or cells from another vertebrate species. Bordet also made other high-class scientific contributions to investigations of the mechanisms of coagulation of blood. Furthermore, together with Octave Gengou, he discovered the bacterium causing whooping cough. His textbook *Traité de l'immunité* was a classic in its time.

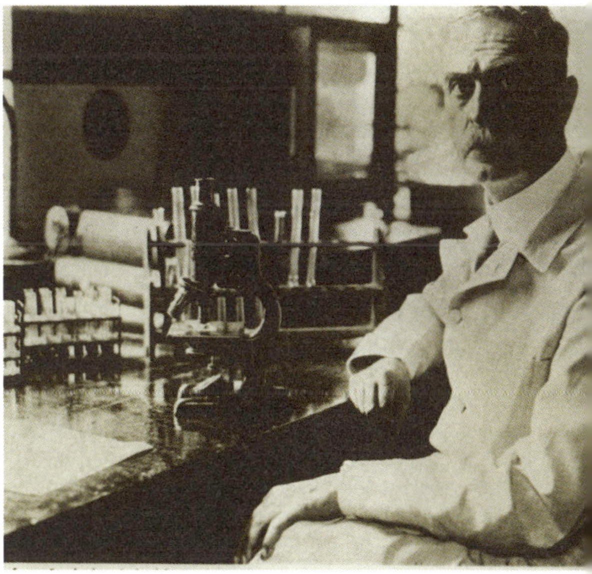

Karl Landsteiner (1868–1943), recipient of the Nobel Prize in physiology or medicine 1930. [From Ref. 31.]

The discovery as early as 1901 by Karl Landsteiner of naturally occurring antibodies capable of agglutinating red blood cells of humans laid the ground work for distinguishing human blood groups, A, B, AB and O. It took time to recognize the importance of this finding, not the least for the evaluation of possibilities for safe transfusion of blood between humans. Landsteiner did not receive his Nobel Prize in physiology or medicine until 1930 after having been nominated for some ten years. The prize motivation was "for his discovery of human blood groups". Landsteiner was a very influential scientist contributing an impressive number of discoveries. He was the first one to recover poliovirus from a patient by infection of monkeys in 1908 (Ref. 2, Chapter 5). His early work was done in Vienna where he was born and also received his medical education. He became engaged in biomedical sciences at an early stage and spent five years in Germany to learn biochemistry, partly in the laboratory of H. Emil Fischer, the recipient of the 1902 Nobel Prize in Chemistry. In 1919 he left Vienna and after a few years in The Hague he moved to New York and the famous Rockefeller Institute. There he continued his high class research even after he became an emeritus professor in 1939. Late in his career, in the 1940s, he demonstrated another important blood group system. This was the Rh system, from *Rh*esus monkeys, which can play an important role during pregnancy.

It might be noted in this context that a pregnancy represents a particular potential source of immunological complications. The cells of the embryo carry antigens both from the mother and from the father and hence it contains foreign antigens that potentially can result in an immunization of the mother. There are of course mechanisms that have evolved since the emergence of vertebrates which prevent a pregnant mother from mounting an immune response against the embryo she is carrying. Surprisingly, in spite of the amazing advances of immunology to be discussed below, it is still not clear what the nature of these important protective mechanisms are. There is a particular problem with circulating cells of foetal origin that might be transferred to the mother. This is where the Rh system becomes important. If a mother is Rh– and the fetus Rh+ — antigens from the father — the leakage of blood that normally occurs from the foetus to the mother over the placenta will cause an immunization of the mother. This will not lead to any problems during the first pregnancy, but repeated exposure of the mother to Rh+ cells in connection with later pregnancies potentially can give a mild to severe haemolytic disease in the newborn and even lead to stillbirth. Today these complications can be prevented by giving the mother an immunoglobulin preparation containing antibodies against the Rh antigen.

Landsteiner also made yet one more fundamental discovery during the last years of his life. He laid the foundation for forthcoming extensive studies of cell-mediated immunity. In a classical 1942 publication Landsteiner and Merill Chase examined the quality of immunity in guinea pigs immunized with Mycobacterium tuberculosis. They collected lymphocytes from the immunized animals and transferred them to non-immunized — naïve — animals. When the latter animals were immunized with the same bacterial antigen they mounted an accelerated and recollected — *anamnestic* — antibody response as if they had already been immunized before. This was not seen in control animals who had received antiserum from previously immunized animals. Landsteiner died in 1943, literally with a pipette in his hand.

It would take 30 years after the award of the prize to Landsteiner until further advances in our understanding of immune functions in 1960 were recognized by a Nobel Prize in physiology or medicine. At that time there were two fundamental questions concerning adaptive immunity waiting for an answer. The first, central question was

> Which are the mechanisms that allow a vertebrate organism to develop and memorize a specific immune response against essentially any foreign structure?

Connected to this was another important implicit question and that concerned

> How can an organism (a body) distinguish between its own components and foreign components and ensure that it does not develop (immune) reactions against itself?

The prize in 1960 to Burnet and Medawar only concerned discoveries addressing the second question and the Prize motivation was "for the discovery of immunological tolerance". Still Burnet argued that he had answers to both questions. As we shall see he in fact concluded that he was not recognized for his most important discovery in immunology, but only for his second best.

From Virology to Immunology

Self and Non-self

Burnet as we have seen in the previous chapter always took a broad view when he reviewed the different kinds of interactions between infectious agents and the host. As he repeatedly emphasized he was a biologist and an evolutionist. His thoughts through the 1940s and more intensively during the 1950s came to focus on how we defend ourselves against infectious agents, how we could mobilize a specific immune response and how our bodies can retain a memory of the exposure and give protection, often life-long, against a renewed infection with the same agent. The first thing that struck him was that there must be some way that different living systems, even relatively simpler ones, are able to distinguish between chemical entities that are a natural part of the organism — the *self* — and those that are foreign — the *non-self.* Such a distinction is essential to any kind of defence mechanism. It should be noted that at the time of Burnet's hypothesizing it was understood that an antibody like an anti-diphtheria toxin was a globular protein, but little was known about the chemical nature of genes.

It had become appreciated that individual humans could have different representations of "self"-antigens. There are different blood groups in humans, A, B, AB and O, reflecting varying representation of antigens on red blood cells, as mentioned above. These blood groups were demonstrated to be subjected to a regular Mendelian genetic inheritance. The principle is that a person with blood group A has antibodies against red cells with group B structures on their surface whereas the reverse is true for someone with blood group B. In order to avoid serious complications of intravascular aggregation of red blood cells, this needs to be considered in connection with blood transfusions. Homologous blood needs to be used. However, transfusion of red blood cells from an individual with blood group O is without risk since these red blood cells lack structures on their surface that allow them to be agglutinated by antibodies against either the A or B antigens. Such individuals are referred to as universal donors. The absence under physiological conditions of antibodies against the naturally occurring antigens in an individual indicated that there must be some event early in (embryonic) life that for all future blocked the capacity of an individual to react against his own antigens.

This theory was further strengthened during the 1940s by consideration taken of additional observations in other systems. Attempts to immunize chick embryos with influenza virus that was highly immunogenic in adult animals failed. This lack of capacity of the embryo to produce antibodies to an antigen also applied to bacteriophage and sheep red blood cells. A similar phenomenon was also observed under natural conditions in experiments by Richard E. Shope and Erich Traub at the Rockefeller Institute. They studied an infection in mice by a virus with the complicated name — it can give inflammation in the membranes covering the brain — lymphocytic choriomeningitis (LCM) virus. It was found that some stocks of mice were heavily infected since birth, although this persistent infection did not seem to affect the health of the animals. If the virus was transferred by injection into the brain of adult mice that had not seen it earlier, severe disease followed. In rare instances the LCM virus can also infect man and Shope himself did in fact come down with a disease caused by the virus in the late 1930s.

Two particular phenomena were observed in the stocks of mice which were chronically infected since birth. The first one was that they did not produce any immune response and the second that they carried the extensive virus infection without showing any symptoms from the organs where the virus was actively replicating. This led to two conclusions. First that a virus infection initiated already during the embryonic development led to an abrogation of the capacity of animals to respond with an immune reaction to the infectious agent and secondly that the symptoms in the adult animals must be due to a *combined effect* of virus replication and the immune response to the infected cells. Such importance of both virus replication in cells *and* an aroused immune response, necessary to start a healing process by clearance of the affected cells, for the development of symptoms has later been demonstrated to be of more general importance.

Twin Calves

There was one other observation by Ray D. Owen in studies of twin calves that stirred Burnet's interest and made him formulate his hypothesis of tolerance as a mechanism for preventing an organism to mount immune responses to self structures. The synthesis of Burnet's thinking about this problem evolved during the 1940s and was presented in 1949 in a book published together with his colleague Fenner (p. 22). There was an earlier 1940 version of this book providing a synthesis of his first thoughts on the subject. He made an interesting remark on this book in his autobiography, as follows:

> At the time I was considerably crestfallen at the rejection of a paper I had put a lot of thought into, felt a distinct sense of being unjustly treated and began collecting material for a monograph on antibody production which the Institute could publish without risk of veto by editors. A thoroughly immoral attitude, but in a way and another it opened the road that led eventually to Stockholm.

Owen's studies takes us back to the existence of blood groups and what happens when, in a case of genetically distinct (non-identical) twins in calves, the two animals have different blood groups. The reason this is of particular interest in cows is that their placenta has a different structure than in most other vertebrates, including ourselves. Owen found that the placentas in the cow carrying the non-identical twins were fused to a common structure and that therefore the red blood cells of the two foetuses could mix. The result was that both twins had a permanent mixture of red blood cells representing the two different blood groups in their circulation. Because of the shared placenta a condition of tolerance had developed to both kinds of red blood cells in the twin calves.

To make a temporary digression it can be mentioned that in situations of non-identical twin calves of different sexes an interesting situation may arise. This is referred as *freemartin* — a name of unknown etymological derivation — and involves the female part of the twin pair. This calf is infertile because of non-functioning ovaries and displays a masculinized behavior. The reason for this abnormal development is that male hormones from the other twin, because of the fused placenta circulate freely and irreversibly suppress the normal female development. The occurrence of freemartins was noted way back in time and also referred to in folklore. It was also speculated, unfoundedly, to possibly apply to human non-identical twins of different sexes. Aldous Huxley in his famous novel *Brave New World*[5] described how those in power exploit the freemartin phenomenon. By government policy 70% of all women in the society are made sterile by exposure to male hormones during their foetal development.

Taking all these different phenomena together Burnet in the 1949 book on the immune response (Ref. 3, p. 103) arrived at an astoundingly visionary conclusion:

> If, in embryonic life, expendable cells from a genetically different race are implanted and established, no antibody response should develop

> against the foreign cell antigen when the animal takes on an independent existence.

It was this brief statement that served as the basis for his 1960 Nobel Prize! Burnet himself tried to verify his hypothesis by use of different antigens applied during embryonic development. The experiments failed presumably because the antigens he had chosen for the experiments were not suited for the purpose. However, experiments by others soon demonstrated that tolerance was inducible during embryonic life. The establishment of the existence of a tolerance phenomenon provided a reasonable answer to the second of the two questions — the self and non-self phenomenon — posed in the beginning of this chapter, but it remained to answer the first of the two them:

> Which are the mechanisms that allow a vertebrate organism to develop and memorize a specific immune response against essentially any foreign structure?

This question increasingly occupied Burnet's mind during the 1950s and led to the formulation of a hypothesis that he himself considered his own most important contribution to science.

Instruction versus Selection

Already during the early part of the 20th century Ehrlich had speculated about possible mechanisms behind the highly variable specific antigen-antibody reactions. He referred to them as a "key and lock" reaction. His speculations, in the absence of any knowledge about the structure and production of antibodies, of the existence of a so-called "side chain" arrangement, were very tentative and later shown to be wrong. As more was learned about the antibody response and chemists managed to define them as "globular" proteins, intense speculations on how these specific proteins could be produced began to be formulated.

The dominant person in this problem-solving was Linus C. Pauling at the California Institute of Technology (Caltech). He was the leading scientist in the protein field and received the 1954 Nobel Prize in Chemistry. This prize will be discussed more thoroughly in Chapter 7. Pauling reflected on possible mechanisms by which an antigen could instruct the antibody-producing machinery but he had difficulties providing solutions to the "key and lock" problem. Burnet's own feelings after discussion with Pauling during the early 1940s, was that many questions remained unanswered. He intuitively believed that any mechanism based on *instruction* must be wrong. But what was the alternative? If a mechanism was not due to instruction it must be based on *selection*. Burnet's thinking was clearly influenced by his understanding of biology. This discipline taught that the emergence of new characters was made by Darwinian selection and not by inheritance of acquired characteristics as favored by Jean-Baptist Lamarck. And still it was difficult to imagine how the fully developed organism could develop a repository of millions and millions of potential moulds (antibodies) to be individually retrieved for occasional future use. At the time there was simply too little insight into the functions of the genetic material to make a meaningful hypothesis.

Burnet would have to wait until the mid-1950s when a bold Danish immunologist Niels K. Jerne (p. 81), at the time visiting Caltech, developed his experiments and thinking. He studied the antibody response to bacteriophages in horses. It intrigued him that already *before* immunization he could identify a small amount of some kind of antibody molecule reacting with the selected antigen. He then hypothesized that there might exist a huge number of such "natural antibodies" generated by some kind of random process and that these were critical in the first contacts with an antigen. The idea that an antigen could chose an already existing antibody led Jerne to formulate a *natural selection theory*. Burnet took this theory one step further and hypothesized that the natural antibodies were produced by clones of immune cells[6]. The term clone is derived from the Greek *klone* meaning sprout, twig. Inspiration to speculate about such clones of cells was obtained from experiments carried out in his own laboratory. In 1955 Carleton Gajdusek, the forthcoming recipient of half of the 1976 Nobel Prize in physiology or medicine (Ref. 2, Chapter 8), was a visiting scientist in Burnet's laboratory. Gajdusek's unique personality was presented earlier, but it can be noted that on occasions the shy Burnet could be a rather shrewd and incisive reader of human characters. In a letter he presented "this foreign interloper" in the following way:

> Actually, I got on better than I expected with Gajdusek during the 15 months at the Institute. During the last 4 or 5 months he did some first-rate work on autoimmune reaction; and we parted on excellent terms. My own summing up was that he had an intelligence quotient up in the 180s and the emotional immaturity of a 15-year-old. He is quite manically energetic when his enthusiasm is roused, and can inspire enthusiasm in

> his technical assistants. He is completely self-centered, thick-skinned, and inconsiderate, but equally won't let danger, physical difficulty, or other people's feelings interfere in the least with what he wants to do. He apparently has no interest in women but an almost obsessional interest in children, none whatever in clothes and cleanliness; he can live cheerfully in a slum or a grass hut. He is not a first-class scientist in any field, but I doubt whether anyone in the world has anything like his knowledge of children in primitive communities in very many parts of the world.

As was discussed earlier, the later part of Gajdusek's life was shadowed by his conviction for paedophilia in the US in 1996 leading to imprisonment for a year and later a life in exile in many countries outside the US.

Gajdusek's project in Burnet's laboratory aimed at identifying the virus causing hepatitis. Later it was demonstrated that there is in fact more than one kind of hepatitis virus. He looked for possible immune reactions between extracts of livers from patients with hepatitis and sera from patients with this disease. No virus-specific reactions were identified but instead he found that some sera reacted both with potentially infected and also (control) healthy liver extracts. The strongest reaction was seen with sera from patients with the rare malignant disease of certain white blood cells called Waldenström's macroglobulinemia. The reaction was referred to as AICF (*a*uto-*i*mmune *c*omplement *f*ixation). The phenomenon of complement fixation was briefly introduced above. The recognition that tumor cells originating from the lymphatic system could produce antibodies with a restricted auto-immune specificity stimulated Burnet to think along the lines that "if cells produced a characteristic pattern of globulin for genetic reasons and were stimulated to proliferate by contact with the corresponding antigenic stimulus, then ...". The critical interaction thus would be expected to be between an antigen and an antibody structure exposed at the surface of a clone of cells capable of producing only this specific antibody. Such an interaction might result in a proliferation of cells — building up a clone of cells — producing only this antibody. Progressively, new data accumulated supporting the correctness of the *clonal selection theory of antibody production*. In the publication introducing this theory[6] he even specified:

> The theory requires at some stage in early embryonic development a genetic process for which there is no available precedent. In some way we have to picture a "randomization" of the coding responsible for part

of the specification of gamma globulin molecules, so that after several cell generations... there are specifications in the genomes for virtually every variant the can exist as a gamma globulin molecule....

This would turn out to be a very visionary statement!

Clonal Selection

Somewhat unexpectedly Burnet published this revolutionary theory in an Australian journal. His own motive was that, on the one hand, wherever he published his theory he could claim priority and, on the other hand, if it turned out to be wrong he would not have tarnished his reputation too much in the international scientific community by publishing discreetly. In addition he had some good reason to be in a hurry, because there were other scientists, like David Talmage, who were on their way to publishing similar theories. During the subsequent ten years experimental data accumulated which consolidated the clonal selection theory. It was shown for the first time in 1959 that if one blocked replication of cells in an animal which just had been immunized, the development of an antibody response was prevented. Thus division of cells, the expansion of a clone, was an absolute requirement for this event to occur. These early experiments paved the way for the later development of *immune-suppressive drugs*, the introduction of which made it possible to carry out heterotransplantations in man. This will be discussed in Chapter 4. It was further documented that a single clone of immune cells could only produce one kind of antibody. The very first experiments documenting this were performed in 1958 by Nossal (p. 8), at the time a visiting scientist in Joshua Lederberg's laboratory at Caltech. Lederberg who received his Nobel Prize in physiology or medicine that year (Ref. 2, Chapter 6) had visited Burnet's laboratory the year before and become captivated by the new thinking about mechanisms of antibody production.

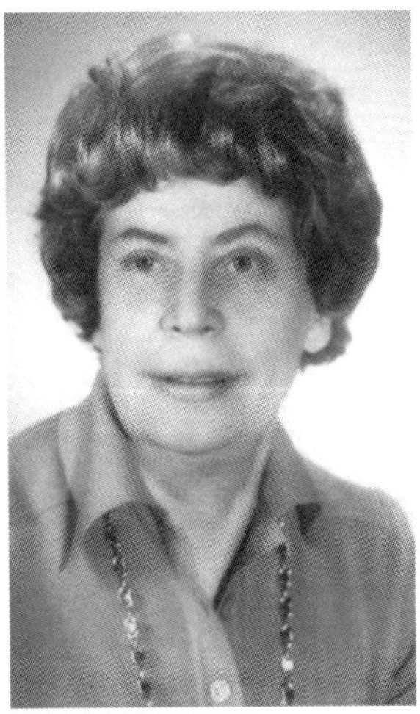

Astrid Fagraeus (1913–1997). [Courtesy of Renée Norberg.]

Already in 1948 a Swedish pathologist/immunologist Astrid Fagraeus in a pioneering PhD thesis had postulated that the *plasma cell*, a special kind of lymphocyte, was responsible for production of antibodies. Occasionally this kind of cell may develop into a tumor, called *myeloma*. Such tumors have been known since the late 1930s to be associated with an increase of gamma globulin, the fraction of serum later shown to contain antibodies. Eventually it could be shown that a spontaneous myeloma in a patient produced only one kind of antibody, the specificity of which could rarely be identified, whereas a myeloma from another patient produced a massive amount of a different antibody. The studies of myeloma proteins came to be very important for the understanding of the structure of antibodies and for the development of a technique to produce clonal antibodies with a predetermined specificity in the laboratory as we shall see in the discussion in the following chapter on Nobel Prizes in immunology after 1960.

In 1967 there was a state of the art conference on immunology at Cold Spring Harbor Laboratories. Jerne summarized this symposium. He had a considerable respect for Burnet's development of his selection theory for antibody formation which was apparent by his formulation "I hit the nail, but Burnet hit the nail on its head." Jerne's concluding remarks at the symposium were as follows:

> Sir Macfarlane Burnet must have been pleased not only to witness at this symposium the vindication of his Clonal Selection Theory of Acquired Immunity, but also to see how his stimulating ideas have led to a great proliferation of immunologists and to know that the fate of immunology is deposited in so many capable hands.
>
> As this younger generation of professionals is pressing rapidly towards the definitive solution of the antibody problem, we older amateurs had better sit back Waiting for the END.

Of course this was not the end, even though Burnet had a tendency to refer to the end of different disciplines of science as already discussed, and there came to be many more major additional discoveries in immunology to be recognized by Nobel Prizes in physiology or medicine. One of them in fact also recognized Jerne's pioneering theoretical contributions, although he had to wait until 1984.

It Takes Two to Tango

The Nobel Prize in physiology or medicine in 1960 was awarded jointly to Burnet and Medawar and it is now due time to introduce the latter scientist. This presentation can be pre-empted by recognizing that Medawar was another rare example of a uniquely imposing personality in science, a very energetic polymath. Not only was he a brilliant, imaginative scientist and an impressive leader of prestigious academic institutions, he also had a unique capacity, like Burnet, to present in a written form his insights into science and views on its development. In fact his well formulated perspectives on various issues also extended, like in the case of Burnet, into wide reflections on human affairs in general. The two of them were very different as individuals, but together they represented a rare combination of minds and characters among the exclusive club of Nobel laureates. Medawar has summarized his life in an autobiography called *Memoirs of a Thinking Radish: An autobiography*[7] and his wife Jean has given rich personal insights into their long life together[8]. Medawar was 22 years old when he married his fellow zoology student in 1937.

A Multicultural Background

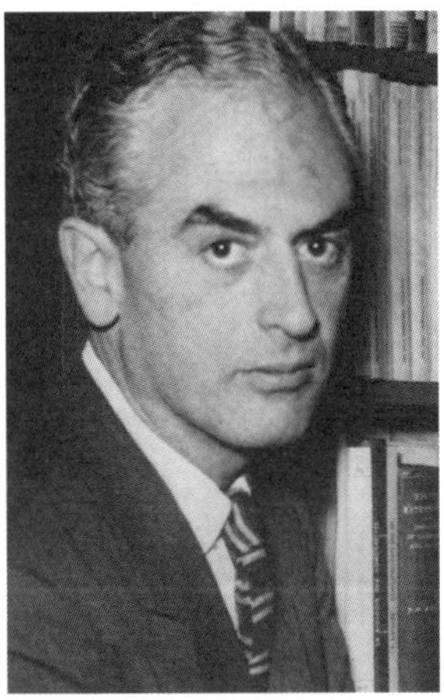

Peter B. Medawar.
[From Ref. 31.]

Medawar was born in 1915, and was thus a little more than 15 years Burnet's junior. He had a British mother and a Lebanese father. In a radio interview he emphasized the cultural heritage through his father. The Lebanese people count the Phoenicians, the seafaring people who first developed the Mediterranean ("mid world") human culture as their ancestors. In addition to, or perhaps connected to, their success as business people they came to be responsible for one of the most important advances in human civilizations, the introduction of an alphabet. The cultural impact of moving from pictures illustrating whole concepts — *ideograms* — like in old Egyptian and in Chinese writing, to individual letters — *phonetics* — is comparable to the much later introductions of the printing press and the world wide web. As would be expected the individual letters introduced originally had their roots in stylized depictions of objects: A (at the time a consonant), an inverted head of an oxen, B, a house, C, a camel, etc. The use of letters instead of ideograms was a revolutionary invention which immediately allowed the creation of a limitless number of written words. The key term in this context is *combinatorics* in which a random permutation of letters, numbers and other symbols (modules) — like in a lottery or a zip code — is used. Such an arrangement allows an endless number of different specific terms (products) to be formulated (created). The reason for this digression is to emphasize that also the success of biological evolution has its basis in a number of combinatorial events; in the dawn of life various primitive replication competent systems were most likely combined; the genetic code is combinatorial using only four letters combined into triplets (Chapter 8 and Ref. 2, Chapter 7); and, as we shall see, the potential generation of a limitless number of antibodies in our body is due to combinatorial events in lymphocytes during an early phase of their embryonic development.

Medawar was born in Petrópolis in Brazil, a country where his father made his living as a business man. The family moved to England only three years after his birth. Medawar and his brother were educated in England in boarding schools and when they had started their first term their parents returned to Brazil. He had mixed experiences during the early school years but early on he became an omnivorous reader and in particular a lover of music, especially operas. If early schooling was difficult it was nothing compared to what he experienced when he moved to Marlborough College, the same place where a grandfather on his mother's side had also been educated. In his own words: "After more than fifty years I still feel resentful and disgusted at the manners and mores of this essentially tribal institution."[7] Bullying, sadism and paedophilia were frequent ingredients in the day-to-day experiences. In this harsh environment the biology master Ashley G. Lowndes provided some consolation. Although a crude person, he was passionately devoted to biology and was an excellent experimentalist. This had a contagious effect on young Medawar and he decided to become a scientist.

The Appeal of Oxford

After four years in Marlborough College he could move on to Magdalen College at Oxford University. This provided a dramatic change. He thoroughly enjoyed the tutorial system and John Young, who was appointed to supervise him, was ideally suited for the purpose. Incidentally in the lineage of British intelligentsia it can be remarked that Young himself was a pupil of Gavin de Beer, who in turn was a pupil of Julian Huxley. His great-great-grandson Francis, the son of another Julian Huxley, happened to become the pupil of Medawar. Although Medawar's studies focussed on zoology, he got a wide exposure to mathematics and philosophy which he thoroughly enjoyed. He built up a considerable confidence in his own talent and on occasion of being invited to dine at High Table he referred to himself as "a good-looking young man in a Latin or Levantine way, getting a reputation for being intellectually bright …". In the zoology department Medawar was instructed by a Dr John Baker about how to prepare slides for histological examinations as a part of the cytology course. Medawar's training in zoology was very successful and, inspired by his future wife, he finished by winning a senior scholarship at the college which in fact secured a good financial situation.

The time had come for Medawar to start his own research. It focussed on some problems in embryology with an attempt to apply tissue culture techniques. It was difficult to manage this technique in the zoology building and Medawar was therefore introduced to Professor Howard W. Florey, a future Nobel Prize recipient (Ref. 2, Chapter 6). He generously offered a laboratory space for the work. Progress was slow and the results were meagre. Medawar summarized his findings after two years of work and showed them to Florey. He was not appreciative of the draft and said "It sounds more like philosophy than science to me." In other studies Medawar engaged himself in evaluating the mathematics of organ and body size development. These data were published and even accepted as a PhD specimen, but eventually he decided not to apply for this degree. While in Florey's laboratory Medawar became involved in studies relevant to the Second World War situation. These concerned treatment of war wounds by topical application of sulphonamides and also the early preparations of penicillin.

It was a particular incident which encouraged Medawar to get engaged in transplantation research. One Sunday afternoon when he was sitting with his wife and young daughter in the garden of their house a large two-engine bomber approached over the treetops and crashed into the neighboring garden and exploded. Still it was possible to extricate the young British airman, who was taken to the nearby Radcliffe Infirmary with third-degree burns on 60% of the body. Medawar was called on to assist in providing ideas about how to manage the wounds. His immediate thought was to consider transplantation of skin from a voluntary donor, but he was aware of the limitations of this technique. Such transplantations were known to be possible only between identical twins. In other cases there was some undefined barrier. It was reflections on this problem that came to define Medawar's future engagement in science. By his own words:

> This conjunction of events that had first made me aware of the body's exquisite powers of discrimination also fixed my career as a scientist. I was henceforward to devote the greater part of my time, thought, and creative energy to discovering how the body discriminates between its own and other living cells — the "self and non-self" substances, according to Macfarlane Burnet.

However, at the time of choosing his new direction in research Medawar was not aware of Burnet's evolving philosophical conjectures.

His first studies involved collecting skin from plastic surgical operations and trying to grow the tissue in cultures. At the time growing of cells in the laboratory was cumbersome and in particular it was important to use techniques that as far as possible prevented contamination by microorganisms. A modification of the original techniques of keeping whole pieces of tissues alive by providing a suitable nutritional medium was to break them into pieces by treating them with trypsin. This technique had been introduced already in 1937 by two American pathologists Henry S. Simms and Nettie P. Stillman. Trypsin is an enzyme that splits protein chains and it has a critical function in our intestines to digest food into smaller pieces that can be transported into our blood stream. Much later, in the 1950s, the trypsin treatment came to be very important for the development of the discipline of virology. It was Julius Youngner who in his work on polio vaccine in 1954 (Ref. 2, Chapter 5) developed a technique for practical use of this enzyme for establishment of a single mosaic cell layer — a *monolayer* — on the bottom of tissue culture vessels. This monolayer technique allowed the identification of the major part of viruses causing disease in man during the 1950s (Chapter 1 and Ref. 2, Chapter 3).

To go back to Medawar's wartime experience of using trypsin treatment, he found that it separated different layers of the skin, the cells of the continuously renewed epidermis from the underlying tougher layer, the dermis. He made a suspension of the epidermal cells and tried to apply this solution to the raw surface of the wounds of the pilot. The attempt was not a success. Eventually the patient was helped by the use of an already recognized technique, the so-called "postal stamp" grafting procedure, using tissue taken from undamaged areas of his own skin, a so called *autograft*. Medawar persisted in reflecting on possibilities of using skin from relatives or other voluntary genetically non-identical donors, a *homograph*, to treat extensively damaged skin. He wanted to understand what the physiological barriers were. This led to a proposal to the War Wounds Committee of the Medical Research Council, which caught their interest. Medawar got a grant to study the problem. In order to pursue his studies he established collaboration with the Burns Unit of the Glasgow Royal Infirmary.

Tissue Rejection Is an Immune Reaction

Together with a Scottish surgeon, Tom Gibson, he decided to analyze the difference in changes in the transferred and the surrounding/underlying tissues upon transplantation of autografts as compared to homografts by use of human volunteers. At various time intervals the transplants were removed. Histological samples were prepared and examined in the microscope. After a few days certain differences became discernable. The main one was that the homograft was invaded by white blood cells of the kind called lymphocytes. This kind of cell has a normal defence function in managing intruders in our body, like viruses and bacteria. Could it be that there was an immunological reaction against the foreign, allograft tissue? If that was the case one would expect that a second homograft should be rejected faster than the first one, because of the immunity — the sensitization — developed after the first transplantation. To the satisfaction of the scientists this prediction turned out to be true. A second-set homograft from the same donor was promptly rejected by an intense inflammatory reaction. These were indeed conceptually important results, published in 1943[9]. For the first time it now became apparent that rejection of grafts could and should be studied as an immunological phenomenon.

This is what Medawar set out to do when he returned to Oxford. He used rabbits and could confirm and considerably extend the concept of homograft rejection as an immunological phenomenon. He started to reflect on the nature of the immunity-provoking factors of the graft — the "antigens". The work became totally consuming doing experiments during the day and reading and writing at night, a pattern well recognized from Burnet's engagement in science. Besides his intense work Medawar also had some energy and strength to progressively enlarge his intellectual contacts in Oxford. As one of the different engagements he was a member of the Theoretical Biology Club, which included three generations of university teachers. Thus his own mentor

John Young was a member as were his own two pupils, Francis Huxley and Avrion Mitchison. Eventually Medawar became a Fellow of Magdalen College. He thrived in the fertile Oxford environment.

After the war Medawar was uncertain about his future directions in science and he even had an offer from Burnet, whom he had met for the first time in 1946, to work at the Walter and Eliza Hall Institute. Instead of going to Australia he accepted a Chair at Birmingham. It was his previous colleague Solly Zuckerman who tempted him to come to Birmingham and he was interviewed for a Professorship by Norman Hawarth, who received one half of the Nobel Prize in chemistry in 1937 "for his investigations of carbohydrates and vitamin C". Medawar was appointed as the Mason Professor of Zoology in the University of Birmingham. He was only 32 years old and therefore frequently referred to as "the young professor". Medawar brought along his first graduate student at Oxford, Rupert Everett (Bill) Billingham. He was a very important collaborator throughout many years. In particular he played a central role in managing the experiments that led to the discovery selected for the Nobel Prize in 1960. However, it took some time before they returned to the homograft rejection problem. This occurred after another chance encounter.

A Visit to Stockholm

In 1948 Medawar participated in an International Congress of Genetics in Stockholm. At this meeting he met a New Zealander by the name of Hugh Donald. Donald was the Head of the Agricultural Research Council's Animal Breeding Research Organization in Edinburgh and the two of them came to discuss the problem of distinguishing between fraternal (non-identical, two egg) and identical cattle twins. Medawar in a cocky way stated that there was no problem distinguishing the genetic identity or non-identity of such twins. All one had to do was to simply graft skin from one twin to the other. He agreed to help Donald to do this. A few weeks later the experiment was performed. Medawar's predictions fell flat. All cattle twins accepted the skin graft from the other, although some of the pairs obviously must have been non-identical since they were of different sexes. The answer to this conundrum came when Medawar hit upon Burnet's and Fenner's book on antibody production, the 2nd edition of 1949[3]. In this book he learned about Owen's demonstration of shared placentas in heifers carrying twins. This sharing of circulating blood in non-identical twin calves as already discussed, in some way during embryonic differentiation must have induced a state of tolerance. It could be shown that the tolerance was specific, since a graft from an unrelated sibling or a parent was effectively rejected by the calves. The data were published in a well recognized journal of genetics[10].

Medawar travelled to the United States for the first time in 1949, where he gave a number of lectures. He also met one of his heroes Dr Peyton Rous at the Rockefeller Institute, the scientist studying virus-induced tumors who had to wait the longest for his 1966 Nobel Prize in physiology or medicine (Ref. 2, Chapter 3). On his return to England Medawar learned to his dismay that he had been selected to become Dean of Science. He did not look forward to this responsibility and therefore took advantage of an opening for a professorship at University College London. In 1951 he moved to this College to shoulder the Jodrell Chair of Zoology, the longest established chair in this discipline in England. He was joined by Billingham and also a talented student called Leslie Brent. The three of them brought the work on tolerance to a climactic conclusion. The project they selected for their main engagement was to try to induce tolerance experimentally. For this purpose they expanded the facilities to house experimental animals and acquired a number of inbred mouse strains. The importance of inbred mouse strains for experimental work furthering the advance of immunology including the genetic basis of transplantation deserves some special comment.

Inbred Mice

The potential use of inbred mice had already been appreciated by the beginning of the 20th century. Brother-sister mating of mice leads after some twenty generations to a strain of animals which all are genetically comparable to identical (monozygotic) twins. Different kinds of such inbred mouse strains were used to define rules for transplantation of normal and tumour cells. This field had been established by Dr Clarence Little, who also founded the Jackson Laboratories, Bar Harbor, Maine in the US. It was discovered that the transplantability was governed by the Mendelian laws of genetics and it became possible to map the different cell surface antigens involved[11]. They were later referred to as the *major histocompatibility complex* (MHC), a term we will meet frequently in the next chapter. In 1980 a Nobel Prize in physiology or medicine was given with one third to George D. Snell for his contribution to "discoveries concerning genetically determined structures on the cell surface that regulate immunological reactions". He had spent his whole professional life at the Jackson Laboratories using mouse strains to map the major MHC loci that decide the fate of a transplanted tissue. Many of the inbred mouse strains used by scientists all around the world had been developed by Snell. The genetic inbreeding can lead to the development of particular disease traits, as also seen for example in various breeds of dogs. In an essay *Animal Experimentation in a Medical Research Institute* written later in life[12], Medawar has illustrated the enormous value of properly cared for and experimentally used animals in clarifying human disease processes.

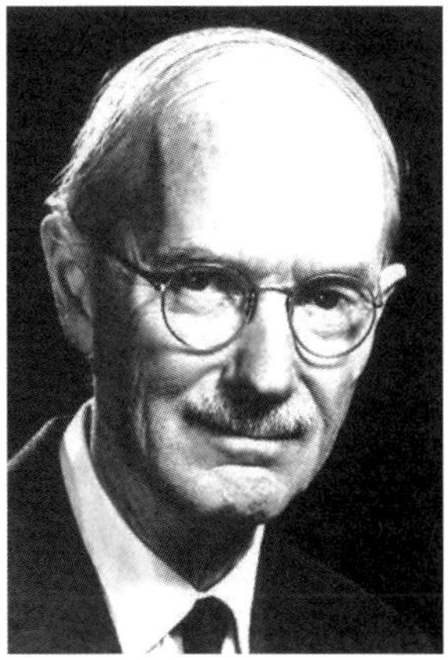

George D. Snell (1903–1996), recipient of the shared 1980 Nobel Prize in physiology or medicine. [From *Les Prix Nobel en 1980*.]

Tolerance Unraveled

In a genetically homogenous inbred mouse strain tissue can readily be moved from one animal to another. If one inbred mouse strain is crossed with another mouse strain it is still possible in the first — the F1 — generation to transplant tissues from representatives of either parental mouse strain to the offspring. In the next generation — F2 — the genetic differences become too large and transplantation is not possible. After a number of preliminary experiments, Medawar and collaborators elected to use brown mice of strain CBA and white mice of strain A for their experiments. In order to attempt to induce tolerance, cells from one strain were injected through the abdominal wall of a mother, representing another strain, directly into the unborn foetal mice at different times of gestation. The relatively simple technique worked well and soon it was possible to demonstrate that a state of tolerance had been induced in the injected animals. Tolerance was induced most effectively by use of lymphoid cells. Skin from the brown CBA mouse was accepted by a "tolerized" white A animal, whereas in controls there was a significant inflammatory reaction rejecting the tissue in 10–12 days[13]. Burnet's prediction, which he himself had not been successful in verifying experimentally, finally was documented to be true.

In parallel with Medawar and collaborators the Czech scientist Milan Hašek obtained data also illustrating phenomena of induced tolerance[14]. However, the motives for his experiments were entirely different from those of Medawar and collaborators and he did not make a correct interpretation of his experimental findings until after reading the publication from the London group. The motivation for Hašek's experiments was somewhat exceptional. He was a staunch communist who wanted to provide experimental support for Lysenko's genetic doctrine. This said that environmental experiences could be inherited and hence that the proper "communistic" environment would improve the quality of man. In order to study this Hašek developed a model in which two chicken embryos of different genetic origin were manipulated to share blood flow. A situation like in Owen's calf twins was artificially established. Hašek referred to the experimental conditions as parabiosis. Although his experiments originally were not performed to study immunological problems, the presence of antibodies against the red blood cells of the two chicken embryos was determined. There was no formation of antibodies to any of the two kinds of blood cells. A situation of tolerance had been induced, but this was not understood until after publication of the data.

The solidarity with the prevailing authoritarian political system gave Hašek considerable advantages in mobilizing resources for his research. These political favors were counterbalanced by the ideologically motivated bias in data interpretation. This is a situation of special — and fortunately rare — dogmatic influence in modern secularized and non-politicized science. At the present time the dogmatic influence of prominent non-visionary, influential scientists who are in error represents a much larger problem. Hašek eventually had to pay a price. In 1970 at a mature age he was expelled from the Party, and removed from the directorship of his laboratory, managed by the Czech Academy of Sciences, and also the Council of the Academy.

At this point it may be appropriate to pause and ask if one can really say that the outcome of an experiment demonstrates a hypothesis to be true. This question has been considered in depth by the philosopher Karl Popper. Medawar has written about the essence of his scientific philosophizing in one of his essays[12]. The result of an experiment can clearly give support to a hypothesis and increase the likeliness that it may be correct. The caution needed to be introduced is that the chances of correctness must be judged within the framework of knowledge available at the time. Newton came as close as possible to the truth at his time but later Einstein introduced corrections improving the predictability of the theory. The emphasis in Popper's theories is on results that do *not* support a theory. He prefers to discuss the impact of experimental data contrary to the hypothesis appearing to *falsify* it. Whatever the situation, one needs to evaluate the strength of the evidence. Possibly data that appear to negate a certain hypothesis may force it to be rejected or possibly modified.

It was a very fundamental principle that Medawar and colleagues had found experimental support for. Later on a number of findings have amplified the original observations. Three examples will be mentioned here. Beatrice Mintz working in Philadelphia in the mid-1960s was interested in the properties of cells derived from the very first divisions of a fertilized egg. It had been demonstrated that if one collected a mouse embryo which had undergone the very first three divisions to eight cells, and separated these cells, each one led to the development of a complete mouse after implantation into a surrogate mother. Embryonic cells with such a capacity are referred to as *pluripotent*. Mintz took this experiment one step further and collected early embryonic cells from both an inbred white mouse strain and also another strain that was black. After dissembling the *pluripotent* cells from the two mouse strains by mild treatment by trypsin they were mixed. The mixture was then reimplanted into a surrogate mother. The offspring animals displayed "zebra-like" fur patterns. In this case it is a question of a genetically derived tolerance of the same kind seen with non-identical calf twins.

The second example involves the use of modern techniques that allow an effective destruction of selected genes and production of so called "knock-out" animals, for example mice. This technique was considered of such an importance that it was counted as a discovery and in 2007 a Nobel Prize in physiology or medicine was given to Mario R. Capecchi, Martin J. Evans and Oliver Smithies "for their discoveries of principles for introducing specific gene modifications in mice by the use of embryonic stem cells". It was used for critical experiments elucidating the mechanisms of prion diseases (Ref. 2, Chapter 8). Mice in which the host-cell gene directing the synthesis of the endogenous (mouse-specific) prion-related protein (PrP) had been destroyed were shown to be completely refractory to infection with high doses of prions. There was no replication of the prion protein and no disease developed. Furthermore these animals were capable of producing a variety of antibodies against the prion protein, something which it had not been possible to achieve before. Animals without the PrP gene were no longer tolerant to production of the normally host-specific prion protein.

Finally it should be added that it was found in 1962 that the induction of tolerance was not exclusive to the prenatal state. In studies with adult animals it was found that by use of sublethal doses of irradiation followed by injection of selected donor cells it was possible to induce tolerance even at this late stage.

A Graft Can React Against the Host

The reaction of a host to a homograft is due to activation of the host's lymphocytes. However transplanted tissue, be it a kidney or in particular bone marrow, contain lymphocytes representing the donor and they can, in their own right, react against the tissues of the host. Therefore, the tables being turned, the graft can attack the host, hence the term *graft versus host reaction* or *runt disease*, as Billingham named it. This phenomenon was discovered and studied in parallel in several laboratories. Besides Medawar's group, Morten Simonsen working in Copenhagen made important observations regarding this phenomenon using a chicken system. Also Burnet was involved in the same kind of studies for some years using his chicken chorioallantoic membrane system. The observations made had an obvious influence on the developments of future transplantations of bone marrow materials between humans. As we shall see in Chapter 4 it is of particular importance to match donor and recipient when this kind of treatment is used.

The Nobel Committee Reviews the Discovery of Immunological Tolerance

In 1958 Medawar was nominated for the first time for a Nobel Prize in physiology or medicine by Professor F. Albert, Liege for his work on the biology of transplantation and in particular the actively acquired tolerance. The committee considered this extensive nomination in French to be important and asked Malmgren to make a full evaluation.

A Bacteriologist Reviews Immunology

Malmgren with his background as a bacteriologist perused the literature at the time about the field of tissue transplantation and his 17 page review, including two pages of references, is very thorough. It gave a good presentation of the history of transplantation and the recent insights into immunological phenomena of relevance for the results of attempts to transfer tissues. He introduced the terminology used. Tissues transplanted between different parts of the body of the same individual were named *autografts*. If the donor instead was a genetically identical, homozygotic twin one used the term *isograft*. Tissues transferred from genetically non-identical individuals were called *homografts*. Today one prefers to name them *allografts*. Finally there is the situation when tissues are transferred between two different species. Then one talks about *xenografts* or sometimes *heterografts*.

Before it was understood that the immune system was responsible for identification of non-self tissues there were very vague and conceptually fuzzy ideas about the mechanisms of rejection of tissues from individuals other than a person himself or from an identical twin. Well into the 20th century it was argued, mainly by surgeons, that it was all a matter of technical proficiency. It is interesting that Malmgren described this part of the history of transplantation without mentioning Alexis Carrel, the 1912 recipient of a Nobel Prize in physiology or medicine (Ref. 2, Chapter 6). There had been speculation that the allograft rejection had an immunological basis and that it originated either in surface phenomena involving cells in the transplanted tissue or had a more systemic background using humoral factors produced by the host or the transplant. Attempts had been made to take into consideration blood groups about which a lot had been learnt during the 1920s and 1930s. However, careful matching of blood groups between donor and recipient in skin transplantations in man did not improve survival. The postulated set of antigens determining the possibility of transplanting tissues encompassing nucleated cells must be different from, or significantly supplementary to those that regulate survival of red blood cells. However, these different speculations about immunological mechanisms of transplantation were not put on a firm basis until the results of the Gibson and Medawar studies with human skin were published in 1943. These early data were consolidated by experiments with rabbits and much later with inbred mice. Taken together the data demonstrated that humoral factors were not sufficient to explain the tissue rejection. Specific *cellular* reactions were of importance and these had a considerable complexity. It was not possible in the early experiments to divide individual animals into "transplantation" groups by some immunological typing. Additional critical observations by Medawar and his group concerned the growth of blood vessels into the transplant — vascularization and the inferred importance of access of the hosts' immune cells for the rejection process. When tissues were transplanted into sites in the body lacking effective immunological drainage — immunologically *privileged* sites — like the brain or the anterior chamber of the eye, a much prolonged survival of the transplant was seen.

The importance of different types of lymphocytes in various kinds of immunological reactions including the transplantation reaction continued to be elaborated during the 1950s. Cell-mediated immunity was coming of age. Malmgren noted this in his report. He underlined the possible similar role of cells involved in so-called delayed hypersensitivity reactions, like the tuberculin reaction, and in transplantation rejection reactions. Medawar and collaborators had shown that the accelerated rejection in "immune animals" could be transferred to another animal of the same inbred mouse strain by lymph node cells, collected from a draining site of a transplant under rejection, but not by use of antibodies. This finding was confirmed by others enclosing the transplant in a chamber which only allowed the access of antibodies but not intact cells. Under these conditions the foreign cells could survive, as in the immunologically privileged sites just referred to. This phenomenon of immunity transfer by cells was referred to as *adoptive acquired immunity* a term cited by Snell in a review article in 1957[11].

In further studies Medawar and collaborators tried to define the chemical nature of the critical antigens. Their tentative conclusion in 1957 was that the antigen was deoxyribonucleic acid (DNA), a molecule coming into a particular focus of interest at the time (Chapter 8). However very soon they had to abandon this proposal. In his continued evaluation Malmgren returned to the experiments with calf twins and the chimerical nature of heterozygote pairs of animals. He appropriately highlighted their importance in formulating new concepts for the understanding of tolerance. The concluding part of the evaluation departed from Burnet's and Fenner's hypothesis about the immunological naïveté of the embryo and how this, by exposure to different antigens during a certain period of its development might acquire a lifelong tolerance to such antigens. Malmgren also cited Burnet's own attempts to validate his theory by experiments in which he used influenza virus as antigen. The discovery by Medawar and collaborators that tolerance could be induced in inbred mouse strains, described in detail in the review, was critical to a completely new understanding. The new term introduced was "*actively acquired tolerance*"[13,15]. This phenomenon was confirmed by the Czech scientist Milan Hašek in studies of embryonic parabiosis between birds, as already mentioned. Similar observations were also made in experiments using bacteria or tumor cells as antigens. It can be added that neither Owen nor Hašek were ever nominated for a Nobel Prize and hence their possible candidatures were never evaluated.

A Discovery Worthy of a Prize

In the final judgement of Medawar's contributions Malmgren noted that his studies of the nature of the homograft reaction did not by themselves qualify for a Nobel Prize. However, when his observations of actively acquired tolerance, implying the introduction of a new biological law of fundamental importance, were considered he was clearly prize-worthy.

Malmgren then turned to the problem of judging the relative importance of Medawar and his collaborators Billingham and Brent. In all their joint publications the order of the names was Billingham, Brent and Medawar. The reason for this was that Medawar celebrated the principle of using alphabetic order of authors in a joint publication. By doing so he avoided the problem of ranking the relative qualitative and quantitative contributions of different authors. Although an honorable approach, this way of presenting authors poses a problem in different contexts. One, which is more trivial, is that transferring an English alphabetic order from one language/cultural group to another may cause confusion, but the other is that the withheld information about the relative contributions of different co-authors may cause problems in particular to a Nobel Committee, which as one of its primary responsibilities has to determine who has priority to a discovery.

To discuss the minor spelling problem first it can be noted that the English language has 26 letters, whereas the Swedish until recently had 28. The reason is that Swedish has three additional letters Å — originally AA-, Ä — originally AE — and Ö — originally OE. Since a few years the Swedish language has had 29 letters. The reason is that W has been added. Originally V and W were categorized as the same letter, although it was more prestigious to have your surname spelled with W. Recently W has been added to the Swedish alphabet because of the importation of many English words — weekend, workout, etc. This means that a Swedish author by the name of Åsjö would move from one of the very latest to one of the earliest alphabethical positions in shifting from a Swedish to an English publication. In fact the use of these extra vowels is not consistent even among the Scandinavian languages. In Danish the Å, which exists as the 29th and last letter in this alphabet can also be spelled AA. Hence if your name was Aaby, you can be sure to be first in an English publication but in a Danish one you would be at the tail end. In essence there must of course be a solution to this problem. It is a question of agreeing on general rules for name indexing, something that already exists. Still, the problem of ranking individual contributions remains. Therefore alternative arrangements of sequence of names in an authorship list are in general use.

In the business of giving credit for contributions of different authors at least in biomedical sciences specific rules have evolved long since. An example of the discussion of these rules can be found in the book by the Nobel Laureate Peter Doherty[16]. The usual convention is to give the first place on the name list to the junior scientist, who has had the greatest experimental and coordinating/writing responsibility in the group. The last place is given to the leader of the group, frequently referred to as *principal* investigator. Not infrequently it is the latter who has arranged for the availability of a good part of the resources needed for the study. There are of course many situations when the identification of the proper arrangement for the first and last author position is complex. In more modern times one sometimes sees an asterisk on the first two or three names stating that their contributions are of equal size. Then there is the question of the names of additional co-authors, who in these days of large research consortia can number in the hundreds. The situation becomes particularly complex when one starts to add an explanatory footnote explaining the relative contributions of all co-authors in the experimentation, the discussions of the data and the writing of the manuscript. As a member of a Nobel Committee one often has the very delicate task of discreetly finding out what really has happened in a laboratory in which a major discovery has been made. This requires a considerable diplomatic talent and one need to be aware of the fact that it is generally recognized by the people one interacts with that one has an involvement in the Nobel Prize work. By definition there are situations when it is difficult to find the "truth" and another complication is that sometimes it may turn out to be essentially impossible to distil the main contributors to a discovery to three persons or less.

In the case of Billingham, Brent and Medawar Malmgren did not hesitate to define Medawar as the leader of the group and this was obvious already from the nomination. But Malmgren had another problem. He wrote:

> In my opinion Medawar's research concerning immunological tolerance should be considered as the most important event (discovery) in (the field of) immunology since Ehrlich's and Behring's days and (it) is to a high degree prize-worthy. However one cannot escape from the fact that Medawar in his works has originated in a hypothesis previously

> formulated by Burnet and Fenner. The credit of this hypothesis needs without hesitation be allocated to Burnet. It therefore seems to me, under these circumstances, that in the context of decision of prize-worthiness it is inevitable to also discuss Burnet's name.

This conclusion is reiterated in the final paragraph:

> In conclusion I would like to express as my opinion that Medawar's publications concerning actively acquired tolerance are prize-worthy. When it comes to the question of awarding a prize one can (should), however, not neglect to discuss Burnet's name. Since Burnet has not been included in a nomination in this context (this year) the consequence must be that the discovery under evaluation cannot be the (a selected) subject of the award of the 1958 Nobel Prize.

The committee concurred and noted in its recommendation to the College of Teachers that Medawar's discoveries concerning immunological tolerance were prize-worthy. Burnet had two nominations in 1958 for his work on viruses and following the formulation for many years past the committee in his case noted that his discovery of a method of making cells insusceptible to infection with certain viruses was prize-worthy, as already mentioned.

In 1959 the discovery of the phenomenon of tolerance was not discussed by the committee in the absence of any nominations of contributions in this field. Burnet remained prize-worthy for his work on viruses.

Nominations in 1960

In the critical year of 1960 there were three nominations for Burnet and two nominations for Medawar, one of them including both of them. Burnet was nominated by R. Lovell for his work on animal virus genetics and by Jorgen M. Birkeland, Columbus, Ohio, not for his virus work, but for the first time for his involvement in immunological problems. Birkeland cited his very recent (1959) publication of the book *The Clonal Selection Theory of Acquired Immunity*[17]. In particular he referred to the further elaboration in this book of the prediction that it should be possible to induce tolerance during embryonic life. It was noted that this prediction had been substantiated by the findings made by Billingham and Medawar who, however, were *not* nominated by him.

Regarding Burnet it was stated that his "critical analysis and syntheses have stimulated others to do so much good work that (it) sets Burnet in a class by himself". Professor Sverre D. Henriksen, Oslo, Norway made a comprehensive three-page nomination, with attachments, of Billingham, Brent and Medawar. This proposal did not mention Burnet. A thoughtful nomination came from Lederberg, mentioned above. It included both Burnet and Medawar, but the nomination of the two of them was essentially separate. Burnet was cited for his work on viruses reflected in the concepts he had formulated in his book *Virus as Organism*[18] and was also proposed for his approach to the problems of immunity from a modern point of view. Lederberg stated that it is difficult to focus on a single discovery among Burnet's many contributions, but suggested, highlighting the work on genetic recombination, phenotypic mixing and heterozygosis demonstrated in studies of influenza virus, that these discoveries "justify a favorable attention of the Nobel Committee". Medawar was recommended for his experimental demonstration of induced immune tolerance. Lederberg stated:

> They are also fundamental observations for any comprehensive biological theory of immunity (as, for example, the clonal selection theory advanced by Burnet). From a practical standpoint, the phenomenon of induced tolerance furnishes the principal basis for optimistic efforts at rational use of homotransplanted tissues as a surgical procedure, and in replacement therapy in the treatment of cancer and of radiation injuries.
>
> Two questions will undoubtedly arise in this evaluation. One is that Medawar has been associated with several co-investigators in these studies, and their relative contributions must be sorted out. The second is that not all of his studies have had such a constructive outcome, for example, those dealing with "infective transformation" of non-pigmented cells in guinea pig skin, purportedly by granules endowed with hereditary continuity and derived from pigmented cells; also the premature identification of the homograft antigens with DNA, rather than mucoids of the cells' surfaces as now appears more likely. The Committee will doubtless give careful study to these considerations. For my own part, the importance of Medawar's main contribution far outweighs the detriment of these evidences of human fallibility; further, while giving due and ample credit to his colleagues, Medawar's role stands out clearly in my own view.

In sum, I would be proud to be associated with either or both of the candidates herewith submitted.

None of the nominations proposed a combined Prize to Burnet and Medawar for their discovery of acquired immunological tolerance, but this was to become the conclusion by the Nobel Committee, a decision supported by the Faculty. In order to understand how this came about we need to review the investigations made during the year and also consider the composition of the Committee. As discussed earlier (Ref. 2, Chapter 7) new winds were blowing at the Karolinska Institute during the late 1950s. There was a changing of the guard with young dynamic professors added to the Faculty and the new fields of molecular biology and microbial/viral genetics were beginning to expand rapidly, infringing on the turf of the traditional disciplines of medical chemistry and physiology.

Sven Gard's Busy Summer

The late summer of 1960 was a very busy time for Gard. Normally it is a full commitment to make one in-depth Nobel investigation in a particular year, but he made *four*. One of the investigations concerned Albert H. Coons who, in the early 1940s, had introduced a new technique to demonstrate specific antigenic material in cells, the so-called *immune fluorescence technique*. It could be used to demonstrate the presence of foreign material in cells, e.g. the occurrence of viral or bacterial products in connection with an infection, but also individual cell-specific components. The technique took advantage of the specificity of antibodies. The proteins of an immune serum containing a selected specific antibody were coupled via a chemical reaction to a fluorescent compound. This reagent was then allowed to react with cells in a thin slice of tissue or with cells in a culture, treated to make them permeable to the labelled proteins. The presence of labelled antibody that had attached to its specific target, be it a virus or a cell component, was then identified by fluorescence microscopy. This technique immediately became widely used for diagnoses of microbial diseases and for studies of normal and abnormal proteins in cells. Gard wrote an 11-page review and praised the technique and its value for many different applications. However he did not recognize it as a discovery and therefore did not recommend that it should be declared prizeworthy. The conclusion of the Committee was that Coons's contribution should not at the moment be considered for a prize.

Gard's second full investigation in 1960 concerned Heinz Fraenkel-Conrat, Alfred Gierer and Gerhardt Schramm, who had discovered that ribonucleic acid (RNA) isolated from tobacco mosaic virus (TMV) was infectious and could initiate the production of complete virus particles. This observation, which already had been evaluated for a prize in Chemistry in 1956 and in Physiology of Medicine in 1959, was of considerable importance in the understanding of nucleic acids as the carriers of genetic information as has been discussed extensively (Ref. 2, Chapter 7) and will be examined again in Chapter 8. Gard made another thorough 18-page review and concluded that the three nominated scientists deserved to be recognized by a prize. Again the conclusion by the committee concurred with the recommendation given in the review. This special field of research will be further discussed in Chapter 8.

The remaining two reviews made by Gard in 1960 were devoted to Burnet and to Billingham, Brent and Medawar. This was the fifth time that he reviewed Burnet. Still he was very thorough and gave an in-depth analysis of his major contributions, but now for the first time the review also included Burnet's theoretical discussions of the fundamentals of immunology. In fact the latter was the main emphasis of the review. Revisiting Burnet's impressive and many-faceted contributions to virology for which he had been considered prizeworthy by the committee for more than ten years, Gard, with a certain stubbornness, highlighted in particular his development of the influenza virus receptor concept and the genetic studies of this virus. However, the other strong candidate in this area, Hirst, had not been nominated in 1960 and Gard used this as an excuse not to push for a prize in virology to Burnet this year.

Gard's extensive discussion of his theoretical reflections on fundamentals of immunology departed from Malmgren's conclusion in his review two years earlier. A prize to Medawar could not be discussed without simultaneously considering Burnet's theoretical contributions. All his theories had their origin in the simple statement that they "have to make biological sense". Burnet used this formulation not only in his discussions of viruses as an organism, being an actor in evolutionary processes[18], but also extensively in speculations on the principles[3] and possible mechanisms of antibody production[17]. Gard referred to Ehrlich's template theory as applied by Pauling and it was noted that the mechanism he proposed would require that the critical antigen needed to remain in the organism for the future in order for a memory to be preserved. However, experiments to demonstrate the fate of injected antigen using the above-mentioned immune fluorescence technique for antigen detection or radioactively labelled antigen had provided evidence that the antigen was broken down and disappeared. The only exceptions to this were certain complex sugar compounds (polysaccharides) which, however, by their nature induced a different kind of antibody responses.

In the absence of persistence of antigen the logical way of explaining production of antibody with any kind of specificity was to postulate that there must be some mechanism by which the organism can generate a limitless number of antibodies, a minute fraction of which may be of value for future use as discussed above. Burnet further speculated that this repository for production of antibodies with any kind of specificity must rely on genetic mechanisms in cells and that division of cells should be a prerequisite for an antibody response. Already at the time there were some experimental data showing that blocking of replication of cells at the time of immunization by exposure to X-rays or treatment of animals by cytotoxic drugs delayed or prevented the mobilization of an antibody response. Burnet even conjectured that the first interaction between an antigen and a pre-existing antibody, postulated to be critically localized at the surface of a potentially antibody-producing cell, need not be very precise, and that it might be improved by extended contact with the specific antigen during subsequent division of the selected cell into a clone. These speculations led to the formulation of the clonal selection theory of antibody production, which, as has already been discussed above, introduced a critical modification and extension of Jerne's theory for generation of specific antibodies. One consequence of Burnet's theory was that there must be a mechanism by which clones producing antibodies against the organism's own tissues — the self — were eliminated. It was this prediction that led to the formulation of the postulate of the existence of acquired immune tolerance, which received support from the experiments by Medawar and collaborators. Gard's many-faceted discussions of Burnet´s speculations also included his thoughts regarding different stages of maturation of macrophages-lymphocytes and his recognition of a distinction between an antibody response and delayed responses of the tuberculin type.

The Support for a Prize Amplified

Gard's summary of his review expressed a deep admiration for Burnet's uniqueness as a biological philosopher. He wrote:

> Burnet characteristically tries first to define the central problem and hereafter gradually approach more peripheral problems. This means that

> he has to spread in many directions and cover broad grounds. It (this approach) requires a considerable general introduction to the subject, (and) to be well read and to have exceptional practical experience. To Burnet all problems within biology in the first place are biological; as he himself has expressed it in his discussions; they are "weighted by a strong biological bias." This (attitude) helps him never to lose sight of the wider contexts which may have been hidden in the jumble of details.

Somewhat later in the text Gard wrote:

> This conclusion is in my opinion an impressive intellectual achievement. Medawar's and his collaborators discovery of the acquired immunological tolerance was a direct consequence of their attempts to test the validity of Burnet's theory. Prof. Malmgren in his review in 1958 has characterized this discovery as the major event in immunology since the days of Ehrlich and Behring, a statement which I would like to concur with. According to my opinion it is — without reservation — prize-worthy and Burnet's contribution has been of decisive importance.

Gard finished his review in the following way:

> During this process of development he (Burnet) has not needed to change the core concepts of his theory and the (its) details have been gradually chiselled. As an example one can select his firm conviction that the synthesis of globulin of a certain kind needs to have a genetic background. In 1949 he expressed this view in a way acceptable at the time. In 1956 he attempted to bring the theory up to date without himself being fully satisfied by the result. In his theory of 1959 he finds a point of view that can more smoothly be adjusted to the original concept.
>
> It is still too early to judge which one of the many different interesting ideas in the latest monograph will lead to interesting (new) discoveries. However, the results that have been gained so far are, without hesitation, according to my opinion prize-worthy.

The last of Gard's four reviews concerned Billingham, Brent and Medawar. He referred back to Malmgren's extensive review of 1958 and then provided certain supplementary remarks. The term "immunological unresponsiveness" was discussed and he noted that this can have different meanings. With certain antigens a tolerance or "paralysis of the immune response" can also be induced in adult animals. He further discussed the maturation of the immune system and noted that there may be certain variations in the stages of development when acquired immune tolerance may be induced (with intact cells or fragments of them) in different strains of mice. In one paragraph he discussed the separate observations by Simonsen and by Billingham and Brent that immune cells in a transplanted (adult but not embryonic) tissue can develop a graft-versus-host reaction. Towards the end of the review Gard cited some recent experiments by one of Burnet's recruits Gus Nossal (p. 8) working at Caltech with Lederberg, which gave the first indications that an isolated lymphocyte can give rise to a clone of cells producing only one kind of antibody, as already mentioned. Towards the end, the six page review provided support for the conclusions already arrived at by Malmgren in 1958:

> The importance of the discovery for experimental research in immunology, transplantation and tumour research is obvious and easy to appreciate from the flow of important publications that now pour forth. One can also assume that it will prove to have a great practical importance for transplantation surgery and at (in connection with) treatment of irradiation damages and leukaemia even if the results of the few attempts at practical applications so far obtained do not allow the deduction of any clear conclusions. I would therefore, without hesitation like to consider the discovery as prize-worthy.
>
> When it comes to evaluating the relative contributions of Brent, Billingham and Medawar in their joint publications it should be underlined that Brent in 1953 was a graduate student and one of Medawar's students. Billingham has an M.D. and is skilled at doing experiments. However, there is, according to my firm conviction, no doubt in my mind that Medawar not only has been the leader of the group because of his seniority but also the one who has taken the initiatives and been the brain (behind these). It is my view that among the three only Medawar should be considered for a Nobel Prize.
>
> In agreement with Prof. Malmgren, however, it is my view that one cannot pass by Burnet, who already in 1949 very firmly predicted the existence of the tolerance phenomenon, although he himself did not manage to prove it experimentally. Thus a prize according to my opinion should be divided between Burnet and Medawar.

Harmony but Breach of Consensus

It is not surprising that the conclusions of Malmgren's and Gard's evaluations were in harmony. They had close contacts both professionally and privately, living as next-door-neighbors in link houses at Solna Kyrkväg. Gard was appointed to the chair in bacteriology at the Karolinska Institute in 1948, but he left this in 1949 when he received a personal chair in virus research from the Swedish Parliament. This opened the way for Malmgren to become professor of bacteriology at the Institute. The two of them argued successfully for Burnet and Medawar in the committee, but it was not possible to reach a consensus. Besides Gard and Malmgren, a further five of the 12 members of the committee supported their recommendation, but the chairman Ulf von Euler, who was to share a Nobel Prize in physiology or medicine in 1970, and four additional members preferred two other candidates. They voted that one half of the Prize should be awarded to John C. Eccles for his discoveries concerning synaptic transmission and the mechanism for excitation and inhibition and the other half to Horace W. Magoun for his discoveries concerning the stimulating and inhibiting influence of *formatio reticularis* in the brain stem. It appeared that there must have been some leak of these discussions. It was said that Eccles brought out the chilled champagne only to learn that it was another Australian, who had been recognized by the prize in physiology or medicine in 1960. He brought his team back to work and their achievements were not recognized until three years later when Eccles, together with Alan L. Hodgkin and Andrew F. Huxley, received the Nobel Prize in physiology or medicine "for their discoveries concerning the ionic mechanisms involved in excitation and inhibition in the peripheral and central portions of the nerve cell membrane". However, Magoun´s work was never recognized by a Nobel Prize.

It is not unlikely that there was some additional discreet support for the Burnet and Medawar proposal from the non-voting secretary of the committee Göran Liljestrand, who in 1960 served his last — and 42nd! — year in this function. He had had repeated opportunities to become acquainted with Burnet´s outstanding capacity as a scientist. This was apparent from the presentation of Burnet to the class of medical sciences at the Royal Swedish Academy of Sciences in support of the nomination of him as a foreign member of the Academy in 1957. The text gives a deep insight into Burnet's research and the first signature on the submitted nomination is Liljestrand's.

The Nobel Events in 1960

Burnet and Medawar and their families happily came to Stockholm and both of them and also Medawar's wife Jean have vividly described their experiences[4,7,8]. The yearly fairy-tale celebration was done with a "dazzling, fresh, imaginative elegance". At the ceremony the men wore tails and top hats whereas the women provided colors in their beautiful dresses. Female Academicians, rare at the time, but exemplified by the "mother of plasma cells" Fagraeus, mentioned above, carried a top hat, according to Burnet "remarkably becoming". Burnet and Gard knew each other well and formed a pair in the procession entering the Concert Hall at the prize ceremony, whereas von Euler escorted Medawar.

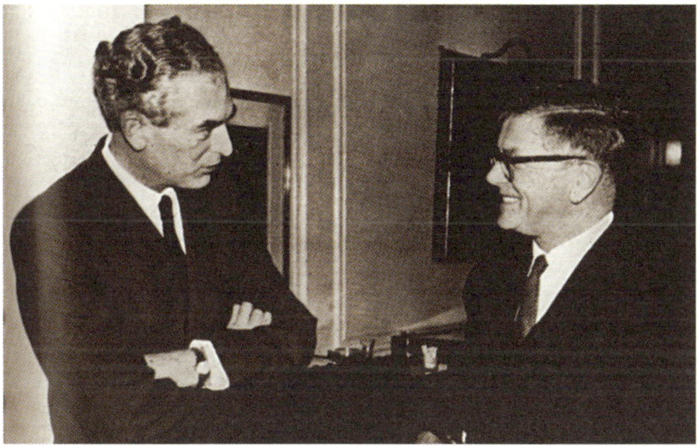

Medawar and Burnet in conversation in 1962. [Photo from Ref. 31.]

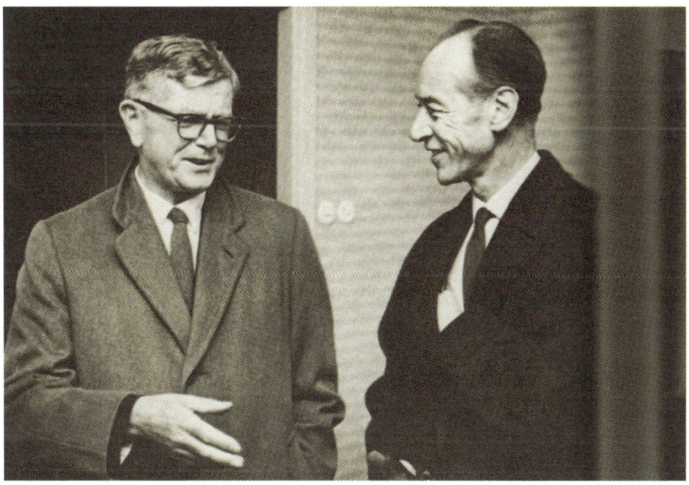

Burnet and Gard in conversation in 1962. [Photo from Ref. 31.]

Gard introduced the two prize recipients without referring to any notes and hereafter they, one at a time, received their diplomas and gold medal from the gracious Gustaf Adolf VI. The diplomas were beautifully bound and included a calligraphic presentation of the recipient and of the prize motivation. In 1960 the left-hand side of the unfolded diploma also included a selected piece of art. The right-hand side presented the prize motivation and was signed by *all* members of the Faculty. The Karolinska Institute changed this design in 1964 and replaced the piece of art with a picture of the Nobel medal. Furthermore the diploma was signed only by three main officials and not all professors of the Institute. The other prize-awarding bodies have retained the original design including a piece of art. The gold medal had the front a portrait of the testator and the years of his birth and death in Latin numbers. On its reverse it had a symbolic image illustrating the art of acquiring medical knowledge and a citation in Latin "Inventas vitam juvat excoluisse per artes" meaning "Let us improve life through science and art". The medal weighed approximately 200 gram and was originally made in 23-carat gold. After 1980 the gold content was reduced to 18 carat. Considering the present value of gold it is not a medal you keep on your office desk. Copies containing a core of copper instead of gold can be provided for the purpose of display.

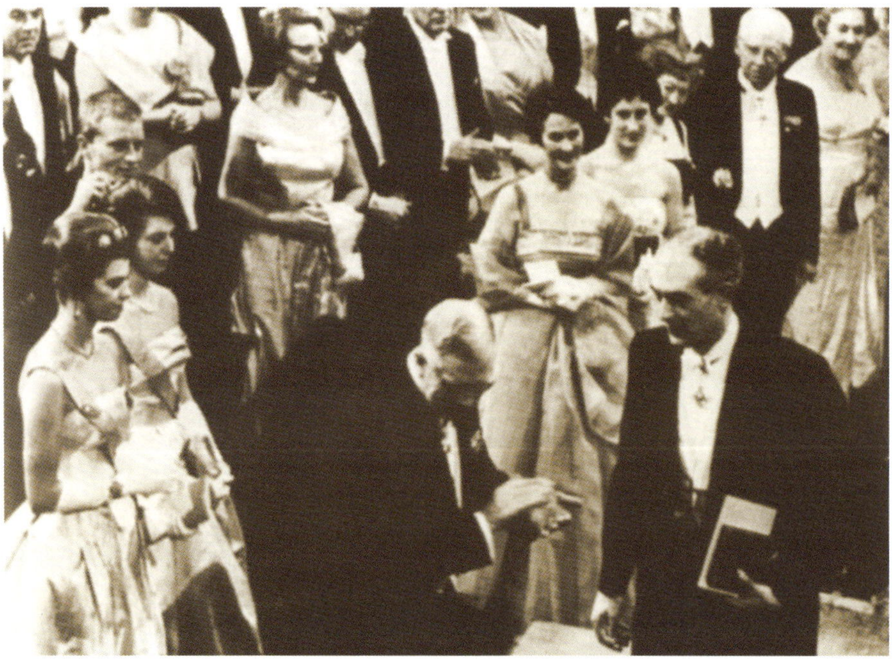

Medawar after having received his Nobel insignia from His Majesty Gustaf VI Adolf. [Photo from Ref. 31.]

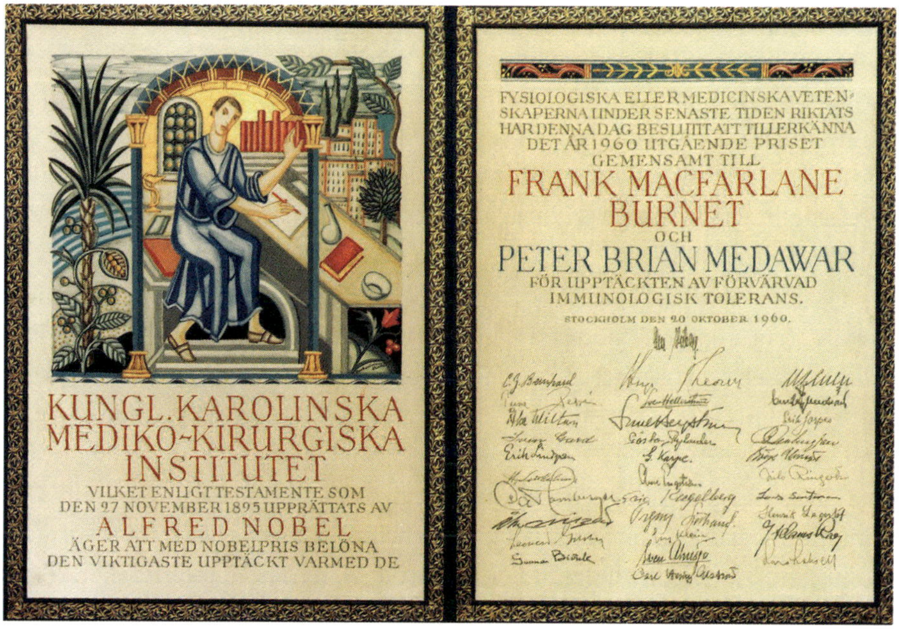
KUNGL. KAROLINSKA
MEDIKO-KIRURGISKA
INSTITUTET
VILKET ENLIGT TESTAMENTE SOM
DEN 27 NOVEMBER 1895 UPPRÄTTATS AV
ALFRED NOBEL
ÄGER ATT MED NOBELPRIS BELÖNA
DEN VIKTIGASTE UPPTÄCKT VARMED DE
FYSIOLOGISKA ELLER MEDICINSKA VETENSKAPERNA UNDER SENASTE TIDEN RIKTATS
HAR DENNA DAG BESLUTAT ATT TILLERKÄNNA
DET ÅR 1960 UTGÅENDE PRISET
GEMENSAMT TILL
FRANK MACFARLANE
BURNET
OCH
PETER BRIAN MEDAWAR
FÖR UPPTÄCKTEN AV FÖRVÄRVAD
IMMUNOLOGISK TOLERANS.
STOCKHOLM DEN 20 OKTOBER 1960.

Burnet's Nobel diploma. 1960 was the second to last year when the diploma included a piece of art and was signed by all members of the College of teachers. [From Suzanne Cory, courtesy of the Walter and Eliza Hall Institute.]

When Burnet died his diploma and gold medal were taken care of by the Walter and Eliza Hall Institute. The question of what happens to the personal insignia of a Nobel laureate after his death presumably is solved in many different ways. In Burnet's case it was a good arrangement for the future to have his diploma and medal in his mother institution. Georg de Hevesy's family donated his Nobel medal to the Hungarian Academy of Sciences as we shall

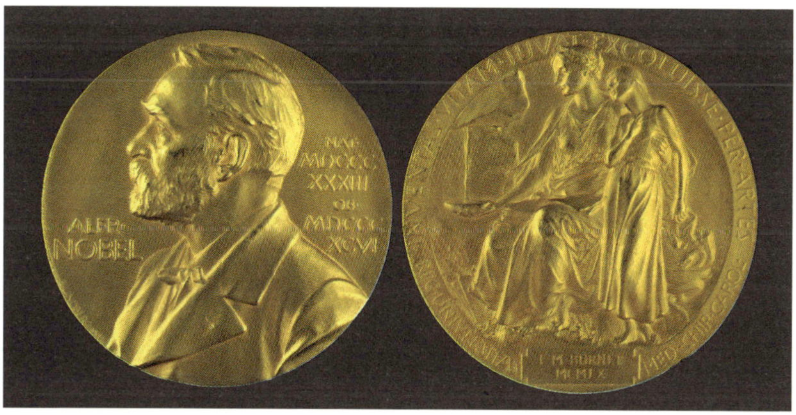
ALFR. NOBEL
NAT. MDCCC XXXIII OB. MDCCC XCVI
F M BURNET
MCMLX

Burnet's Nobel gold medal. [From Suzanne Cory, courtesy of the Walter and Eliza Hall Institute.]

see in Chapter 5. I met Baruch Blumberg (Ref. 2, Chapter 2) in Philadelphia in the autumn of 2011 at a meeting of the American Philosophical Society. He was its president at the time. During a walk in a neighboring park he asked for advice about what he should do with his Nobel medal. Should he give it to one of his four children or should he perhaps will it to the Society? My advice was to do the latter and this is also what happened after his unexpected death only a few months later.

When Burnet and Medawar had received the insignia of their new dignity at the ceremony there followed a musical interlude, Vaughan Williams' *The Wasps*, which Burnet interpreted both as a tribute to Medawar's homeland and also to his own early interests in entomology. Following traditions since many years the prize ceremony in the Stockholm Concert Hall was followed by a dinner in the Golden Hall of the magnificent red brick Town Hall. The dinner was described by Burnet in the following way: "The Hall glitters in gold mosaic with the heroic figure of a Norse goddess in colored mosaic at one end. With the (candle) lights, the silver and glass, the white napery and the formal attire of the guests, a Nobel banquet is a magnificent sight." To this might be added that the walls of the Golden Hall are covered by as many as 18.6 million mosaic pieces, bought from Germany for a bargain prize in connection with

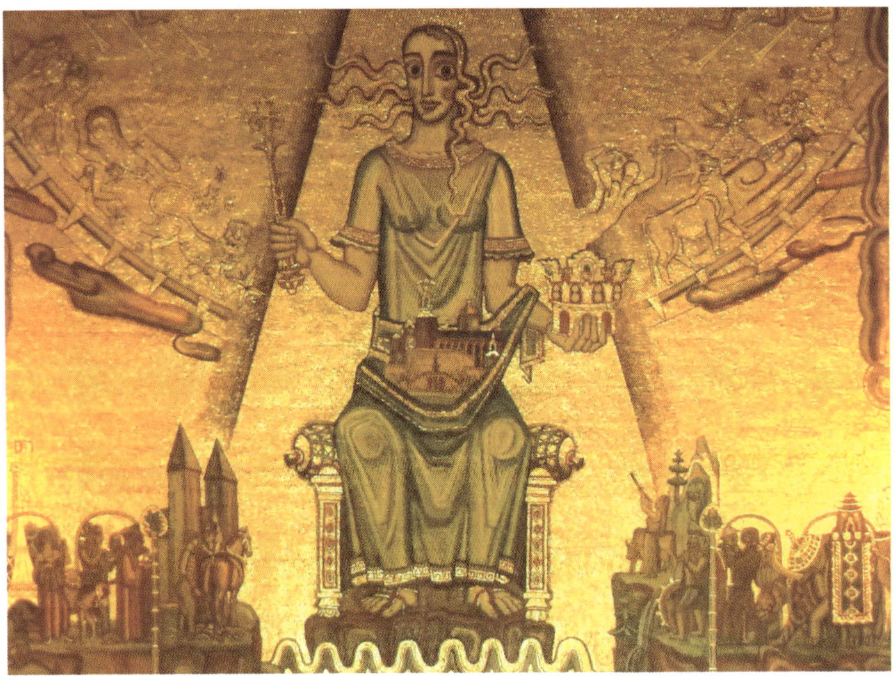

The Mälar Queen at the Golden Hall of Stockholm City Hall.
[Credit: Holger Ellgaard/CC-BY-SA-3.0]

World War I. The figure Burnet alluded to does not depict a Norse goddess but a symbol of Stockholm called Mälardrottningen — the queen of the Lake Mälar(en) — carrying a sceptre and crown in her hands and in her lap a model of the City Hall itself. Her appearance with exophtalmic eyes, medusa hair and oversized arms was very much criticized for a number of years. Today she is an indispensible part of the unique ambiance of the Golden Hall. The Byzantine-inspired mosaic art was designed by Einar Forseth and he was only 30 years old when he reached this peak of creativity in his life. Like many scientists who are fortunate enough to make a major discovery early in their life he had problems later in life carrying the yoke of his own expectations on himself. Forseth had a long life (1892–1988) which gave me an opportunity to meet him in person. On one occasion we had a discussion about acedia, the listlessness that can restrain the creativity of both artists and scientists.

After the festivities it was time for Burnet and Medawar to give their Nobel lectures. The titles were "Immunological recognition of self"[19] and "Immunological tolerance"[20], respectively. Burnet not unexpectedly took the opportunity to discuss his recently-proposed clonal selection theory, which he considered his most important theoretical contribution to science and the one for which he would have liked to get a Nobel Prize. However, it would be a long time until this advance in the understanding of fundamental immunological mechanisms was recognized by a Nobel Prize. It was in 1984 when the 73-year-old Niels K. Jerne shared a prize with the motivation "for theories concerning the specificity in development and control of the immune system and…". When this happened Burnet sent him a letter of congratulations which included the following passage:

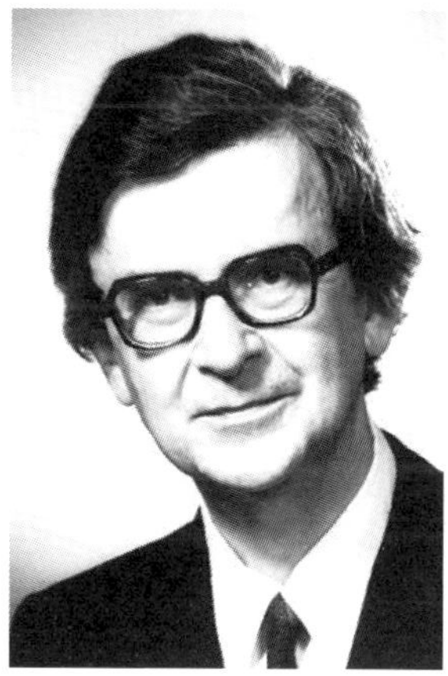

Niels K. Jerne (1911–1994), recipient of the shared 1984 Nobel Prize in physiology or medicine. [From *Les Prix Nobel en 1984.*]

> I have often thought that you and I should have had a joint award for putting antibody production on the right track rather than the one I shared with Medawar. Anyway we are now both on the list.

During his visit in Stockholm I had the pleasure of meeting Burnet and his wife at a dinner in Gard's home two days before the prize ceremony. It was a memorable experience for me as a 23-year-old medical student, who had just started to do experimental virological research, to meet one of the absolute giants in the field. I remember him as a gentle person, but open to conversation with a young person like myself. We discussed the importance of a certain manual dexterity in laboratory work and Burnet exemplified the importance of this from his own development of the embryonated egg technique. He did many of his experiments himself together with a skilled, often female, technician. He never worked with a large group of collaborators and he was not excited about the new more advanced biochemical techniques that started to become available during the end of the 1950s as discussed at the end of the previous chapter.

When Medawar had returned home he split a part of his Prize money with his close collaborators Billingham and Brent to emphasize the significance he attributed to their contributions. He also gave a large share to his mother and the rest was used to buy "a good refrigerator and a good Bokhara rug"[8].

The Post-Prize Engagements of Burnet and Medawar — Two Exceptional Statesmen of Science

At the time when they received their Nobel Prizes, Burnet and Medawar were respectively 61 and 45 years old. According to T. S. Eliot echoed by Samuel Beckett — prizes in literature 1948 and 1969 — receiving the Nobel Prize could be likened to being issued a ticket to one's own funeral. This was certainly not the case for Burnet and Medawar. Both of them were to live for another 25 years and they remained very active to the end of their lives. In Medawar's case this was possible in spite of some very crippling medical problems. We know a lot about their whereabouts since both of them enjoyed presenting their ideas and experiences of life in print. Their talents for writing have been appropriately praised and their list of published books is impressive. As personalities they were very different. According to Sexton's formulation[21] "Burnet, the reticent and somewhat unworldly Australian, Medawar, the supremely articulate and urbane Englishman." In spite of this they entertained a deep respect for each other. Their outlook on the future of man and forthcoming human civilizations differed, with Burnet representing the more pessimistic perspective.

Burnet, the Dystopian Visionary

Although enthusiastic about the achievements of experimental science during his active time he was gloomier when it came to the possibilities for future scientific advances, in particular in the field of molecular biology. As discussed in the previous chapter he declared the end of the science of virology towards the late 1950s when a large number of the essential human pathogens had been identified. Because of this belief he reoriented the research at the Walter and Eliza Hall Institute from virology to immunology in 1957. Ten years later he declared the end of the discipline of immunology, but at that time he was no longer the Director of the Institute. As will become apparent in the next chapter his doomsday prophesy about the end of immunology was, like his judgement of the end of virology, wrong. Burnet retired from the Director's position in 1965 but continued to do some research in the field of autoimmune diseases in another academic setting. His main occupation however was writing. An endless number of articles debating or reviewing various topics stemmed from his energetic pen.

Of course he could not receive a Nobel Prize without reflecting on the future of this kind of prize[4]. He said that he had "sufficient resemblance to Alfred Nobel" to speculate on how Nobel would have allotted the prizes if the will had been written in the mid-20th century. His conclusion was that Nobel would have provided for four annual prizes to the man or woman who

(1) "had done the most to increase the understanding of the bases of human conflict and its control"
(2) "had contributed most effectively to the understanding and control of human population levels"
(3) "whose work had the greatest significance for the conservation of world resources in such fields as reforestation, extraction of low grade minerals, correction of soil deficiencies, agricultural education of primitive populations"
(4) "whose work had done most for the understanding of human genetics and of ways by which that understanding could be applied to maintain the genetic health of our species".

This is just one of many examples of how he addressed in his writing most of the important issues in what is often referred to as *La condition humaine*, used in 1933 both as a title for a novel by André Malraux and a painting by

René Magritte. It appears that Burnet had developed into a committed ecologist way ahead of the developments that were later to come in our present society. The tone of Burnet's concerns for the future of man can also be appreciated from the last paragraph of one of his books of the 1950s[22]. It read:

> Famine, pestilence, and war are the three great evils from which men have always prayed to be delivered. Within a 100 years the second of these evils has been removed almost in its entirety by the work of a few thousand men guided by the ideas of six men of genius: Koch, Pasteur, Ehrlich, Theobald Smith, Dubos, Goodpasture. Only a medical bacteriologist who has seen with understanding the last 25 years of that greatest of social revolutions could be expected to dream that one day war might similarly be dealt with. Human behavior is as much a subject for scientific study as influenza or yellow fever, and sooner or later an adequate understanding of the processes by which one man dominates another will emerge. That understanding represents the only substantial hope of curbing the malignant concentration of power that seems to lie ahead of us. I believe that there is no other approach to effective knowledge than the scientific method, and I believe that only knowledge can counter evil that makes use of knowledge.

This is a testimony that invites serious reflections.

The tone of general pessimism of this secularized Presbyterian came to prevail in his forthcoming books colored by expressions like "a dismal unappealing view of humanity". His total production was impressive encompassing about 500 scientific publications and more than 30 books and monographs. His last two books were *Endurance of Life: The Implications of Genetics for Human Life*[23] and *Credo and Comment*[24]. The unrestrained dark views he presented generated considerable controversy. He was referred to as a rationalist, meritocrat and an elitist and his overemphasis on the role of genetics in the balance of nature and nurture leading to a flirting with eugenic ideas evoked particularly strong reactions.

Burnet was bestowed with many honors and awards and became the most decorated scientist to have worked in Australia. As early as 1942 he became a member of The Royal Society and in 1959 he received its most prestigious award, the Copley medal. In 1951 he was knighted and in 1958 he was awarded the prestigious Order of Merit, which is limited to only 24 holders. Because of his long life he eventually became the Doyen of this exclusive group, something he enjoyed at his last visit in 1982 to London and Buckingham Palace. At that time his indispensable life partner Linda had died painfully from lymphoma back in 1973, which led to major adjustments in Burnet's life. For years to come he wrote her a mock letter every Sunday evening. In spite of this, a few years later Burnet did in fact engage in a new marriage to a widow, Hazel Jenkin. She gave enrichment to the final years of Burnet's life. When Burnet turned 80 years old there were major celebrations in his home town Melbourne. The Walter and Eliza Hall Institute established the Colin Syme Lectures in his honor and the first speaker was the Nobel laureate Gajdusek (Ref. 2, Chapter 8), who had been instrumental in generating data inspiring Burnet to formulate his clonal selection theory. During Burnet's long active life a large number of honorary doctorate degrees were bestowed on him, but the question is if Medawar did not receive an even larger number. In the latter's memoirs[7], in the context of noting that he never received his PhD, he jokingly referred to the fact that he was showered with more doctorates *honoris causa* than he knew what to do with. He was close to having such recognition from countries with initial letters representing all those used in the English alphabet, except Y and Z. His own comment was "... and shrewd observers will have observed that Yale and Zimbabwe are unaccountably dragging their feet".

Burnet eventually died from colon cancer three days short of his 86th birthday at his son´s farm near Port Fairy.

In 1999 a symposium was arranged in Melbourne to celebrate the centennial of Burnet's birth. The first page of the program cited the engraftment on Burnet's tombstone. The text was taken from Plato and read "A man who threw off ideas like sparks, which caused a blaze that leapt across to the minds of others." According to Sexton the original text by Plato is "... a spark may suddenly leap, as it were, from mind to mind, and the light of understanding so kindled will feed itself." In this vein one might transmute the crest *Fiat lux* of the Walter and Eliza Hall Institute into "let there be sparks".

Seven Nobel laureates representing the fields of virology and immunology were present, as were nine Australian scientists, many of whom had careers markedly influenced by Burnet's sparks. There were also a limited number of other invited scientists including myself. My lecture was entitled "The new biology and the global society" and into this I had woven the inspiration for future scientific endeavours proffered by Burnet's legacy. I had had previous reasons to familiarize myself with Burnet's life contributions, since I had been chosen to present the eulogy for him as a foreign member of the Royal Swedish

Academy of Sciences after his death.

After the meeting my wife and I visited Canberra, where Fenner (p. 22), one of Burnet's closest scientific friends, was our host. He had the most charming personality with a capacity to blush even into his 80s. On a Saturday morning he handed over the hosting of us to a colleague because he was going to play his weekly tennis. I commented that it was admirable of him to keep up his physical activities and to maintain contacts with his friends. He agreed, but noted that one problem was that his friends had started to die. Fenner had a rich life and did not die until 2010 at the age of 94 years. Besides Burnet, he is one of the most admired Australian scientists to have lived and the two of them stimulated each other's academic concerns and thinking.

Medawar — The Years of Hubris and the Rich Aftermath

Two years after receiving the Nobel Prize, Medawar was appointed director of the National Institute for Medical Research, which had moved from inner London, where it had been located when Burnet worked there in the 1930s, to Middlesex north of London. Medawar had considerable ambitions for the Institute and managed over the years to develop it into a stronghold of immunology. At the same time he remained actively engaged in experimental research. He was a very much sought after lecturer and travelled worldwide, frequently just for a few days, often returning home from trans-Atlantic flights to be at his desk at 8.30 in the morning. His boundless energy covered both the intellectual and physical realms. He could challenge his colleagues to a violent game of squash or rush up three stairs and then whistle a familiar tune. He also smoked American cigars, after having felt that he was morally obliged to give up cigarette smoking when he became director of the institute. Considering himself invincible he disregarded his high blood pressure and his wife even used the word hubris to describe his attitude to life[8]. He clearly burnt his candle at both ends and eventually he had to pay a price.

Medawar's handicapping illnesses started in 1969. On a Saturday he gave an address entitled "On the effecting of all things possible" in Exeter Cathedral as President of the British Association for the Advancement of Science

followed by another lecture as a substitute for a colleague who could not make it to the meeting. The day continued with engaging social activities and a swim in the cold water of the river Dart. This was too much and Medawar did not feel well the following morning. As he was reading the Lesson at the divine service in the cathedral his speech became slower and he started to slur. As it turned out there was a major haemorrhage at the right side of his brain. His lust for life and sense of humor carried him through the forthcoming months of many challenges and even life-threatening events. When he woke up from his unconsciousness he said, referring to having read the Lesson "Human beings simply don't realize the risks they run when they meddle with the supernatural." But there was more to come and eventually a clot had to be removed surgically. Waking up from the anaesthesia his first comment, seeing his wife was "Entire visual field agreeably occupied." It was such stamina that allowed him to gain further rich life experiences. Still it would take many months for him to recover to the extent that he could walk with a stick, and a certain paralysis remained on the left side.

Fortunately his intellect remained untouched. His wife Jean had to take on extra responsibilities helping him to overcome his life-long physical handicap. By 1980 additional health problems developed. There was a blood clot in one of the brain stem vessels. Two years later there was another blood clot in a retinal vessel making him blind in the left eye. Throughout all these health challenges he kept his spirit and sense of humor. And he remained impressively active. After 1969 he had to leave the directorship of the National Institute for Medical research, but he continued to be involved in the pursuit of experimental research at a separate building of the Institute, the Clinical Research Centre. The Institute remained in good hands, since James L. Gowans, an outstanding immunologist to be discussed in the next chapter, took over the Directorship.

Medawar's major activities turned towards writing for which he had a highly admired proclivity. His talent as a writer was already apparent by the late 1950s when he published a collection of essays under the title *The Uniqueness of the Individual*[25]. In 1967 this was followed by another collection of essays *Pluto's Republic*[26], *The Limits of Science*[27], the popular *Advice to a Young Scientist*[28] and his already-mentioned memoirs[7]. Together with his wife he wrote a book on aphorisms and short stories called *Aristotle to Zoos*[29]. A number of his most famous essays and also some previously unpublished essays and lectures were published posthumously in the book *The Threat and the Glory. Reflections on Science and Scientists*[12]. In the foreword Lewis Thomas, a highly respected essayist in the field of biological philosophy in his own right — see, for example, *Late Night Thoughts on Listening to Mahler's Ninth Symphony*[30] — wrote:

Something that I hope will not be missed: the electromagnetic energy of this spectacular man, his exuberance, his outrageous disrespect for so many canons (of all stripes and definitions), and most important of all, his own pleasure in life, his immense respect for Jean, and all the fun he had all his life, with his astonishing and capacious mind.

In the introduction of the book the editor David Pyke emphasized Medawar's own recipe for good writing. This was "Brevity, cogency and clarity are the principal virtues and greatest of these is clarity." His love for words and their etymological origin is obvious. Just a few examples from his biography[7]; panjandrum — a pompous personage in a small place; gobbledegook — involved, pedantic, repetitious, and pompous jargon, relying heavily on Latinized expressions and meaningless clichés; gormenghastly — too many arguments, too much fancruft (of importance only to a small population of enthusiastic fans); ratiocination — the deduction of conclusions from premises; solecism — any impropriety or incongruity etc. He also forged formulations that promptly caught the reader's attention, like "One should not study tomatoes with blue eye glasses." Medawar also coined the term "obsessionalist" to describe this particular trait of his devoted fellow scientists. In his view there was no middle ground between engagement and estrangement for the committed researcher.

Medawar received many honors during his lifetime. His large number of honorary doctorates has already been alluded to. In addition he was knighted in 1965 and in 1981 he received the prestigious Order of Merit and therefore for four years, together with Burnet, came to represent two out of the 24 most royally honored of all British citizens at the time. On Medawar's tombstone there is a sentence taken from Thomas Hobbes, *Leviathan*. It reads: "There can be no contentment but in proceeding." His life was an illustration of this credo. The citation represented the last sentence in Medawar's lecture in Exeter cathedral the day before he had his major stroke that forever changed his and his family's life.

Chapter 3

More Nobel Prizes in Immunology

Networks of Signals
A Rich Twitter between Cells
and Harmony Still

The discipline of immunology has advanced in a very powerful way during the more than 50 years that have passed since Burnet and Medawar received their Nobel Prize. Seven separate Nobel Prizes have been awarded in this field, the latest one in 2011 (Table 3.1). They serve as excellent departures for a discussion of the impressive developments in the discipline. Due to the 50 years secrecy rule the progress of the field will have to be presented without access to the precious information provided by Nobel archives. However, my own engagement in the Nobel Committee work for about 20 years in the 1970s and 1980s is a repository for a possible use for comments on procedures but not on discussions of candidates. Furthermore my own studies of viruses have relied heavily on the use of immunological methods and on insights into immune defence mechanisms.

The development of immunology has been and continues to be very strong and the different Nobel Prizes each recognizing particular advances only represent a sample of the major discoveries made. After all there is only one prize each year in the wide area of physiology or medicine and the competition between different (sub) disciplines is fierce. As we shall see additional fundamental findings in immunology might have been recognized by Nobel Prizes.

Table 3.1. Nobel Prizes in physiology or medicine (1961–2011) recognizing advances in immunology.

Year	Awardee(s)	Motivation
1972	Gerald M. Edelman Rodney R. Porter	for their discoveries concerning the chemical structure of antibodies
1977	Rosalyn Yalow (shared)	for the development of radioimmunoassay of peptide hormones
1980	Baruj Benacerraf Jean Dausset George Snell	for their discoveries concerning genetically determined structures on the cell surface that regulate immunological reactions
1984	Niels K. Jerne Georges J. F. Köhler Cesar Milstein	for theories concerning the specificity in development and control of the immune system and the discovery of the principle for production of monoclonal antibodies
1987	Susumu Tonegawa	for his discovery of the genetic principle for generation of antibody diversity
1996	Peter C. Doherty Rolf M. Zinkernagel	for their discoveries concerning the specificity of the cell mediated immune defence
2011	Bruce A. Beutler Jules A. Hoffman Ralph M. Steinman	for their discoveries concerning the activation of innate immunity for his discovery of the dendritic cell and its role in adaptive immunity

The Origin of Lymphocytes Engaged in Immune Responses

As discussed in the previous chapter it started to become clear during the 1940s that there were two principally different categories of immune responses, one operating by use of antibodies — the humoral immunity — and the other that had a more immediate dependence on cells — the cell-mediated immunity. Of course antibodies had to be produced by specialized cells and the pioneering work by Astrid Fagraeus (p. 52) had already highlighted the particular role of plasma cells in this context in 1948. It was speculated that these cells with their eccentric nucleus displaying a cartwheel appearance were derived from immature parental cells in the reticuloendothelial system — the spleen, the lymph nodes, the liver, the bone marrow and the thymus — but their true origin was not known at the time. Then during the 1950s and 1960s it was recognized that white blood cells — *lymphocytes* — like the red blood cells, circulated widely in the body. The main contributor to this understanding was James L. Gowans. He obtained his scientific training at Oxford, where he later

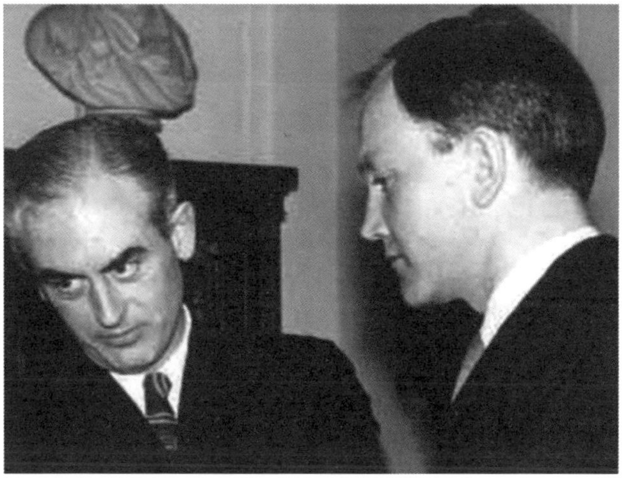

Medawar and James L. Gowans. [From Ref. 25.]

became professor of experimental pathology. Gowans used isotope labelling of the genetic material of the cells, a technique pioneered by Georg de Hevesy (Chapter 5), to trace their movement in the bodies of small experimental animals. A new and difficult technique of cannulation of the thoracic duct was developed. By use of this technique it could be demonstrated that large amounts of lymphocytes — about 1000 million cells per day — circulated via lymph vessels into the blood and back again. The existence of a separate system to transport white blood cells had already been discovered in the 17th century by the Swedish anatomist Olof Rudbeck the elder. He referred to them as *vasa serosa*. Gowans found that the main transport from blood to lymph occurred within lymph nodes, the lymphoid follicles of the spleen and the Peyer's patches of the intestine. No involvement of the thymus was observed.

It would take many years to understand how lymphocytes could differentiate and what their range of diversity might be. In particular it took time to understand that the thymus was a central organ in the processing of lymphocytes. It had been observed for a long time that this organ contained small lymphocytes but no signs of activation of these cells were observed in connection with generalized immune responses. It was therefore believed that the thymus was a vestigial organ that had become redundant during evolution, like the lymphocyte-containing appendix. In my worn-out 1965 edition of a college dictionary the thymus was described as "A lymphoid organ of glandular character and *unknown function* (my italics)". The main reason why the central role of the thymus in the immune defence system was not appreciated was the experience that removal of this organ from adult animals seemed to have no

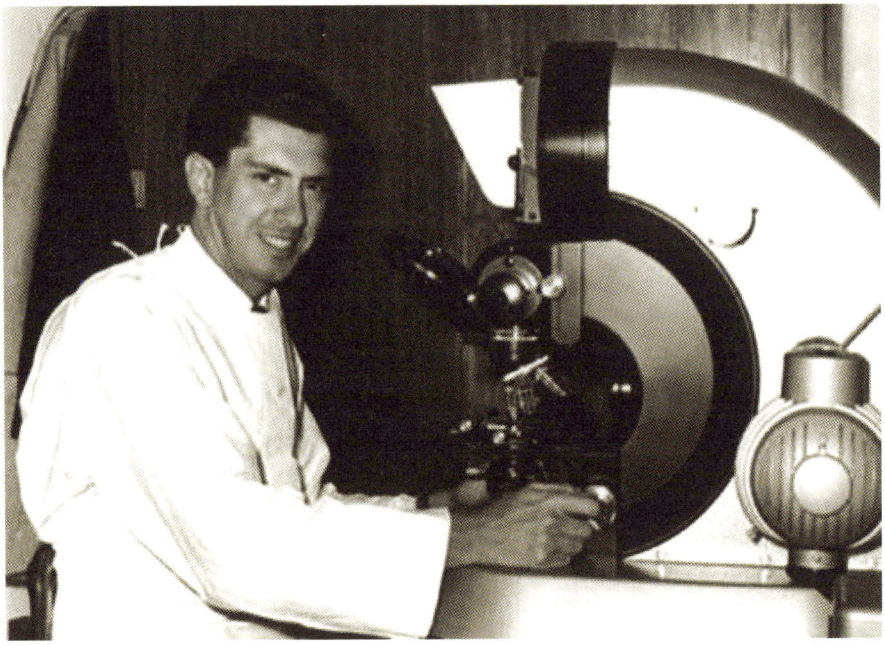

Jacques F. A. P. Miller. [From Ref. 25.]

serious consequences. It was first when the organ was removed from newborn mice that its central role became apparent. These experiments were performed by Jacques F. A. P. Miller and collaborators in the early 1960s. Miller was born in France but moved with his family to Sidney in 1941. In connection with that move the original name of Meunier was changed to Miller. At St. Aloysius' college where he studied he met Nossal, his future colleague. Miller received a scholarship that allowed him to develop his research in the United Kingdom. He received his PhD from the University of London based on work performed at the Chester Beatty Research Institute of Cancer Research. In 1963 he continued his pioneering work at the National Institutes of Health in London, before finally returning to Australia, where he joined Nossal at the Walter and Eliza Hall Institute.

Originally the purpose of Miller's studies in the UK was to examine the effect of the Gross leukaemia virus in newborn mice. It had been found that virus-induced tumor development was prevented if animals injected with the virus at birth had had their thymus removed after weaning. The question therefore was what would happen if this intervention had already been made at birth. Removal of the thymus in newborn animals was a technically much more complicated procedure than the corresponding operation in more adult animals. Eventually the technical problems were solved and the experiment could be performed. The newborn animals without the organ fared well until weaned but thereafter they deteriorated and wasted away. They had a markedly reduced number of lymphocytes in the blood and lymphoid tissues. If the animals were grafted with skin from a different mouse strain before the weaning there was *no* rejection of the transplanted tissue. The only way of allowing the animals to survive after weaning was to graft a new thymus tissue. Taken together these findings demonstrated that the thymus had some central role(s) in the development of immune functions. These data were published in 1961 (reviewed in Ref. 1). Later it could be demonstrated that the thymus played a role also in adult animals. If the removal of the thymus in such animals was combined with X irradiation to destroy cells of the haematopoietic system and then followed by a transplantation of bone marrow cells the recovery of immune functions was markedly delayed.

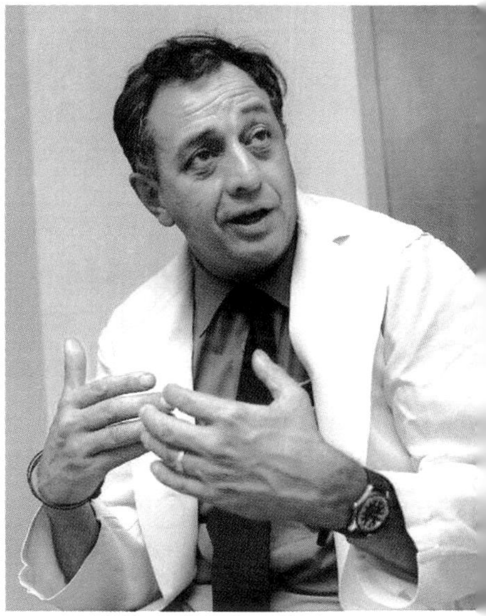

Henry Robert A. Good (1922–2003).

The central role of the thymus was also identified by Robert A. Good and collaborators using a different system. His early training as a physician and his later development as a scientist engaged in research on the immune system was at the Medical School of the University of Minnesota. He observed in the early 1950s that a patient with a large tumor originating in the thymus — a thymoma — had very low numbers of circulating lymphocytes and only small amounts of antibodies in his blood. Since this original observation, similar cases of thymoma and hypogammaglobulinemia have been referred to as Good's syndrome. Because of these early observations in patients Good tried to prove the role of the thymus in rabbits. These experiments failed and only several years later could evidence of the role of the thymus be documented in tests with mice. Good claimed to have made his discovery independently and at the same time as Miller, but his results were not published in a regular scientific journal until in 1962[2]. There was still a third group of researchers including Branislav Jancovic, Barry Arnason and Byron Waksman at the Harvard Medical School, Boston, who had also made important experiments providing evidence for the role of the thymus. After some delay their data were published, also in 1962[3]. The fact that three groups in parallel made the same important discovery is not uncommon in science. It would seem that in some way the time had become ripe for the formulation of a fundamental new concept. The critical question in this situation was to try to tease out who had priority. It must have been a delicate task for Nobel committees to allocate priority after reviewing proposals for the discovery of the central role of the thymus in the immune system.

In 1956 Bruce Glick, a PhD student at Ohio State University, had made a serendipitous finding. He demonstrated that removal of the *bursa of Fabricius* — lymphatic tissue located by the cloacae named after the 17th century naturalist Hieronymus Fabricius — in newly hatched chickens led to that the birds became unable to produce antibodies. These data were confirmed by Good and others. The equivalent of the bursa of Fabricius in man was later shown to be the bone marrow. By about 1968 it had become clear that there were two major classes of lymphocytes one originating from the bursa of Fabricius/bone marrow and the other from the thymus. With time they came to be named by Ivan Roitt at Balliol College, Oxford University, simply *B* and *T cells.* B cells were responsible for the *humoral immunity*, whereas the T cells were involved in different kinds of *cell-mediated immunity*. The story of lymphocyte differentiation and maturation into cells serving different functions has developed to reveal a considerable complexity. In order to discuss the different Nobel Prizes in physiology or medicine focussing on immunology after 1960 the following highly condensed summary of the present state knowledge needs to be given, but first a short notice on the inflammatory process.

A local infection is managed by inflammatory reactions. Inflammation represents a local mobilization of an immune response. It is characterized by four easily registered phenomena; in musical Latin, calor — heating; dolor — pain; rubor — reddening and tumor — swelling. The swelling which is due to a local accumulation of fluid allows transport of cells to the site of inflammation, but it also leads to pain. The reddening is the result of influx of cells of different kinds including the erythrocytes in the blood. The increased temperature allows an accelerated metabolism to favor cleaning efforts, which involve the participation of many different kinds of lymphocytes and a wide range of signalling substances. The aim of the inflammatory process is to restore the tissue to its original condition —*restitutio ad integrum.*

When our body is exposed to a foreign antigen such as an invading bacterium or a virus infecting, for example mucosal cells and potentially spreading to neighboring tissues, many defence mechanisms are activated. They were briefly alluded to in the previous chapter. There is a first line of defence, the so called non-adaptive innate immunity. Hereafter the adaptive immunity involving both antibodies and cells make a specific attack on the foreign antigens. Toward the end of the 1960s it was demonstrated, again by Miller, now in collaboration with George F. Mitchell that there was a certain kind of T cells that assisted the B cells in the development of an antibody response. These T cells were named *helper T cells*.

Certain lymphocytes were found to carry immunoglobulin molecules at their surface. Some early pioneering work in this area was made by the Swedish immunologist Göran Möller[4]. His findings became a part of a PhD thesis presented at Georg Klein's Department of Tumour Biology at the Karolinska Institute. Göran was a classmate of mine in medical school and one of the most talented students of his vintage. He had a broad general education and stimulated me to further engagements in the canonical literature, including reading among other books Thomas Mann's *Buddenbrooks* during our joint military service. Göran became a special friend and was the best man at my wedding in 1959. His career in science was powerful and developed rapidly for a decade, after which the trajectory of his rising star levelled off. During the intermission after our second year of medical studies at the Karolinska Institute his identical twin brother Gunnar was killed in a car accident in Germany. This must have been a deep emotional and even "physical" trauma and I have always wondered to what extent this may have explained his impeded career. Could the loss of an identical twin be like losing one's shadow, a metaphor frequently used in the arts, like in Richard Strauss–Hugo von Hofmannsthal "The woman without a shadow".

In 1975 it could be demonstrated that there existed a kind of T cells that differed from the helper T cells. This newly identified kind of T cells had a capacity to destroy cells and was therefore referred to as *cytotoxic T cells*. The two kinds of T cells had different surface characteristics. The various forms of T cells were found to differentiate and mature in the thymus. To summarize a lot of data accumulating during the 1970s it can be said that whereas B cells can recognize antigen in a soluble form this is not the case for T cells. The latter can only recognize antigen displayed at the surface of cells; specialized antigen-presenting cells (APC) such as macrophages, dendritic cells (from Greek dendron for tree) — further presented on page 34 — or virus-infected cells. The helper T cells have a surface marker called CD4 whereas in cytotoxic T cells the corresponding structure is CD8. To add to the complexity these surface structures act as receptors *in coordination with* still one more surface structure, the *T cell receptor*. The nature of this receptor remained enigmatic for a long time. Eventually scientists were able to demonstrate that it was the MHC, introduced in the previous chapter, but that again there were differences between the two kinds of T cells. The MHC molecules were of class II in the case of helper cells and class I in the case of cytotoxic cells. We will leave these complex relationships for the time being but will come back to them in connection with the discussion of the particular Nobel Prize awarded in 1996.

The Lack of Recognition of the Discoveries of B and T Cells by a Nobel Prize

In his autobiography[5] Medawar discussed the golden age of immunology towards the end of the 1950s giving insights into tolerance and graft versus host (GvH) disease. He referred to this period as "abounding in synthetic discoveries". In a footnote, briefly alluded to in the previous chapter, he explained what he meant by a synthetic discovery.

> An *analytic discovery* is a mapping of territory already known to exist — for example, the elucidation of the crystalline structure of a molecular species which is known *a priori* to have a crystalline structure. By contrast, synthetic discovery is an entering upon territory not until then known to exist. Immunological tolerance was a *synthetic discovery*, so was GvH disease, and so was Dr James Gowans's discovery that lymphocytes were circulating cells as red corpuscles are. Another example would be the discovery by Jacques Miller and Robert A. Good that the thymus gland is crucially important for the maturing and development of those lymphocytes responsible for the transaction of many immunological reactions.

Medawar frequently returned to the point that the discovery of the role of the thymus in the education of T cells should be recognized by a Nobel Prize in physiology or medicine. In an essay *The "ultra-élite" of science*[6] he said "I, for example, think it quite amazing that the elucidation of the functions of the thymus gland should not have been worthy of an award." Thus one may wonder why this was not the case. Certainly there must have been proposals for a prize in this area, both by Medawar and others, but since this concerned a time period of the 1970s and 1980s, when I personally was active in the Nobel committee I must refrain from any comments. It must be left to future historians of science to review this matter. Medawar's essay was a review of Harriet Zuckerman's book on successful US scientists[7]. This book listed important scientists, including Nobel laureates, but also others who had not been recognized by any Nobel Prize. The latter group was referred to as occupying the 41st chair in science. This figure of expression was proposed by her late husband, the authority on social sciences Robert Merton. It had its origin in the fact that the "immortals" of the French Academy — like the original Platon's Academy — occupied 40 chairs. Thus number 41 represents the non-existing chair for those who never made it. It may appear regrettable that the fundamental discoveries in immunology during the 1960s were never recognized by a Nobel Prize in physiology or medicine.

In the historical and sociological analysis of discoveries in the biomedical field other prizes and citations than the Nobel Prizes in physiology or medicine and in selected cases chemistry have been used[8]. Examples are scientists cited as worthy of a prize in the Nobel Prize archives and those who have received one, for example, the Albert Lasker Basic Medical Research Award, the Louisa Gross Horwitz Prize for Biology or Biochemistry and the Holger and Greta Crafoord Prize in Biosciences (with the emphasis on ecology), the latter like the Nobel Prizes in Physics and Chemistry awarded by the Royal Swedish Academy of Sciences.

Of course the scientists involved in the synthetic discoveries in immunology mentioned above were recognized by other prizes than the Nobel Prizes. In 1970 Good (alone!) received the Lasker Award in the area of Clinical Medical Research "for his uniquely important contributions to our understanding of the mechanisms of immunity". Four years later Gowans and Miller received the Paul Ehrlich and Ludwig Darmstadter Prize. The following year Miller's collaborator Mitchison also received the same prize together with two other immunologists. The question is often asked if receiving other prizes will facilitate recognition by a Nobel Prize, the ultimate accolade for scientific achievements. Because the Nobel Prizes have developed to be in a league by themselves, other prizes of more recent date have a natural ambition to recognize individuals who will later receive such a prize. However it seems fair to state that other prizes do not give a push towards a Nobel Prize. My experience from working in the Nobel committee at the Karolinska Institute is that it almost never happened that a reference was made to prior recognition by other prizes. The discussions focussed on the individual and the originality and magnitude of his discovery and that the question of priority had been unequivocally clarified. It could be added that concerning relations between prizes there is a paradoxical reverse effect, as mentioned previously[9]. A person who has received a Nobel Prize generally does not receive any other prizes.

Another essay by Medawar in the collection of his writings already referred to[6] has the title *The strange case of the spotted mice.* It dealt with a very special situation of fraud in science that he himself was engaged in uncovering. This case was also referred to as the Summerlin affair from the name of the scientist responsible for the misconduct. Very briefly William T. Summerlin, who was working in Good's laboratory at the Sloan-Kettering Institute for Cancer Research in New York and supported by him, argued that his experiments showed that if allogenous skin tissue was cultivated in laboratory vessels for some time they became transplantable. He showed that a piece of skin from a black inbred mouse could survive in the skin of a strain of mice that was white. In the end it was found that Summerlin had simply painted the black spot on the white mice! "Mouse-painter" later became a general term of reference to someone who had committed a fraud in science. The revelation of Summerlin's misconduct of course had a disastrous impact on his own career, but it impacted also on the head of the laboratory, Good. His tenure was marred by the disclosure of this fraud in 1974. Since his reputation was tarnished, one may ask what impact this may have had on him as a candidate for a Nobel Prize and on other candidates in the field.

Fraud in science is rare and the explanation is simple. One absolute requirement of scientific results is that they can be reproduced by other scientists knowing the trade. Thus there is a big and qualified jury of fellow researchers in the total scientific community and anyone who tries to cheat will be relentlessly disclosed. Someone behaving like Summerlin will be doomed forever, but as mentioned his mentors/advisors will also be stigmatized, because one of the absolute fundamentals in training of a scientist is to infuse rock solid honesty. As in any good work as defined by Howard Gardner and collaborators[10] there are three critical words starting with e to be highlighted — excellence, ethics and engagement. They are particularly applicable to scientific pursuits.

The Basic Structure of an Antibody

The development of chemical techniques allowed a deeper insight into the structure of antibodies during the early 1960s. By use of the electrophoresis technique developed by the Uppsala professor Arne Tiselius the antibody containing gamma fraction of serum proteins could be isolated. An extensive presentation of Tiselius will be given in Chapter 7. The chemistry of the most common and smallest kind of antibodies, the 7S IgG (immunoglobulin gamma)

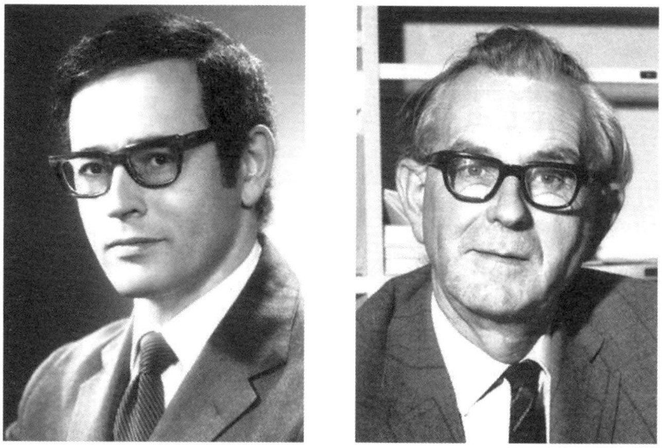

Gerald M. Edelman and Rodney R. Porter (1917–1985), recipients of the shared 1972 Nobel Prize in physiology or medicine. [From *Les Prix Nobel en 1972.*]

proteins was elucidated by Gerald M. Edelman at the Rockefeller University, New York, and Rodney R. Porter, Oxford University. The unit S is taken from the first letter in (The) Svedberg, another Uppsala professor. He was the father of high speed centrifugation techniques and the recipient of the 1926 Nobel Prize in chemistry and we will encounter him again in Chapters 5 and 7.

Edelman had his original education in New York public schools. After this he attended Medical School at the University of Pennsylvania where he graduated M.D. He did his internship at Massachusetts General Hospital and got further clinical training at the American Hospital in Paris. For a long time he was uncertain if he should spend his life in music or in medicine. His final choice was science and not the violin. In 1957 he started at the Rockefeller Institute in Henry Kunkel's laboratory. Kunkel had made pioneering studies of myeloma proteins, a critical material for the unravelling of the structure of antibodies as it turned out. Edelman presented his PhD thesis in 1960 and then he developed his own research group and rapidly became a rising star in molecular immunology.

Porter received his training as a scientist in the laboratory of Frederick Sanger, the only two-time recipient of a Nobel Prize in Chemistry (Ref. 9, Chapter 7). Porter was Sanger's first doctoral student. Because of his involvement in the Second World War Porter had become delayed in his studies and he was in fact slightly older than Sanger. At the time, Sanger had already developed techniques to sequence insulin, the achievement that brought him his first Nobel Prize and the use of these techniques was important in Porter's PhD thesis presented in 1948. In that same year he initiated studies of the

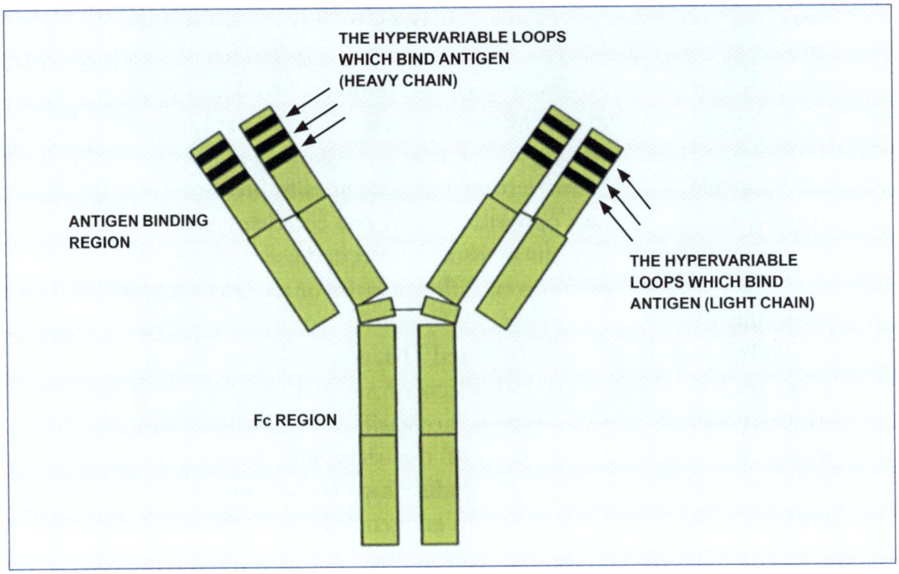

Schematic illustration of the structure of an IgG antibody.

structure of antibodies, something that led to fruitful engagements for the years to come. He described in his Nobel lecture[11] how he had become inspired to undertake these studies by reading Landsteiner's book, *The Specificity of Serological Reactions*[12].

These two prize recipients had revealed the structure of the IgG antibodies and demonstrated that they were composed of two pairs of protein chains, one pair with a larger molecular weight — the *heavy chains* — and one pair with a lower molecular weight — the *light chains* . The chains were kept together by multiple disulphide bonds. The N-terminal ends of the four chains showed considerable variability and combined pair-wise to form two *antigen binding sites*. This implied that the IgG antibody was bivalent. The rest of the chains had a constant structure. The two scientists had provided critical information about the structure of IgG antibodies by use of different approaches. Edelman had separated the chains by breaking the disulphide bonds[13]. He also took advantage of an accident of nature. Patients with myelomas had long been known to excrete a special class of proteins in their urine. This phenomenon had originally been observed as early as 1847 by Henry Bence Jones and the protein was accordingly referred to as Bence Jones protein. In elegant experiments Edelman and collaborators demonstrated that this protein represented isolated, presumably excess light chains of the myeloma IgG. Porter used another approach and cleaved the antibodies with proteolytic enzymes. It was the combined data obtained by Edelman and Porter that clarified the principal structure of IgG. The citation for their joint Nobel Prize was "for their discovery concerning the chemical structure of antibodies".

Later it has been shown that there are four additional classes of antibodies. They are formed by use of similar building elements but serve different functions. One example is a very large structure called IgM (M stands for macro) combining five IgG-like molecules. This antibody is the dominating class in an early phase of an original (primary) immune response. Another example is an antibody called IgA, which is a dimer of the principal four-chain structure of IgG. It appears in the secretion at mucosal surfaces and serves a particular role in the establishment of a local immunity.

Apparently some rumor about the forthcoming prize to Edelman and Porter had leaked because, just prior to the decision on the prize, I received an international telephone call from a colleague arguing that a prize should not be given without including Kunkel. However, I did not have any influence on the processing of the prize at the time, since 1972 was the last year that my predecessor Gard was in charge. Throughout the 24 years he was professor of virology at the institute he had a deep involvement in the work of the Nobel Committee. Kunkel was not included in the 1972 prize and it was Gard who introduced Edelman and Porter at the prize ceremony. This was the fifth and last time he carried this prestigious responsibility, probably a record of sorts.

In my presentation at the Burnet centennial symposium in Melbourne in 1999, mentioned above, I cited an anecdote which I had heard directly from Edelman. In the mid-1960s Burnet was visiting Edelman in his laboratory at the Rockefeller Institute or University (the name was changed in 1965) and was shown the advancing insights into the chemistry of antibodies. According to Edelman Burnet's comment was "Why do you do that? I know that the clonal selection theory is right. Chemistry only makes things more complicated."

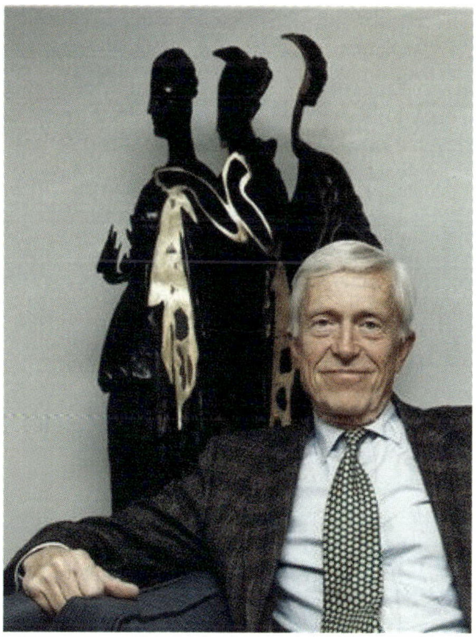

Baron Stig Ramel (1927–2006).

Baron Stig Ramel was appointed executive director of the Nobel Foundation in 1972, a responsibility he was to carry for 20 years. We will meet him again in Chapters 6 and 9. Edelman and Porter were his first recipients of the prize in physiology or medicine. He developed a particular friendship with Edelman and gave an extensive description of him in his biography[14]. Just prior to the section to be cited, Ramel had discussed the remarkable overrepresentation of prize recipients with a Jewish ethnic background with a geographical origin in the ghettoes of the original Eastern Europe, which he referred to as the "original home" of the Nobel Prizes. The citation from Ramel's Swedish text read:

> The natural scientist who has made the strongest impression on me is Gerald Edelman, who received the prize in medicine in 1972 and whom I am glad to count as a personal friend. His parents came to the USA from this original home. Besides the fact that he is one of the leading scientists of his time and according to many is on his way towards a second Nobel Prize for his revolutionary contributions to the field of brain research, he is an expert on French literature and he could have become a professional virtuoso on the violin if he had chosen to continue in the field of music. Gerry is a splendid speaker — and he loves to talk. But he is a speaker (participant in a conversation) who elevates his less gifted conversation partner to his own level. He does not crush them by his knowledge. He enlightens difficult questions with a never-ceasing flow of Jewish stories and parables. At present he has the appearance of an elegant and sophisticated New York citizen. But he could have been a teacher in a Rabbinic school in far away Eastern Europe, had not the ghettos been shattered once upon a time.

Whereas Porter remained true to immunology in his continued work Edelman left the field of immunology and switched to neurosciences. Porter continued his career as professor in Oxford. For some time he was the President of the Royal Society. In one of his speeches in this role he made the frequently-cited statement "There are two kinds of science, applied and as yet not applied." Porter died prematurely in a car accident in 1985.

Edelman's involvement in the neurosciences began in the late 1970s and in 1981 he started a separate institute for this purpose at Rockefeller University. In 1993 this institute was moved to La Jolla first in provisional quarters but then in a newly constructed complex on the campus of The Scripps Research Institute. The new buildings were inaugurated in 1995. Ramel was one of the keynote speakers at the spectacular event and I was privileged to participate.

There was considerable praise for the architecture and of particular interest was the attached auditorium with its great acoustics. This could be appreciated from the unique chamber performance by the Juilliard string quartet from New York, which I among others had the great pleasure to listen to. To Edelman only the best was sufficient. The auditorium has become a favored place for music and performing arts in the La Jolla area.

It has been a very enriching experience for me to interact with Edelman over a number of years[9], in particular since 1997 when I became a visiting scholar at his Neuroscience Institute. At this institute he and his collaborators have pursued many different aspects of the neurosciences aimed at understanding the physiological basis of consciousness. As mentioned by Ramel, discussions with Edelman always mean that one had to stretch one's mind. His broad insights into essentially any subject and remarkable memory made every discussion an adventure.

Characterization of antibodies against an antigen by electrophoresis showed that they had heterogeneous migration properties. Baruj Benacerraf, whom we will meet later, had prepared antibodies against very small chemical groups, so called *haptens*, attached to a carrier structure when used for immunization. In a collaborative study Edelman and his co-workers analyzed the light chains of such anti-hapten antibodies by electrophoresis. This analysis showed that the light chains had a restricted heterogeneity, appearing as 3–5 sharp bands. The migration characteristics of the few bands varied with the nature of the hapten. The conclusion, as given in Edelman's Nobel lecture[13] was that "These experiments showed not only that antibodies of different specificities were structurally different but also that their heterogeneity was limited." This finding had a bearing on the homogeneity of the antibody product of individual immune cells.

In 1977 half a Nobel Prize in physiology or medicine was awarded to Rosalind Yalow. She had developed a highly sensitive technique to measure the concentration of antibodies by use of radioactive isotopes. This prize will be further discussed in Chapter 5.

One Cell — One Antibody

Burnet's clonal selection theory predicted that an immune cell can only produce an antibody with a single specificity, but it took some time before this could be experimentally demonstrated. Electrophoresis analysis of the products of B cells showed a smear of proteins with different mobility. Isolating clones of B cells supported the idea that they had a restricted antibody-producing capacity and tumors originating from this kind of lymphocyte, the myelomas, produced a single protein product carrying some, generally unknown, antibody activity as already referred to.

As also mentioned briefly in the previous chapter the brain is an immunologically privileged site. Under healthy conditions there is only a limited transport of lymphocytes in and out of the brain. This has a consequence for the qualities of a local immune response in the brain. In very rare instances a lethal brain infection by a defective virus may occur many years after regular case of measles. This very uncommon complication essentially has disappeared in the present era of extensive vaccinations. The disease is called subacute sclerosing panencephalitis (SSPE), a name we may leave unexplained in this context. In patients who had this disease a defective virus, for unknown reasons, had managed to persist. Electrophoresis analysis of the antibody-containing fluid in the brain — the cerebrospinal fluid — revealed a different pattern than an analysis of serum from the same patient. The proteins in the gamma globulin region did not represent a smear but showed a restricted heterogeneity and appeared as multiple bands, referred to as *oligoclonal IgG*, oligos — Greek for *few*.

Together with a precious friend and scientific colleague Bodvar Vandvik, professor of neurology in Oslo, I was curious to see the distribution of different virus-specific antibody activities in samples of the bands of oligoclonal IgG from patients with SSPE. We found that antibodies reacting with different virus components were unevenly distributed[15]. This suggested that individual bands might carry different specific antibody activities. On the side it can be noted that we published our data in the *Proceedings of the National Academy of Sciences*, USA, a prestigious journal. If one is not a member of this academy a manuscript to be considered for publication must be submitted by a *bona fide* member. We asked Jan Waldenström, professor of medicine in Malmö in the southern part of Sweden, who was a foreign member of the academy, to consider our manuscript. He graciously agreed to introduce it to the journal. His own pioneering scientific contributions made him particularly suited to do this. He was the discoverer of the disease that came to be named Waldenström's macroglobulinemi, referred to above in the presentation of Gajdusek's studies in Burnet's laboratory. This disease is caused by a special form of myeloma, with the unique characteristics of producing a homogenous population of the large form of antibodies, IgM. The understanding that a clone of immune cells only could produce a single antibody became well consolidated with time

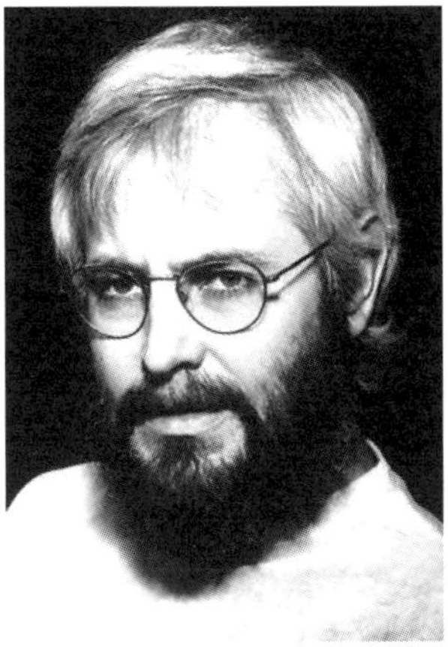 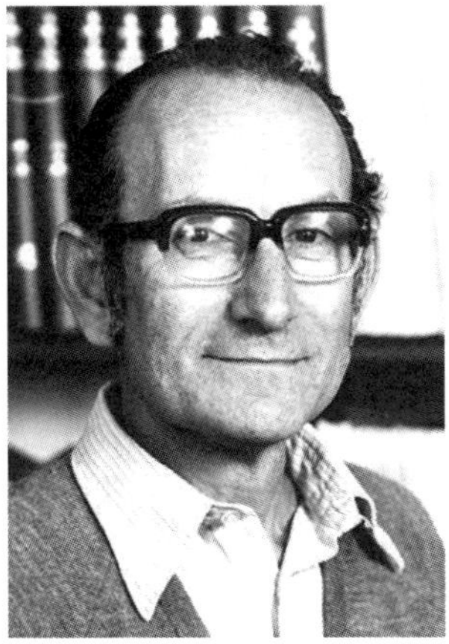

Georges J. F. Köhler (1946–1995) and César Milstein (1927–2002), recipients of the shared 1984 Nobel prize in physiology or medicine. [From *Les Prix Nobel en 1984.*]

but the possibility to take advantage of this for a production of monoclonal antibodies with a predetermined specificity remained a pipe dream — until just a few years later.

In 1975 Georges J. F. Köhler, a visiting scientist at the Medical Research Council, Laboratory of Molecular Biology, Cambridge together with César Milstein, a researcher of Argentinean origin heading the laboratory, published a paper[16] that came to revolutionize the field of immunology and other branches of research using immunological techniques. Mouse myeloma tumor cells, selected to no longer be capable of producing any immunoglobulin of their own, and spleen cells, collected from a mouse immunized with a selected antigen, were fused by a simple procedure using polyethylene glycol. The fused cells were diluted and seeded into wells as single units and provided nourishment so that they could divide to establish a clone. Each clone was found to produce only one kind of antibody with a single specificity. Those that were identified to produce an antibody against an antigen of particular interest, like a certain virus protein, were selected for further characterization. The lines of immortalized cells producing specific antibodies were called *hybridomas.* This technique provided a very important tool to be used in many different fields of research, not the least in our own studies of the antigenic property of building blocks of different viruses.

The introduction of the hybridoma technique was considered so spectacular and revolutionary that it was equal to a discovery and this was recognized by a Nobel Prize in physiology or medicine in 1984. The committee and the Nobel Assembly took the opportunity on this occasion to also recognize Jerne's contributions (p. 81) for several years back. The combined prize motivation for the three scientists became "for theories concerning the specificity in the development and control of the immune system and the discovery of the principle for production of monoclonal antibodies."

Köhler presented the development of the hybridoma technology in his Nobel lecture[17]. He had had his original training with the renowned immunologist Fritz Melchers in Freiburg. After his successful postdoctoral time with Milstein he spent ten years at the world famous Basel Institute for Immunology. Finally he returned in 1984 to Freiburg as Director of the Max Planck Institute of Immunology and Epigenetics. But his golden days in immunology were not to return and he died only 49 years old in 1995 from severe cardiac disease. Milstein, his postdoctoral mentor, had a much longer life. In his Nobel lecture[18] Milstein presented his broad involvements in the field of immunology, of which the development of the hybridoma technique represented only a part — albeit the most spectacular one. The main part of the lecture focused on his work with myeloma proteins and his studies of the genetic origin of antibody diversity, a topic we will shortly return to. Milstein ended his lecture with an acknowledgement, the first paragraph of which deserves to be cited. It read:

> The hybridoma technology was a by-product of basic research. Its success in practical applications is to a large extent the result of unexpected and unpredictable properties of the method. It thus represents another clear-cut example of the enormous practical impact of an investment in research which might not have been considered commercially worthwhile, or of immediate medical relevance. It resulted from esoteric speculations, for curiosity's sake, only motivated by a desire to understand nature. It is to the credit of the Medical Research Council in Britain to have fully appreciated the importance of basic research to advances in medicine. We are delighted to belong to the small, lucky group of those who are at the window-dressing end of the justification for the wisdom of that policy.

Many supplementary remarks might be made to these insightful reflections, but it suffices to note that the hybridoma technology was never patented! Clearly greed — fortunately — is *not* a driving force of high quality science.

One Antigen Selects a Swarm of Antibodies

Köhler began his Nobel lecture in the following way: "A mouse can make ten million different antibodies, each synthesized by its own B-lymphocyte. About 1000 different antibodies are able to recognize one single antigenic determinant." The figures given should not be taken at their face value. No one knows how many millions of antibodies a single kind of mouse can produce and the absolute number is not the essential information. The critical insight is that any kind of antigen can be recognized at least with some degree of precision and that only a very minute fraction of this enormous antibody-producing potential needs to be exploited for example for defence against invading infectious agents. As for the number of antibodies that can react with a certain determinant, this number will also vary depending on the nature of the antigen. Again, it is not essential to know the number as long as there are a single or a few of the antibodies produced that can interfere with some important biological activity of the antigen. This critical antibody activity may be focussed on blocking the replication of a bacterium or of a virus.

Antibodies can be produced against essentially any kind of chemical entity. For simplicity a protein antigen has been chosen for the following discussion. The size of polypeptide chains representing different protein products varies enormously. They may contain a few or several thousand amino acid residues. If the protein contains less than forty residues it is generally referred to as a *peptide*. When the diversity of antibodies produced after immunization with a protein was studied by use of the hybridoma technology it was found that there was an enormous variation in their specificity of reaction. Only rarely did two hybridomas react with exactly the same site — the identical amino acids in the polypeptide chain representing the protein. Some sites of a protein have been found to elicit an antibody production more efficiently than others and such sites were referred to as *epitopes*. Techniques have been developed to characterize the immunodominant epitopes in a protein and to determine the biological importance of antibodies identifying such sites, as for example their capacity to block replication — *neutralize* — the infectious activity of a virus.

Originally it was believed that the capacity of a protein to stimulate the production of specific antibodies was dependent on a proper folding of its polypeptide chain into a complex three-dimensional structure. This has turned out not to be true. Surprisingly it was found that shorter fragments of the chain could function both as immunogens — stimulating production of antibodies — and as antigens — reacting with antibodies produced as a result of a previous immunization in connection with for example an infection with a virus. This understanding made it possible to introduce a technique which permitted an even more refined characterization of antigen-antibody interactions when a protein was involved as antigen. This was the *synthetic peptide technology*. A prerequisite for the use of this technology is that the sequence of the amino acid building blocks, sometimes many hundreds, in the long chain representing the unfolded form of a particular protein is known. For many years this has been generally determined in an indirect way by characterizing the nucleotide sequence of the gene (Ref. 9, Chapter 7) responsible for the production of the protein in the focus of interest. Once the amino acid sequence has been deduced it is possible to produce a selected set of partly overlapping peptides with a length of for example 10–15 amino acids. Such peptides can be used as antigens or even as immunogens, although the latter use generally requires that they are coupled to some neutral carrier to induce antibodies. Using peptides for measuring antibodies, referred to as *site-directed serology*, has a very wide application and the following is just one example. The case to be presented is also an illustration of the global cooperation in science.

In the early 20th century two separate epidemics of HIV infections emerged in Africa. The most familiar and the one responsible for the tragic global situation, with more than 30 million individuals infected with this potentially lethal virus, is the pandemic caused by HIV type 1. This virus has its origin in chimpanzees living in the equatorial central parts of Africa. Surprisingly there is a parallel second epidemic, developing over a similar time span, with a related kind of virus called HIV type 2. This virus has a completely different origin. Its natural host is a kind of Old World Monkey called Sooty Mangabey living in the west of Africa. This type of monkey may carry a generally harmless infection with simian immunodeficiency virus (SIV) as the virus is called in its natural host. Transmission of this virus to man may cause disease. HIV type 2, like HIV type 1, can spread from man to man, but it causes a somewhat less aggressive infection. Infection with one type of HIV does not give a complete blocking of a subsequent infection with the other type, but possibly there might be a mutual influence on the intensity of the disease process. In particular it appears that a primary infection with type 2 might mitigate the subsequent replication of type 1. It therefore became important to distinguish infections with one type of HIV from the other and also to separately identify antibodies against each of the two types of viruses. We approached the latter problem in the following way.

In 1986 I was responsible for a full day AIDS conference in San Francisco and all the luminaries — Robert (Bob) C. Gallo, Luc Montagnier, Jay A. Levy to mention a few — were there. At this time I was familiar with the synthetic peptide technology which we had employed in collaborative experimental work with Richard Lerner, who a year later became president of The Scripps Research Institute in La Jolla. By use of this technique a uniquely antigenic site had been discovered in an HIV-1-specific transmembranous protein. The question was whether the analogy of this epitope could be identified in the corresponding HIV-2 protein. I had just heard through the grapevine that colleagues in Gallo's group very recently had finished the nucleotide sequencing of the genome of SIV, the virus which was the source of HIV-2. Gallo was willing to share with me the new information prior to publication. I took this information from San Francisco to La Jolla and together with Lerner and Elliot Parks, Johnson & Johnson Biotechnology Centre, La Jolla, we searched out a sequence homologous to the one found earlier to be a preferred target for antibodies in the transmembraneous membrane protein of HIV-1. A corresponding site in the homologous HIV-2 protein was found. Two overlapping 15 amino acids long peptides representing this site in each of the two types of viruses were produced and these reagents were carried back to Stockholm, where their capacity to react with sera from patients infected with HIV-1 or HIV-2 were tested. This was carried out in collaboration with Gunnel Biberfeld, a classmate in medical school and a qualified HIV researcher with a broad field experience from work in Africa. The results of testing antibodies in the sera she provided were spectacular. The peptides could categorically distinguish antibodies against the two types of viruses. Within a week a manuscript was prepared and sent off to the journal *Nature*, where it was published[19]. A curious twist of our finding was that the amino acid sequence of a part of one of the peptides used to detect the HIV type 2 antibodies encrypted the West African geographical origin of the virus. The particular sequence of amino acids was alanine-phenylalanine-arginine-glutamine-valine which by the conventional letter code reads AFRQ V!

The Richness of Antibodies Is Created by a Lottery System

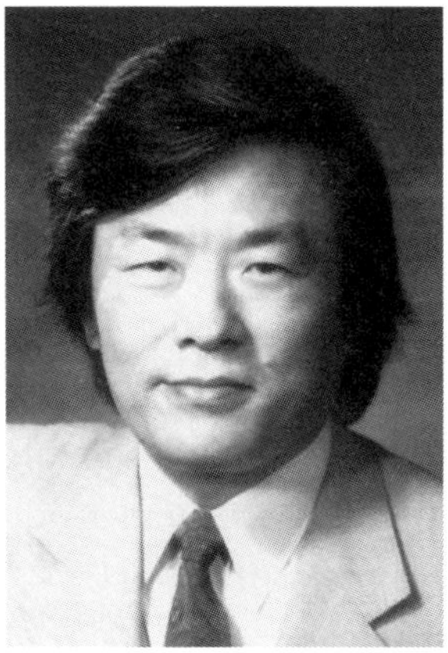

Susumu Tonegawa, recipient of the 1987 Nobel Prize in physiology or medicine in 1987. [From *Les Prix Nobel en 1987*.]

Once techniques had been developed to characterize the structure of genes (Ref. 9, Chapter 7) it became possible to examine the origin of antibody diversity. Studies of this kind were referred to in Milstein's Nobel lecture[18]. This field was pioneered by the Japanese scientist Susumu Tonegawa and the development of his involvements in science is quite enlightening. Like many other Nobel Prize recipients he received inspiration from indirect or direct contacts with other Nobel laureates. Tonegawa's parents wanted him to get a high quality education and eventually he aimed for the Department of Chemistry of the University of Kyoto to which he was admitted in 1959, 20 years old. This was a time when the Japanese nation was highly divided between conservatives accepting the temporary American hegemony and idealistic leftists wanting Japan to manage on its own. When the USA–Japan treaty was prolonged for another ten years, Tonegawa, like many others of his generation, had a feeling of defeat and felt that he had to engage in academic life instead of becoming a chemical engineer, presumably because he thought that this might give him a larger influence on the developments in his home country. By an irony of fate he ended up making his academic career in the USA and also Europe and not in Japan.

Tonegawa became enthusiastic about molecular biology from his reading of François Jacob's and Jacques Monod's publications on the operon theory, the discovery that led to a Nobel Prize in physiology or medicine in 1965. He started his work in Itaru Watanabe's laboratory at the Institute for Virus Research in Kyoto. It did not take long before Watanabe told him that if he was serious about learning molecular biology he should not stay in Kyoto but try his future in the USA. Tonegawa was accepted at the graduate school of the Department of Biology of the University of California at San Diego (UCSD). He learnt molecular biology techniques studying bacteriophages in Masaki Hayashi's laboratory, where he also received his PhD in 1978. After some post-doctoral work in the same laboratory he moved to Renato Dulbecco's laboratory at the Salk Institute, the renowned animal tumor virologist and co-recipient of the 1975 Nobel Prize in physiology or medicine (Ref. 9, Chapter 3). Since he had supported his stay in the US by a Fulbright grant, Tonegawa for visa reasons had to leave the US for two years. This turned out to be a fortunate complication because Dulbecco advised him to go to the Basel Institute of Immunology, headed by Jerne, where he stayed for two years.

The institute offered an intellectually inspiring milieu with many qualified scientists, like Jerne and Köhler. Tonegawa's original idea was to continue his work with the animal tumor virus SV40 (simian virus) that he had started in Dulbecco's laboratory. This did not happen and as he himself said in the introduction to his Nobel lecture[20]. "In the winter of 1971, I found myself surrounded by immunologists in this small town located in the middle of Europe". Thus he became an immunologist. Some enthusiastic colleagues introduced him to the great debate on the genetic origin of antibody diversity. The laboratory work attacking problems in this field advanced rapidly between 1974 and 1981 and to cite Tonegawa again "We all worked hard and had a great deal of fun." In this environment and with the staunch support of Jerne, Tonegawa became the leading scientist in this sub-field of immunology. Invited by Salvadore Luria, the 1969 recipient of a divided Nobel Prize in physiology or medicine (Ref. 9, Chapter 3), he moved back to the US to the Center for Cancer Research at the Massachusetts Institute of Technology (MIT) in Boston in 1981, where he widened his interest in immunology to also take in the genetic basis for the diversity of the recognition structures — the receptors — on T cells.

In 1987 Tonegawa was awarded the Nobel Prize in physiology or medicine. The motivation was "for his discovery of the genetic principle for generation of antibody specificity". In simple terms what he had found was the following.

As progenies of immune cells matured during embryonic differentiation or even during the very early parts of independent life, the part of their genomes responsible for production of future antibody components were modified. Certain gene segments were multiplied and became represented in a variable number of slightly different copies. When an antibody molecule is to be produced a single representative of each one of these homologous copies in each segment combines — in a random way and with imprecise junctions — with fragments representing other segments required for the synthesis of the final chains of immunoglobulins. It is this arrangement that gives the organism a potential to produce hundreds of millions of different antibodies. This "lottery" or "zip code" phenomenon is referred to as *combinatorial diversification*[20].

But the system of antibody generation has one additional level of sophistication. The first contact between a previously unencountered antigen and a pre-existing natural antibody generally has a relatively low fitness. This association, involving an antibody attached to the surface of a cell capable of producing it, sends a signal to the genome of the cell. This signal activates a hypermutation system in the cell and further cell divisions lead to the generation of subclones producing antibodies with variable — sometimes much improved — capacity to bind the specific antigen. This situation represents, in a miniature, evolution in action. The clone of cells that produces the antibodies with the best fit is the one to eventually be expanded the most, leading to an optimization of the immune response. Before leaving the phenomenon of combinatorial diversity it should be emphasized that it is not only used to generate the vast variety of antibodies. It is equally important for the production of T cell receptors endowing them with a corresponding rich diversity, as will be further discussed.

Tonegawa's post-Prize developments of his professional involvements show an interesting similarity to those of Edelman. Both of them left the field of immunology seduced by the field of neurosciences. In their continued work they focussed on the Holy Grail of human brain science, an understanding of our consciousness. Tonegawa became a leader of a Center for Neural Circuit Genetics at MIT but later he eventually returned to Japan to spend part of his time supervising activities at the RIKEN Brain Science Institute outside Tokyo.

Antibodies Cannot Penetrate into Cells

The effect of antibodies is limited to material outside cells or exposed at their surface. They cannot penetrate into their interior environment. This limits their range of activities. They can neutralize the infectivity of virus particles present in body fluids or block the activity of a toxin produced by a bacterium. Under special conditions, when attached to their specific membrane-associated antigen, they can also exert an effect on cells and destroy them. This is achieved by puncturing holes in the membrane by which the cells are enclosed, but this requires the assistance of the complex complement system discovered by Bordet as mentioned in the previous chapter. However the immune system needs additional effective mechanisms to attack and destroy for example virus-infected cells. It is particularly important that an attack can be made *before* a (surface antigen modified) infected cell has started to produce new virus particles. In the not uncommon situation that antibodies do not suffice to bring about an immunological effect of this kind, the other arm of defence, the cell-mediated immunity, needs to be activated. Examples of cell-mediated reactions, given in the previous chapter, were transplant rejection and the tuberculin reaction. The expanded studies of T cells have elucidated very complex relationships as briefly summarized above. Two fundamental principles, which deserve to be recapitulated, are:

(a) The hallmark characteristics of the many different categories of cells that belong to the immune system but do not produce antibodies are that they all have different forms of immunoglobulin (Ig)-like molecules integrated into their outer cell membrane (a superfamily of such membrane structures exist);

(b) All forms of T cells recognize the antigen not as a whole but only after it has been degraded into smaller pieces, a phenomenon that has a central importance for *both* humoral and cell-mediated immune responses.

The antibody production, as already emphasized, is dependent on very complex interactions involving the relevant antigen, antigen-presenting cells, helper T and B cells in cooperation. The antigen-presenting cells take care of the target protein and processes it by breaking it into pieces. Each one of these peptide pieces then become associated with a MHC molecule, an immunoglobulin-like structure at the surface of the T cell. It is this peptide-surface structure complex which eventually is presented to a T cell capable of recognizing the particular peptide antigen, thereby activating it. The T cell can then recognize similar peptides presented by MHC molecules on B cells which have taken them up by binding to the native protein form with their immunoglobulin recepter, and then fragmented them intracellularly. It is only hereafter, upon recognition by the helper T cells, that the B cell can start to produce its specific antibody. The finding of a need for a fragmentation of antigens came as a surprise to the scientists. The use of degraded antigen is also the mechanism used for determining the specificity of other forms of T cells with different functions that will be further discussed below.

The Nobel Assembly and an Influential Secretary

It was in 1979 that the Nobel Assembly took over the responsibility for the decision on Nobel Prize recipients from the faculty of the Karolinska Institute (Ref. 9, Chapter 1). In passing it can be mentioned that at the time of the shift all 65 members of the faculty automatically became members of the assembly. Since the eventual number of members of the assembly had been fixed at 50 it took a long time until, as a result of professors being retired or leaving the Institute for other reasons, the number was reduced to below that level. It was in 1985 that for the first time a new member of the assembly was elected.

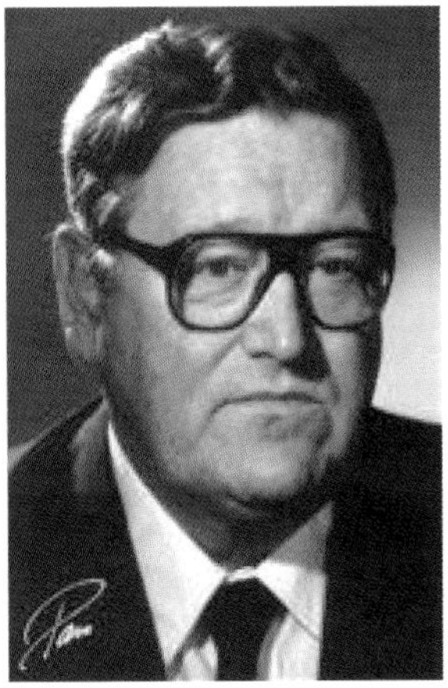

Bengt E. Gustafsson (1916–1986), secretary of the Nobel Committee for physiology or medicine (1966–1978). [Courtesy of the Karolinska Institute.]

Already during the mid-1970s a certain imbalance in the relationship between the committee including its ten adjunct members and the faculty/Nobel Assembly had developed. This problem was caused by the fact that the committee had become relatively dominant in these interactions. It had been led by dynamic and authoritative professors like Börje Uvnäs and the secretariat had developed to become very efficient. When Göran Liljestrand had left the secretariat in 1960 after his exceedingly long term in this position, he was succeeded by Ulf von Euler, mentioned in the previous chapter. In 1966 Bengt Gustafsson, a professor of germ-free animal research, took over the secretariat probably because von Euler's own candidacy for the prize was progressively strengthened. Gustafsson was a very efficient administrator and was often referred to as Mr Medical Science in Sweden at the time. Besides managing and extensively reorganizing the Nobel Committee work, he had the central administrative responsibility for both the Medical Research Council, the major source of Governmental research money at the time, and the Swedish Cancer Society, the main private support for cancer research. In fact I had a career award from the latter society between 1966 and 1972 that gave me free rein to study the immunobiology of adenoviruses, potentially oncogenic viruses, and their structural components.

Gustafsson not only managed the committee and other overriding administrative responsibilities in a skilful way, he also pursued some high profile research of his own requiring very special equipment. He bred mice under conditions that did not allow them any contact with microorganisms — *germ-free animals*. He managed to raise such animals by use of delivery by caesarean section, keeping them in sterile living conditions and feeding them sterilized food. Living under germ-free conditions had many consequences, not the least that the animals were found to have a poorly developed immune system. It deserves to be repeated that we humans are a walking community. We have of the order of a hundred trillion cells in our body, but we have *ten times* more microorganisms localized on our membrane surfaces, like in the gut, on our skin, etc. These organisms have many different functions which have only recently started to become unravelled. One of them is to activate our immune system. The introduction of basic hygienic measures has had a very positive effect on the risk for our exposure to various infectious diseases. This had general positive effects on public health, although there were exceptions like the emergence of polio epidemics during the latter half of the 19th century (Ref. 9, Chapter 5). It has also been argued that excessive hygiene may be a source of an increasing frequency of allergic diseases encountered in modern society. This would be due to a diminution of the original natural stimulation of the immune system.

The absence of microorganisms in the germ-free mice had many consequences, some of which were more curious. Once a new building for Gustafsson's research on germ-free animals at the Karolinska Institute was to be inaugurated and the Swedish King Gustaf VI Adolf had agreed to honour the event by his presence. He was a respected scholar, with a particular knowledge in archaeology, and he was intellectually very curious (Chapter 6). For some reason he had heard that faecal material from germ-free animals had no smell. He therefore inquired about this and Gustafsson could demonstrate to His Majesty that this was true.

An Embarrassed Newly Appointed Secretary

In 1979 the Nobel Committee had decided unanimously to recommend to the Nobel Assembly that a Nobel Prize should be given to Baruj Benacerraf, Jean Dausset and George Snell, the latter already introduced in the previous chapter, for their characterization of surface antigens distinguishing different kinds of cells. Due to very particular circumstances this did not come about. It deserves to be recorded what happened.

In 1979 Gustafsson was succeeded by Jan Lindsten, professor of clinical genetics, and he was to start his 12 years of responsibility by exposure to an unexpected purgatory. The three immunologists selected by the committee for the prize that year were introduced by me during the meeting with the Nobel Assembly at which the final decision should be taken. There was one specialized immunologist in the committee, Peter Perlmann from

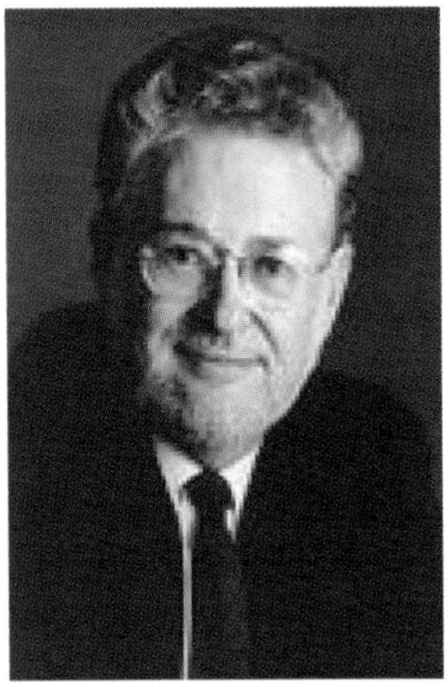

Jan Lindsten, secretary of the Nobel Committee for physiology or medicine (1979–1991). [Courtesy of the Karolinska Institute.]

Stockholm University. His participation in the work exemplified the fact that also scientists not employed at the Karolinska Institute can become adjunct members. The reason I was the spokesperson for the committee most likely was my in-house affiliation. After my enthusiastic presentation of the three immunologists there was a discussion. During this it became clear that the assembly would like to be better informed about the work of the committee and not just be presented with a *fait accompli.* It also wanted to see more prizes in clinical medicine and as an expression of this, Allan M. Cormack and Godfrey N. Hounsfield, pioneers in the development of computer-assisted tomography were proposed as an alternative to the immunologists unanimously recommended by the committee. Cormack and Hounsfield had been thoroughly reviewed by the committee, but they had not been selected for the 1979 prize. Eventually there was a vote with secret ballots. I still remember how I registered each vote as they were announced by the tellers and when they came to the end we had a tie! The chairman, who had the deciding vote in this situation, had selected Cormack and Hounsfield, which thus became the decision of the assembly. Suddenly we also had to take an unprepared decision at the meeting about who should give the laudation speech at the prize ceremony. There was a professor of radiology on the committee, Ulf Rudhe, but this gentleman and humanist declined the responsibility, and eventually we had to call on Torgny Greitz, a professor of neuroradiology. After the meeting we had about an hour until we were to announce the prize at a press conference. All the press releases we had prepared were useless and we did not even have a picture of the unanticipated prize recipients. In some way we managed in an improvised way to prepare a few documents to show to the press. The journalists seemed never to have understood our embarrassing situation and we were actually quite pleased about this. But it was a trying experience and during the coming years there were some adjustments of the interactions between the committee and the assembly.

The Delayed Nobel Prize

The following year the Nobel Prize in physiology or medicine was finally given to Benacerraf, Dausset and Snell "for their discoveries concerning genetically determined structures on the cell surface that regulate immunological reactions". These three scientists had made different contributions to the characterization of membrane surface structures of importance for regulating immune responses. Snell's work with inbred mouse strains was already introduced in the previous chapter. His experimental studies that started by examining immunity to transplanted tumours, progressively came to focus on the critical antigens in normal tissues that decided if a tissue from one inbred mouse strain could be transplanted to another. In painstaking experiments he mapped the diversity of *histocompatibility* genes, from Gr *histos* meaning tissue, abbreviated to H genes. He identified many different H genes, but some of them were found to be much more dominating than others. An example is the H-2 genes — presently referred to as MHC antigens — which Snell characterized in detail.

In the absence of access to inbred humans, Dausset in ingenious studies managed to map the corresponding genes in man. He took advantage of immune reactions that could be identified after blood transfusions. As described in the previous chapter safe blood transfusions can only be made by taking into consideration the blood groups defined by Landsteiner. The red blood cells present a relatively simple surface antigen system, but in the case of other cells in the body, like the nuclei-carrying white blood cells, the system deciding compatibility at transplantation is much more complex. Originally blood transfusions were made without considering the presence of white cells besides the red cells. It is only in recent years that it has been decided to remove white cells from blood to be used for transfusion. This is made for particular reasons, namely to reduce the risk that prions, possibly carried by such cells, would be transmitted (Ref. 9, Chapter 8). When white blood cells were present at transfusion they might elicit an immune reaction in the recipient of the blood, but in practice this did not cause complications.

Dausset characterized the spectrum of such reactions and by this clever approach he could map the genetic diversity in man corresponding to that found by Snell in his studies of the H system in mice[21]. The specific surface antigens on human cells are referred to as HLA from Human Leukocyte Antigens. There are a large number of such antigens, some of them more dominant than others. Mapping of HLA antigens is important in the search for matching

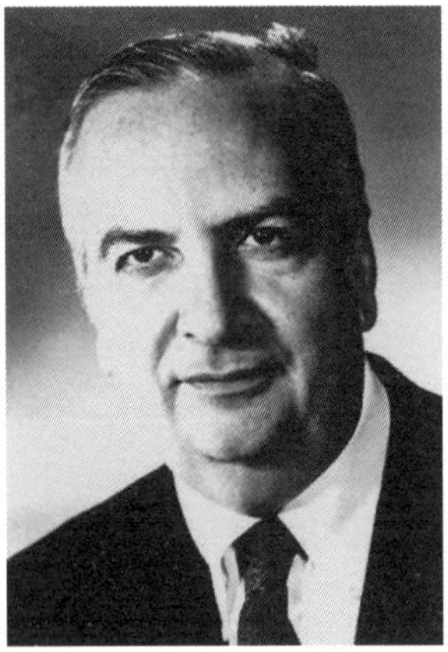
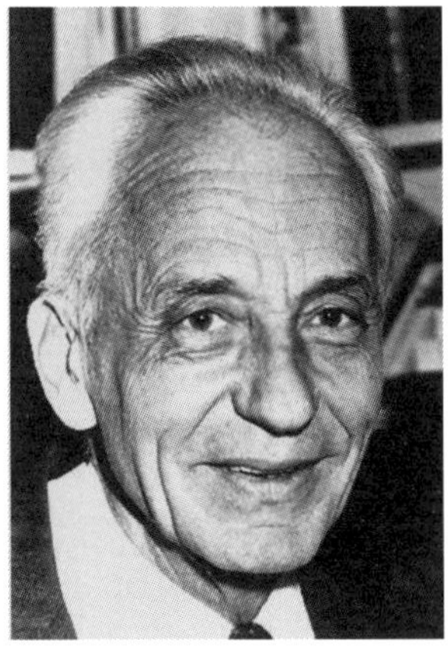

Baruj Benacerraf (1920–2011) and Jean Dausset (1916–2009), recipients of the shared 1980 Nobel Prize in physiology or medicine. [From *Les Prix Nobel en 1980.*]

donors and recipients in transplantation of organs, like kidneys or hearts, and especially of suspended cells like bone marrow, as will be further discussed in the next chapter. Interestingly it has also been found as we shall see that there is a correlation between the occurrences of certain HLA combinations in humans and a propensity to develop particular diseases, not the least those that appear to have an autoimmune background.

Dausset and the third recipient of the divided Nobel Prize, Benacerraf, had very contrasting life experiences. Dausset spent almost his whole life in France except for a year as visiting scientist at Harvard Medical School. His father pioneered rheumatology in France and had by his example a decisive influence on his son's career. Jean Dausset became a haematologist and paediatrician and it was his responsibility for blood transfusion laboratories in Paris that set the stage for his studies. Besides his scientific pursuits his two other interests in life were his family and plastic art.

Benacerraf had a Spanish-Jewish background. Most of his early years were spent in Paris, but when the Second World War broke out, the family moved, first for a year to Venezuela and then to New York to further Benacerraf's education. He had great problems entering medical school in 1942 because of Jewish quota restrictions and had it not been for the contacts of a friend of the family this would not have happened. Benacerraf did well at school and developed a particular interest in immunology partly motivated by his own problems with allergy. He took advice from René Dubos at Rockefeller and John Enders at Harvard Medical School (Ref. 9, Chapter 5) and following their recommendations he started to train with Elvin Kabat at Columbia University

School of Physicians and Surgeons. Kabat was a demanding task-master. In the introduction to his Nobel lecture[22], Benacerraf said the following about him "He taught me immunochemistry and basic immunology, but more importantly, I learned the significance of experimental proof, the need for intellectual honesty and scientific integrity." In the early 1950s Benacerraf for family reasons moved to Paris, but in 1956 the family returned to New York where he was offered a position by Lewis Thomas at New York University School of Medicine. From 1970 he held the chair in pathology at Harvard Medical School.

Benacerraf's contribution was somewhat different than his co-laureates and to a certain extent more in line with the prize motivation given. He mapped genes of importance for the immune response to selected antigens, starting with studies of guinea pigs but then switching to inbred mice. The genes he identified were named Ir genes for immune response. Genetically the Ir genes were located in the region of the genome harbouring the genes directing formation of H2 products, but not in the same loci as those controlling acceptance or rejection of grafts. The Ir genes have their correspondence in the MHC class II genes.

It is now due time to discuss cell-mediated immunity. Dausset's and Snell's contributions belong in this context, but the discovery to be presented in the next section revealed an unanticipated restriction of this kind of immunity.

The Cell-Bound Immunity Has an Unexpected Restriction

Identification of the genetically determined cell surface antigen systems immediately raised the question of what function they may have in the *normal* organism. It is obvious that they are not present in the body to prevent the artificial transplantation of tissues from another individual. They must have some other very central function. With time it has emerged that they are involved in controlling a very elaborate cooperation between cells as they get — or are induced to be — in contact in the complex (multicellular) organism. This can be illustrated by the unexpected finding by Peter C. Doherty and Rolf M. Zinkernagel, which was recognized by the second to last Nobel Prize focusing on the field of immunology (p. 90).

During the mid-1970s Zinkernagel, who is of Swiss origin, went as a junior visiting scientist to the John Curtin School of Medical Research in Canberra to work in Robert V. Blanden's laboratory. Because of shortage of space in this

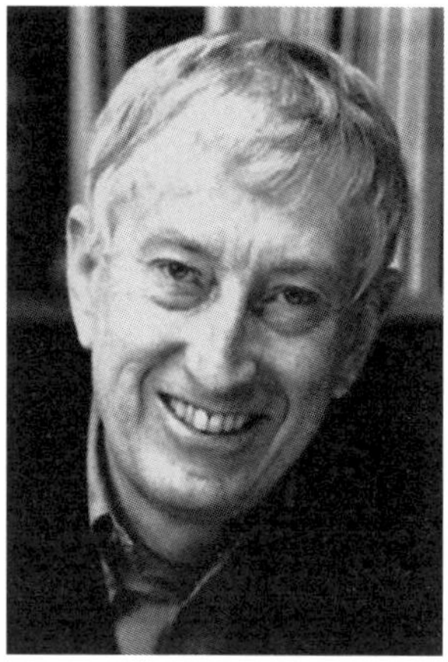 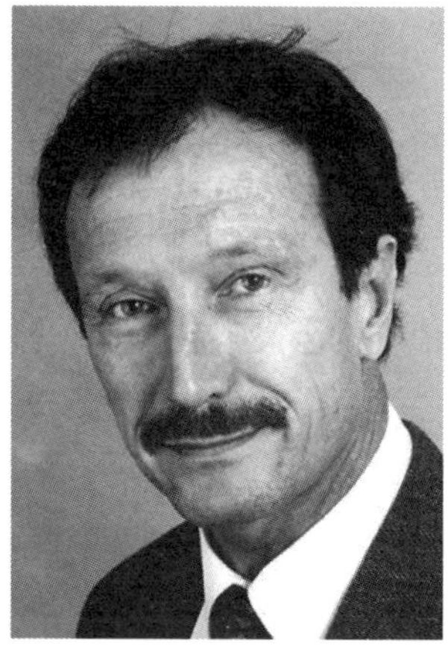

Peter C. Doherty and Rolf M. Zinkernagel, recipients of the shared 1996 Nobel Prize in physiology or medicine. [From *Les Prix Nobel en 1996.*]

laboratory he instead shared a laboratory with Doherty, which led to a very productive scientific collaboration[23]. They decided to evaluate the intensity of a newly developed assay to examine cytotoxic T cells in the LCM virus infection in mice, introduced in Chapter 1. T cells collected from the cerebrospinal fluid of animals with meningitis, an infection of the soft brain membranes, were found to work excellently in an assay using virus-infected mouse cells in cell culture. Doherty and Zinkernagel then decided to test these cells not only in the same strain of mice, but, presumably out of curiosity, also with target cells from a different strain of mice. To their great surprise the virus immune cells were only effective on infected cells of the same mouse strain from which they were derived and not on infected cells of another strain. The studies were extended to include many different mouse strains representing the range of MHC (H) specificities mapped by Snell. What Doherty and Zinkernagel had discovered was the importance of surface antigen characteristics in the interaction between immune cells and the infected target cells, a critical dependence on self and non-self characteristics. The implications of this discovery were profound. Apparently T cells could recognize an antigen only in the context of MHC antigens.

It would take more than another ten years before it was possible to document that the structure of the MHC molecules allowed a unique interaction with fragments of an antigen. Furthermore it had been revealed at that time that the acting MHC was of class I and that the operating cytotoxic cell had CD8 characteristics. By X-ray crystallographic studies it was found that the MHC molecule displayed a groove that could accommodate a fragment of a protein, only about 8–10 amino acids long. Hence it was deduced that a complex protein antigen was digested into fragments in the cell and that hereafter the different fragments associated with the MHC molecule. But the finding by Doherty and Zinkernagel had one more fundamental consequence. There must be a *two signal interaction* between the cytotoxic T cell and the virus-infected target cell. Thus a self-identification was conveyed by the presence of matching MHC molecules in the two interacting cells whereas in parallel a MHC-associated virus peptide gave a non-self signal leading to development of a specific cell-mediated immune response. This principle of double interactions had a general application as already mentioned. The intensity of T cell assisted immune reactions vary between individuals depending on their MHC make-up. This is both a strength and a weakness. Some individuals may be more prone to develop diseases that have an immunological basis, like autoimmune diseases, but on the other hand an individual with some exceptional MHC antigen characteristics may be more resistant to a new, previously unencountered pathogen.

The motivation for the Nobel Prize in physiology or medicine awarded to Doherty and Zinkernagel was "for their discovery concerning the specificity of the cell mediated immune defence". The importance of their discovery can be illustrated by the following excerpt from the laudation speech by Lars Klareskog, professor of rheumatoid diseases, at the prize ceremony[24].

> It became possible to understand that the true function of transplantation antigens is not to provide an obstacle to transplantation. Instead, their function is to bind and present molecules from viruses and other microorganisms to white blood cells in such a way that the white blood cells understand whether they should become aggressive or stay calm. As a consequence it became obvious how each individual, thanks to his/her unique set of transplantation antigens, also carried his/her unique immune system.
>
> It also became possible to understand why evolution has created these large immunological differences between us as individuals within a species. Immunological diversity is advantageous for the single individual as well as for the species. Thus, there will always be some individuals that survive even severe epidemics. In return, individuals carrying a certain variant or transplantation antigens have an increased susceptibility to autoimmune diseases such as rheumatoid arthritis or multiple sclerosis, and this is possibly the price that these individuals pay for the fact that their forefathers survived a severe epidemic.

Innate Immunity Finally Recognized Again

In 2011 another Nobel Prize in physiology or medicine was given in the field of immunology. One half of this prize was given jointly to Bruce A. Beutler and Jules A. Hoffman "for their discoveries concerning the activation of innate immunity". Thus more than one hundred years after the prize to Mechnikov (Chapter 2) in 1908, this important area of first line defence was again recognized. Hoffman and Beutler had completely different approaches to the problems they examined, but in the end they recognized the same critical cell receptor. Hoffman studied how fruit flies can control fungal infections. He found that a so called Toll-like receptor was a critical factor for the rapid host response. Beutler was interested in another kind of problem which is of more direct medical relevance. He studied the imporance of lipopolysaccharides in bacteria causing the life-threatening disease, septic shock. Like Hoffman he independently found that also in vertebrates Toll-like receptors play a special role. Hoffman's and Beutler's findings were quite unexpected since the original discovery of a Toll protein was made in studies of embryological development in fruit flies by Christine Nüsslein-Volhard. A mutation in the Toll gene of the fly had dramatic consequences. The flies looked weird which elicited the spontaneous German exclamation "Das ist ja toll!", equivalent to the English "That's great!". Hereafter this group of genes and their products were referred to as Toll! Names of scientific phenomena or structures sometimes have a strange origin. Nüsslein-Volhard was recognized for her "discoveries concerning the genetic control of early embryonic development" by a shared Nobel Prize in physiology or medicine in 1995.

The other half of the 2011 prize was awarded Ralph Steinman for his identification of a previously unrecognized cell, named the dendritic cell, briefly alluded to above as a critical antigen-presenting cell. His naming of this cell was a way of claiming priority for the discovery. One can say that *to name is to claim*. In many situations one of the major challenges to Nobel committees is to securely identify who has priority to a discovery. The introduction of a new name or concept may be of help in this context, but it need not give a categorical guidance. The proposal of the term prion by Stanley Prusiner (Ref. 9, Chapter 8) was an excellent way of claiming his field of study of atypical infectious agents. Naming in theoretical fields of research may have a particular importance. A mathematician may want to identify that there are different forms of eternity. Thus there is a difference between the endless series 12345... and 33333... in that it is possible to identify a position in the former but not in

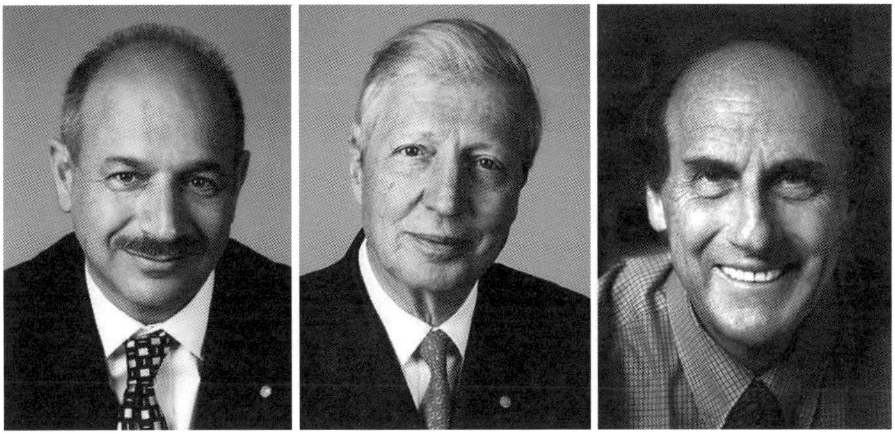

Bruce A. Beutler, Jules A. Hoffmann and Ralph M. Steinman (1943–2011), recipients of the shared 2011 Nobel Prize in physiology or medicine. [From *Les Prix Nobel en 2011.*]

the latter series. It would therefore be possible to give different designations to the two series. On the topic of eternity Woody Allen has provided a very insightful quotation "Eternity is long, in particular towards the end." But let us get back to Steinman.

When the Nobel Assembly at the Karolinska Institute announced on October 3 that Steinman had received the 2011 Nobel Prize in physiology or medicine they very soon recognized a very uncomfortable surprise. It turned out that he had died three days earlier. According to the regulations a Nobel Prize cannot be given posthumously, although a person selected to receive the prize who has died during the time *between* the announcement and the prize ceremony on December 10 will be recognized posthumously. In the case of Steinman the situation was resolved in a pragmatic way. Since apparently no one in the Nobel Committee or the Nobel Assembly was informed about Steinman's impending demise, a fact which in a way emphasized that the focus in the discussions was on the contribution and not on the person to be recognized by the prize, it was decided to make a single exception. Steinman was to be honored by a prize. In a way it was sad that Steinman did not have a premonition of the imminent prize, since it is possible under special conditions to decide one's death day. One of the best examples of this focuses on July 4, 1826. In the morning of that day three persons who had signed the US Declaration of Independence exactly 50 years earlier were still alive. Then one of them, the second president of the country, John Adams died, his last words being "Jefferson survives". However, he was wrong because Thomas Jefferson, its third president, had already expired a few hours earlier.

Steinman's posthumous prize was received by his wife from the hands of His Majesty the Swedish King in a gracious way and as she discreetly withdrew she threw a gentle kiss to her husband in his celestial spheres. It might be speculated that awarding a prize for the discovery of the particular antigen-presenting cell, the dendritic cell, closed the book on possibilities of recognizing the previously discussed pioneers who made the fundamental discoveries of the heterogeneity of lymphocytes, the separate occurrence of B and different kinds of T cells.

Signalling Without Direct Cell Contacts

Before closing this chapter on the Nobel Prizes in physiology or medicine recognizing discoveries in immunology after 1960 a few additional important advances in the field will be mentioned. The consequences of the new insights into the function of the immune system on our interpretation of virus and host interactions will be summarized in the next chapter. As science has advanced we have developed an ever expanding understanding of the complexity of the immune system and its relevance to interactions with other physiological functions in our bodies. Two different large and growing areas of development can be distingushed. One concerns the multitude of cell-to-cell interactions involving many kinds of differentiated cells as already repeatedly alluded to, and the other, the various kinds of signalling between cells by soluble substances. It is the orchestration of signals by direct contacts between cells and on distance that may eventually lead to an effective defence against an invading pathogen.

The network of mechanisms of defence thus also includes many soluble components carrying non-adaptable signals working inside or in particular in-between cells. The complex multi-component complement system assists the antibodies in their attack on viruses and cellular pathogens, as was already mentioned. Other soluble factors are the corticosteroids, the hormones produced by the adrenal gland, under the overriding control of the pituitary gland. Recognition of these hormones and the discovery that they were immunosuppressant and could be used for treatment of the autoimmune disease rheumatoid arthritis was the basis of the 1950 Nobel Prize in physiology or medicine to Edward C. Kendall, Tadeus Reichstein and Philip S. Hench (Ref. 9, Chapter 6). But the orchestra of immune defence functions is even richer in its instrumentation.

There exist representatives of another kind of soluble signal substances, collectively originally referred to as *lymphokines*, but presently instead *cytokines*. Some of these carry signals from cells involved in innate immune responses to those responsible for the adaptive responses. The two defence systems are interconnected. The cytokines are divided into two main categories, the *interferons* and the *interleukins*. A substance called interferon had already been discovered in 1957 by Alick Isaacs, a British virologist, and his Swiss colleague Jean Lindemann. The substance was given its name because in could *interfere* with the replication of viruses. Some of Isaac's original work on interferon was performed in Burnet's laboratory in Melbourne. The substance was discovered to be produced by virus-infected cells and it was interpreted to represent a natural immune defence mechanism against this kind of infectious agent. For a considerable time it was hoped that interferon could be developed as a general remedy for virus infections. Unfortunately this promise has not held up.

Today three kinds of interferon have been identified — alpha, beta and gamma. The latter kind is produced by a subset of helper T cells when they become activated. Thus there is a coordination of a specific cell-mediated response against the virus-infected cell and a suppression of the virus replication by the effect of gamma interferon produced by the activated T cell. The alpha and beta interferons can be produced by a multitude of different cells, like connective tissue cells. These interferons do not only interfere with replication of viruses but in addition they are involved in certain regulations of immune responses. Their practical use has been found to be somewhat limited, but they can suppress certain chronic virus diseases, like hepatitis B virus infections, and mitigate certain diseases of presumed autoimmune origin, like multiple sclerosis.

Interleukins, from Lat. *inter*, between, and *leukos*, white, are soluble small substances that allow communication between white blood cells. They appear in many different forms. To date about 20 numbered interleukins have been described. These different molecules serve many different functions in T cell signalling and their possible use for treatment of different diseases is currently explored. The first T cell growth factor was discovered by Gallo and collaborators in 1976. It was later named interleukin 2. By use of this growth factor it was possible to maintain special populations of white blood cells in culture in the laboratory and this in turn allowed the isolation of the first human retroviruses. Such viruses occur in many forms and we see many traces of them in our hereditary material as will be

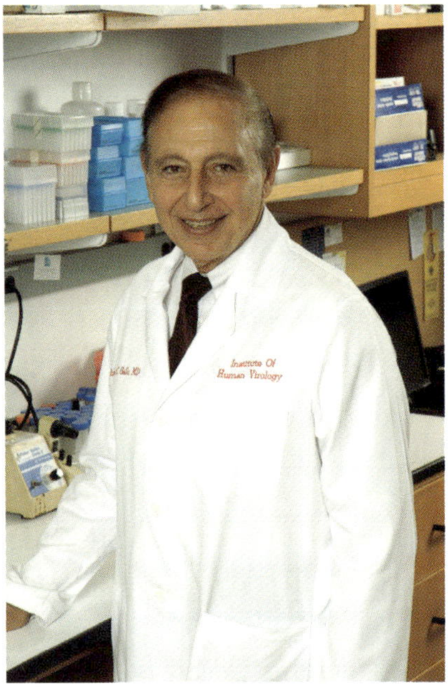

Robert C. Gallo. [Courtesy of the Institute of Human Virology, Baltimore, MD.]

further discussed in Chapter 4.

Two human retroviruses were identified by Gallo and colleagues. They were named human T-cell leukaemia viruses — HTLV — types 1 and 2. If these viruses had been the cause of disease in man with a qualitatively and quantitatively larger impact, Gallo would have received a Nobel Prize in physiology or medicine, but he only got very close to gaining such recognition. It was in his laboratory that Françoise Barré-Sinoussi received training in techniques of isolation of human retroviruses using human lymphocytes stimulated by interleukin 2. Back in Luc Montagnier's laboratory in Paris, she could recover a virus from patients with AIDS, recognized by the divided Nobel Prize in physiology or medicine to the two of them in 2008. Gallo in parallel experiments also isolated viruses from such patients, but originally misjudged their nature and referred to them as HTLV 3. It was soon found that the newly identified agents were representatives of a different genus of retroviruses, which was named Lentivirus, from Lat. *lentus*, slow. Gallo's group pioneered the development of a blood test that could be practically used to identify antibodies in patients and in potential blood donors. Priority issues and rivalry is a recurrent theme in the scientific enterprise. Extended aspects on this theme will be presented and possible means to resolve challenging issues will be further discussed in Chapter 9.

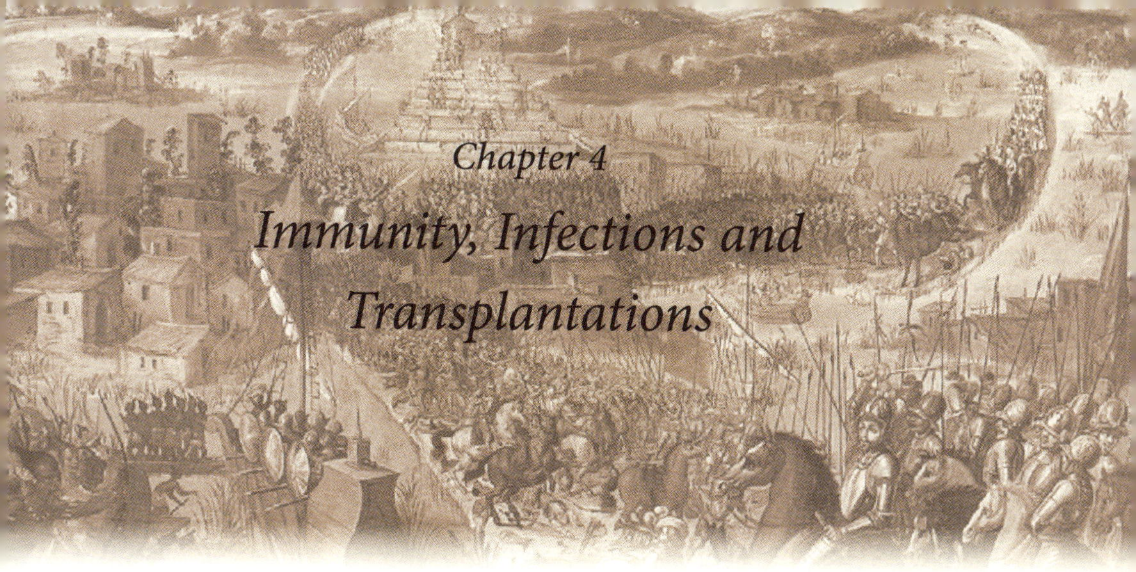

Chapter 4
Immunity, Infections and Transplantations

ON EVOLUTION
BALANCE BETWEEN HOST AND AGENT
SURVIVAL OF BOTH

As should have become apparent by this stage the orchestration of our immune defence is highly complex. In addition its qualitative and quantitative efficacy varies between individuals. Some of us are more susceptible to infections than others and sometimes this pertains to a particular kind of infectious agent. This range of susceptibility among individuals to a certain epidemic disease has served human beings as a species well throughout history. There have always been some survivors even of very aggressive pandemic diseases. Concomitant evolution of newly introduced infectious agents and man has been critical in determining the degree of resistance to such agents in modern human beings. However, in our present day society the situation of interaction between infectious agents and humans has changed. There are several reasons for this. The increased level of hygiene has reduced the circulation of harmful pathogens. The improved state of nutrition contributes to an effective mobilization of immune defence mechanisms. Advances in biomedical sciences have led to the successful development of a number of effective drugs that can prevent the replication of many infectious agents, in particular bacteria, but to some extent also viruses. Finally, the introduction of a number of potent vaccines has allowed us to acquire immunity even without ever having to encounter the disease-causing agent. As a consequence the panorama of infectious diseases has been dramatically changed with time.

Still today the global representation of infectious diseases may change by the introduction of new human pathogens, something the recently emerging HIV pandemic has reminded us of. It should also be added that there are societal changes — urbanization and steadily increasing international travel — favoring contacts between humans in the present day global society that facilitate the spread of infectious agents. At the present time, in spite of all progress, trivial infections like the common cold and other respiratory infections remain responsible for about half of all absenteeism from school and work.

The delicate balance of the immune system is sometimes upset. This can be due to acquired dysfunctions or to inherited genetic defects. The reduced exposure to antigens in our modern hygienic, industrialized society may be one factor contributing to an increased frequency of *hypersensitivity conditions*, the propensity to develop allergic reactions. The altered exposure to particular environmental factors might lead to imbalance of the evolutionary refined self-excluding mechanisms, resulting in reactions with the normal tissues of the host, the *autoimmune diseases*. Burnet prioritized research on autoimmune diseases during his last active period of experimentation and many have followed in his footsteps. The advances in our understanding of immunological phenomena have started to provide new means of managing these important groups of diseases. Another important area besides hypersensitivity and autoimmunity concerns the capacity of the immune system to detect cells with altered and potentially dangerous growth characteristics. The role of this *immune surveillance* in protecting us against cancers will be alluded to briefly at the end of this chapter, but it is clearly a very important field of research, offering hope that new approaches to managing this often life-threatening form of disease might be found.

In the clinical procedure of transplanting foreign tissue the immune system needs to be actively suppressed, as will be discussed in the latter part of this chapter. With time it has become possible to optimize the immunosuppressive techniques used to secure the survival of the graft without causing too harmful activations of quietly persisting virus infections or the development of other complications.

Inherited and Acquired Immune Defects

Because of the complexity of the immune system there are many alternative possibilities for the emergence of genetically defined defects. Such defects may involve many arms of the immune system, the humoral and the cell-mediated defence mechanisms as well as receptors and signalling factors, including those engaged in the mechanisms of the innate system. Sometimes the consequences of a particular genetic change defined by modern time technology can give us insights into additional functional features of the complex immune system. Molecular medicine is a rapidly developing field (Chapter 8) and specific defects in genes may be correlated to molecularly defined functional alterations in known or previously unknown products

There is a rare X-chromosome-linked lack of capacity to generate mature B cells. Because of its genetic association with the X chromosome it is more common in boys than in girls. This *X-linked agammaglobulinemia* was discovered in 1952 and is called Burton's syndrome after its discoverer. The lack of B cells leads to the absence of production of any kind of immunoglobulin and hence the patients are prone to develop serious or potentially fatal infections. The use of antibiotic drugs is critical in managing these infections.

There are also a number of other conditions which cause defects with low or no immunoglobulin production — hypogammaglobulinemia and agammaglobulinemia. They are collectively referred to as *common variable immunodeficiency*. This kind of disease may develop at different ages and both genetic and environmental factors are of importance for its development. One way of helping patients with defects in immunoglobulin production to temporarily control the various infectious agents to which they may be exposed is by injection of pooled immunoglobulin prepared from healthy individuals. The antibodies present in such preparations may substitute for those that these individuals lack. The protective effect only lasts for a limited time, because of the progressive breakdown of the transferred immunoglobulin.

Unsurprisingly genetically determined T cell immunodeficiency diseases also occur in many different forms. They become apparent early after birth and are life-threatening. Two examples will be mentioned. In 1968 the pediatric endocrinologist Angelo DiGeorge described a very complicated syndrome that came to carry his name. It was demonstrated in further studies to be due to the absence of a small segment of chromosome 22. There are multiple symptoms in patients with this syndrome including birth defects, such as congenital heart disease, defects in the palate and differences in facial features, as well as mental disturbances and accentuated susceptibility to infections. There is no cure for this disease. The treatments given aim at alleviating the symptoms. Attempts have been made to transplant thymus tissue in cases when this is absent. The other condition to be mentioned is the very rare disease *severe combined immunodeficiency (SCID)*. This is the most serious of all forms of immunodeficiency, since both B and T cell functions are impaired. It leads to an early death if no interventions are made. The patients need to be prevented from contacts with any infectious agents and are therefore referred to as "bubble children" because of the enclosure used to protect them. The disease is treated by bone marrow transplantation early in life, preferably from a matched donor. In the year 2000 the first attempts to use gene therapy were initiated. Effective immune functions were successfully acquired by the ten patients included in the trial. Regrettably four of them later developed leukaemia. This was demonstrated to be due to triggering of a cancer-forming gene, an *oncogene*, by the transferred gene construct. Attempts are now made to develop a better gene construct which is devoid of such harmful consequences. The deeper the insight into fundamental molecular genetic mechanisms, the more advanced and refined the possible means for interventions will become.

Personal Experiences of Major Health Challenges and Engagement in Research

Sometimes defects of a particular component of the immune defence system may allow an uncontrolled spread of a certain bacterium or some other infectious agent. The spread may be localized and less harmful, but in more severe cases the agent spreads to different parts of the body via infected blood, a *sepsis*. Because of access to antibiotics for more than 50 years we have become much less aware of what a life-threatening situation uncontrolled bacterial infections once represented. However even today there occur particular defects in critical components involved in for example the innate immune system or the complement fixation system that may make certain young individuals highly vulnerable to a sepsis. They may not manage bacteriocidal killing of an invading, generally harmless bacterium like for example *Neisseria meningitis*. This bacterium may spread to cause a severe infection of the soft membrane covering the brain leading to meningitis and also to attack many other organs in the body. The infection develops rapidly and may cause the death of young children mostly teenage boys within hours or a few days.

My wife and I have a personal experience of such a threatening disease. When our oldest son Jacob was two months short of becoming 18 years old, he developed a serious infection leading to a condition of shock in a little more than a day and a night. We were very fortunate in being able to identify the rapid progress of the disease and at the last minute got him by ambulance to the nearby hospital emergency care unit. After one week unconscious in a respirator and being treated with very high doses of antibiotics, he withdrew the foot that was already placed on the other side. His first question when he woke up was "Varför?" — why. It was of course a question reflecting his confused emotions, but on the factual side the background to his severe disease was never identified. It might have been a specific immunological dysfunction — possibly a defect in one of the toll-like receptors of the innate immune system, mentioned in the previous chapter — that could explain why Jacob, among thousands of young people, harmlessly infected by a bacterium that only in rare cases will cause meningitis, would develop this life-threatening disease. It was later demonstrated that he had been infected by a type B meningococcal bacterium. For a number of years a vaccine protecting against the two other types, A and C, of this bacterium has been available, but none against type B. Fortunately developments are now under way that in the future will also allow the production of a vaccine also against type B. Craig Venter and his collaborators characterized the complete nucleotide sequence of the genome of this kind of bacterium in the late 1990s and this knowledge has now been used to generate a new kind of vaccine. A vaccine protecting against meningococcal type B infections was recently licensed for use in Europe.

A severe illness in the immediate family or in a circle of close friends might serve as a stimulus to engagement in biomedical research, in general or focussed on a particular disease. When I see our three oldest grandchildren Heimir, Smàri and Sindri — they have Icelandic names because their Viking mother comes from that country — it often passes through my mind that they would never have been born had Jacob's disease taken another turn. However, it was not exposure to disease in the immediate family surroundings that motivated me to study medicine and later to become a scientist. More likely it was my situation as a minister's son growing up in an environment with a natural emphasis on the responsibility of us humans to help other people combined with a certain proclivity for learning in natural science disciplines that decided my choice. At the age of seven I spent close to a month in a hospital after a double-sided excavation of the mastoid process of the bone behind my ears, performed to facilitate the healing of my severe otitis. Antibiotics had not as yet become available. It was the only time of my life when I could breathe through my ears and overall I found the hospital atmosphere to be positively managed by engaged people. This experience might have been an early encouragement of my future wish to become a physician. After a few years at medical school

I entered the field of virology simply out of curiosity. The stimulus to do this came from Gard's lectures in the field, the impressive early advancement of which was presented in Chapter 1. Although it does not apply to me it still remains to answer the question to what extent scientists engaged in improving the conditions for health have become motivated to do this by exposure to life's vicissitudes, like illnesses, personally or in their neighborhood.

In the previous chapter it was described how Benacerraf became interested in immunological studies because of his own problem with asthma. Gertrud B. Elion, whom we will meet later in this chapter, was motivated to get involved in the development of drugs when she saw her grandfather die of cancer. Gallo has in personal contacts frequently returned to the fact that his original motivation for studying human tumor viruses was his devastating experience of following the course of his sister's leukaemia which eventually lead to her death. Many additional examples could easily have been given, but it should suffice to note that involvement in biomedical science provides unique opportunities to do good to other human beings and to sublimate traumatic medical events afflicting one's nearest and dearest.

The developments in human health during the last hundred years are extraordinary and we can anticipate equally important developments for the coming centennial, not least in the field of immunology. The Nobel Committee at the Karolinska Institute and the Nobel Assembly will have a difficult task prioritizing which single discovery or possibly two separate discoveries, among the many hundred proposed, that each year should be recognized by the prize in physiology or medicine.

The Evolutionary Interplay of Viruses and Their Hosts

Our elaborate immune system has primarily evolved to protect us against various forms of infectious agents, be they viruses or bacteria. Because of my background as a virologist some particular reflections on evolutionary interactions of viruses and man will be given as examples in the following. One important question concerns how the advancing knowledge about the elaborate mechanisms of establishing immunity in an organism has influenced our understanding of different kinds of virus infections in humans. This of course is a very large subject to discuss and only some selected issues will be considered. A particular emphasis will be given to situations when viruses specifically attack certain populations of cells of the immune system possibly even abrogating or enhancing selected distinct functions they carry. It was a central theme in Burnet's biological philosophizing on virus to view it as an organism filling its ecological space by evolutionary adaptations. However since his time so much more has been learnt.

General Remarks

Burnet has taught us that in the examination of the interaction between a cellular parasite and a host, like us humans, the possibilities for survival of both parties need to be considered. What a virus ideally would wish to do would be to find a way to effectively enter the host and replicate, preferably without causing too severe disease. Hereafter the task would be to exit in a way that effectively provides an opportunity to spread to another susceptible host in the immediate surrounding. The challenges to a virus have changed dramatically since the time when humans advanced from living as hunters-gatherers to the formation of settled civilizations as we shall see. In the latter case it is easier to secure transmission to another human being, whereas in the former case the virus needs to have an interaction with its host allowing a long duration. This leads to a categorization into *acute* and *persistent infections*. A further subdivision can be made into *local* and *systemic infections*. Local infections involve superficial parts — the inside or outside — of the body, predominantly mucosal epithelial membranes but occasionally also skin. A typical case of acute local infection is the common cold. Nasal secretions are highly contagious. An acute systemic infection involves not only the tissue(s) at the port of entry of the virus but also many additional organs, exemplified by the disease of measles. Most persistent infections are systemic, with spread of the virus in the body by blood or by nerves. Not infrequently the virus is carried around by circulating lymphocytes.

The viruses have found many different ways of hiding in a slowly replicating or dormant form, as we shall see. A local persistence is also occasionally encountered, as in the case of common warts. The time between infection with a virus and appearance of the first symptoms, the *incubation time*, varies extensively. It ranges from a few days in the case of acute local infections in the respiratory or enteric tract to a few weeks for example in what used to be common childhood diseases such as measles, mumps and rubella. In other virus infections like hepatitis the incubation time may even extend to a few months.

Once an acute infection has been established in an epidemic form among humans it will spread continuously from one infected individual to another susceptible individual. After an incubation period acute symptoms develop from mucosal membranes at the portal of entry or from other parts of the body to which the virus has spread insidiously over some time. The virus can then disseminate by different exit routes to other susceptible individuals in the environment. The mobilization of different arms of the immune system eventually eliminates all the virus from the body, which is quite an impressive feat considering the presence of millions and millions of infectious particles at the height of infection. The individual who has recovered from the infection retains immunity against future infections with the same agent, provided that it, in all essentials, retains the characteristics of its dominating antigen(s).

In the history of human beings the acute infections are recent companions of the developing civilizations. This is due to the fact that they require a sizable population for their transmission and survival. They are *community dependent.* Modern man migrated out of Africa about sixty thousand years ago and started to spread over the different continents[1,2] living as hunters-gatherers and travelling widely. The general flow of migration was from Africa to the Middle East and further on to Europe — Central and Southern Asia — East Asia - Oceania and finally to the Americas. Amazingly there were certain groups of humans who managed as early as ten thousand years after the exodus to reach Australia, presumably travelling as beachcombers. They became the forefathers of the aborigines of that continent. The final step from East Asia to the Americas across the Behring Strait, using temporary land connections between the two continents, most likely occurred some fifteen to twenty thousand years ago. It has become possible to map these historic migrations of man by studies of the individual genomes of representatives of different groups of people all around the world.

It took time for settled civilizations, based on cultivation of soil and raising of livestock, to develop. This occurred in three major regions of the world. Among those three, the most well known and most extensively researched is the Fertile Crescent, the part of Western Asia including Mesopotamia and the Levant[3]. These civilizations were based on the development of the four kinds of cultivable edible grains — wheat, oats, barley and later rye — from their four parental wild grasses. In parallel, advanced civilizations also developed in Eastern Asia, present day China, with rice as a very critical staple food.

A long time later similar advanced settled civilizations also emerged in the Central and South America, the original home of maize and potatoes. It was in these three centers of settled civilizations that a variable separate range of epidemics of acute virus infections first emerged, originally only a few thousand years ago. The origin of what became human viruses in many cases most likely were infections in herd animals. This applies to all kinds of acute human infections; common cold, enteric infections, childhood diseases like measles and mumps, etc. The emergence of the epidemics occurred when the populations had expanded to be large enough to secure continuous access to previously uninfected (non-immune) individuals allowing the chain of infections by the virus in man to remain unbroken. If this chain was broken the virus disappeared. It could not survive outside its host. A highly contagious virus, like the one causing measles, needs about 300,000 people living together to allow continuous spread from man to man. The population of Iceland has been found not to be large enough to sustain ongoing epidemics of measles. The powerful demographic changes during the last century — rapid increase in the global population, progressively increased urban living and rapidly developing global movement of humans — all favor the dissemination of acute infections. Fortunately this kind of disease is the one most effectively managed by preventive health care, by vaccination, a procedure efficiently developed and applied by modern civilization.

The acute infections in man originally came from animals, as mentioned. For example the virus that came to cause measles most likely originated in cattle. Such a transfer of a virus from animals to man is an event that can take place at the present time and will occur in the future. However it is not easy for an animal virus, challenging man for the first time, to display an adaptation allowing it to manage an ongoing spread of acute infections among individuals of this species. This generally requires that a new balance in the virus-host interaction is established. Recently a never previously encountered corona virus — the name derives from the radiating projections on the virus particle — causing SARS was identified as already mentioned in Chapter 1. The source of the virus was the Chinese bushcat, probably infected by a virus carried by bats. It caused a severe disease in man sometimes with a fatal outcome. Fortunately this serious infection which started to spread over the globe could be eliminated by appropriate epidemiological interventions. The virus did not manage to establish a kind of relation to its host that allowed survival for the future under the conditions of modern human civilizations.

The seriousness of an infectious disease transmitted from animals to man is dependent on many factors, both properties of the agent and the capacity of the immune system of its new host to contain its replication. There are a number of severe epidemics afflicting humans that have changed the course of the development of civilizations and influenced the outcome of many wars[4], but they have only been recorded since the description by Thucydides of a plague, most likely of bacterial origin, in Athens in 430 BCE. Man has always reflected on severe epidemics both from the perspective of their origin and spread and also in a religious perspective about their possible importance as a punishment of individuals and of mankind. The infliction of evils by the Gods — the theodicy problem — has been a subject of intense discussions by philosophers through the ages. When reflecting on this problem it might be noted that the need for a balance in ecological consequences of infectious agents attacking man historically from one perspective may be seen to represent a blessing in disguise. It is a disadvantage for the survival of a certain infectious agent if it causes a too severe disease. It needs to become less evil.

It might be that at an early stage in the settled human civilization the first transmission of an animal virus to man may have caused a severe disease. However, with time, as in the case of myxomatosis virus and rabbits discussed in Chapter 1, there has been a selection of an agent giving a relatively milder disease and for hosts that have a better capacity to resist the infection. Individuals that show an increased resistance are those that have been fortunate enough to have been endowed with a relatively better capacity to use the different arms of the immune system and possibly have other inherited qualities that improve their capacity to fence off the specific infection in question.

Interdependent evolution — *coevolution* — of an infectious agent newly introduced to man and its recent host is a very important phenomenon in the history of human civilizations. Such a coevolution of fortuitously introduced new infectious agents and man must have occurred independently in the three centers of human settled civilizations. Two of them, the ones in Western Asia/Europe and in Eastern Asia were connected by a land mass and exchanges of newly emerging infections were facilitated. The historically relatively recent connection of Venice and Xian, a city that more recently has become renowned for its "underground" army of terracotta soldiers, by the Silk Road is an illustration of such contacts between the Occident and Orient. However, the situation was different for settled civilizations in the Americas, like the Incas in present day Peru. There was no connection by land to Europe and when the Europeans developed sea travel[5] dramatic things happened because of the transfer of infectious agents.

Following Christopher Columbus' first contact there was Hernando Cortez and Francisco Pizarro's conquest of present day Mexico and Peru. For example when Pizarro with his 168 men and 27 horses could defeat a population of more than ten million Incas this was only in part due to technical advantages — weapons, armor and horses. The vulnerability of the indigenous Indians to infectious diseases was a much more important factor. Smallpox caused the first devastating epidemic, killing perhaps one third of the Indian population. It was very soon to be followed by measles and several other diseases, which further severely decimated the Indian population. These viruses, with which the Europeans and their ancestors had coevolved to build up a certain degree of resistance, caused very serious diseases in the Indians. They had never before been exposed to these agents. The wipe-out of the Indian populations was of genocidal proportions. Never before had there been a comparable demographic catastrophe in the history of man[6]. The conquistadores may have carried syphilis with them back to Europe, a minor revenge for the Indians. A final era of mixing of all human populations — *homogenocene* — that continues in an ever more intensified way into our present time had been initiated.

There are many different mechanisms that may allow a host, like humans, to show various levels of resistance to a certain virus infection. One possibility relates to the existence of receptor(s) used by the virus to enter the cell (p. 12). Just to give one example it can be mentioned that HIV in order to attach to cells needs two receptors, called CD4 and CCR5. The former is the critical surface structure on T helper cells as described in the previous chapter. CCR5 normally serves as a receptor for humoral factors also involved in inflammatory reactions. However it seems to be relatively less essential and there are individuals that are genetically incapable of producing it. They are resistant to infection by HIV! Individuals with such a resistance would become enriched through consecutive generations in a hypothetical situation of an uncontrollable global epidemic spread of HIV.

Tuning the highly complex immune system as a result of spontaneous genetic changes combined with selection has occurred repeatedly throughout human history. Exposure to new infectious agents has been one important source of selection of progressive modifications of the human genome from the time of our migration out of Africa till today. Two other sources of similar progressive changes of our genomes by selective environmental forces are adaptations to new climatic conditions — the divergence into different ethnic groups; one consequence being that most of us have lost the dark pigment produced by our ancestors — and the other, adaptation to ingestion of new kinds of valuable food materials, like milk. There is one more important factor influencing how the genetic make-up — the hereditary palimpsest — of modern man has evolved. That is powerful natural disasters — like major volcanic eruptions causing climate change and tsunamis — which have randomly wiped out larger fractions of humans during their extra-African odysseys. They have caused genetic "bottleneck" effects.

Certain Viruses Can Evade an Immune Response

The effective immunity following an acute virus infection can be circumvented in two different ways. One way is the evolution of a cascade of different serotypes of the same kind of virus. Rhinoviruses, the agents causing the common cold, provide an example of this. Although individually antigenically stable, the existence of a multitude of types allows the occurrence of repeated yearly infections throughout the lifetime of an individual. Development of a vaccine is essentially impossible because of the rich diversity of types. The best hope is for development of effective antivirals, but so far this has not been a success, as discussed in Chapter 1. In this context it might be mentioned that the term "common cold" is a misnomer. The first symptom of a superficial upper respiratory infection is a contraction of the blood vessels in the periphery of the body. This leads to the patient feeling that his feet or hands are cold, which however is an *effect* and not a *cause* of the infection.

The other way to secure the opportunity for repeated infections with the same agent is to vary its dominating antigenic structures, as in the case of influenza virus — the antigenic drift and shift already mentioned in Chapter 1. Because of these continuous changes the composition of influenza vaccines has to be updated every new season. One may find it surprising that not many other viruses besides those causing influenza and AIDS, to be further discussed below, have acquired the capacity for antigenic variability. One possible explanation might be that the relatively simple constructs of components of viruses imply a close connection between structure and function. Possibly therefore many viruses with modified surface structures might not survive because such changes concomitantly would have negative effects on functions critical for the replication of the virus.

As we shall see it is mostly persistent virus infection which may cause impairments of different functions of the immune system, but there are also some viruses causing acute infections which may lead to a general alteration of the capacity for immune responses. One example is measles virus. An infection with this virus leads to a suppression of cell-mediated immune functions as documented for a long time by a temporary loss of the cutaneous delayed tuberculin reaction. This change of immune reactivity is the explanation for the increased risks of development of other secondary infections in the trail of a full-blown measles disease.

In 1941 an Australian physician and ophthalmologist Norman M. Gregg made the important observation of a temporary occurrence of an increased number of children born with eye changes — congenital cataract. He made the shrewd correlation of this increased occurrence of congenital disease and a recent epidemic of rubella. It was then learned that rubella, generally viewed as a relatively mild childhood disease, could cause severe damage to the developing foetus if a pregnant mother contracted the disease during the first trimester of a pregnancy. Several organs of the foetus could be damaged. This serious complication was the reason for the development and use of a vaccine preventing the disease. Thus the rubella vaccine to a major extent is used to protect a third party, the developing foetus. At present there are efforts underway to achieve a global use of the vaccine with the aim of facilitating a general prevention of this form of congenital disease. Other viruses too can have serious effects on the developing foetus. The rapidly dividing cells of organs being developed and in particular the immunological immaturity of the foetus may contribute to favorable conditions for virus replication. However it is not an efficient means for the virus to survive in nature. Only if there were to be a continuous production of virus allowing spread of infection after birth of the child would it be of survival value to the virus, but this normally is not the case.

Certain spontaneous immune defects of the kind mentioned above may predispose to developing persistent infections with viruses that normally only give acute infection. One example is patients with agammaglobulinemia who can become persistently infected with for example poliovirus. Instead of the normal self-limiting infection these immunodeficient patients can excrete the virus for months and even years. Potentially this might represent a problem in connection with the attempts to eradicate the disease by vaccination (see below), but in the practical situation it has been found not to represent a serious problem. It is now time to discuss naturally occurring persistent virus infections.

Persistent Virus Infections

Whereas acute infections are young in a historical perspective this is not the case in latent/persistent virus infections. This kind of infection can remain associated with the organism, because the immune system of the individual does not manage to clear the virus from the body. There may be many explanations for such persistence. In principle, either the virus may remain integrated into the host genome in a quiet way not revealing its presence to the immune system or it may continue to replicate in some discreet way, undetectable and uncontrollable by this system. A virus may evolve a capacity to block a function of one of the many components of the immune system, for example, a signalling factor like a lymphokine. This may lead to the virus becoming too dangerous to the host, which in turn may increase its defence capacity by improving another arm of the immune system. This evolutionary chess game may result in many draws before a state is reached when the evolutionary consequences for both parties involved are acceptable or even attractive. This parallel evolution of parasite and host may potentially extend over many millions of years and even through successive evolutions of a species, including our own. In fact it may even be traced all the way back to a time before vertebrates diverged from their invertebrate ancestors about 400 million years ago, the first time that immunoglobulin-like molecules emerged in the evolutionary succession of species.

There are a number of different kinds of viruses that can remain for a long time or even throughout the life span of the host under the control of the immune system. One example of viruses with a capacity to persist is papilloma (wart) viruses. Warts on the hands or on the feet can be a major nuisance in children and young adults. They may spread in environments found in sport establishments. I had extensive problems with warts on one heel in the upper teenage years which caused me some trouble when playing handball. Being a medical student at the time I consulted the professor of dermatology Sven Hellerström at the Karolinska Hospital. He prescribed magnesium sulphate (placebo?) to be taken orally. When I took this remedy the warts disappeared. One can only speculate about the reasons for this effect. An effective immune reaction had been mobilized perhaps because I believed that the treatment would work. Also hypnosis has been used to attempt to influence immune functions.

Persistent papilloma viruses, of which there are many types, may initiate differences in cell proliferation that can lead to papillomas on our skin or mucosal membranes, which in some cases, particularly in the genital tract, may eventually lead to the formation of cancer cells. In this case it is viral genes themselves that contribute to the emergence of tumor cells. This relationship was unravelled by Harald zur Hausen, who managed to document the fact that certain types of papilloma viruses, especially types 12, 18 and 31, played a critical role in this context. His identification of the particular role of these specific types has had practical consequences. Vaccines preventing infection with these types of papilloma viruses have been developed and are now used for immunization of girls in the early teenage years with the goal of preventing future cancers. Zur Hausen's pioneering contributions were recognized by one half of the 2008 Nobel Prize in physiology or medicine. The motivation for his part of the prize was "for his discovery of human papilloma viruses causing cervical cancer".

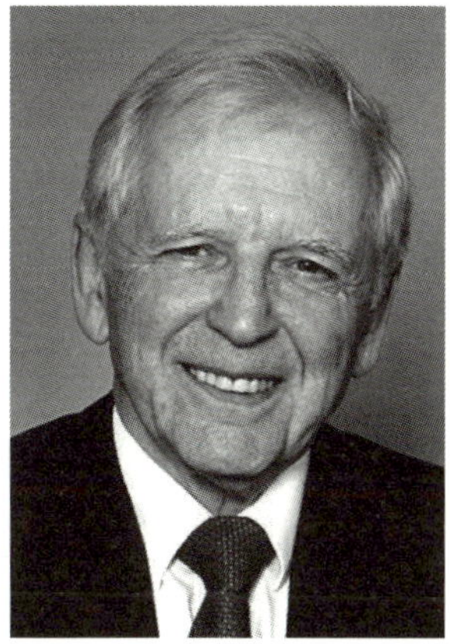

Harald zur Hausen, recipient of the shared 2008 Nobel Prize in physiology or medicine. [From *Les Prix Nobel en 2008*.]

The family of herpesviruses contains many members (Table 4.1), like herpes simplex virus types 1 and 2 already introduced in Chapter 1, and these different members exemplify a wide range of different mechanisms for the persistence of viruses. One example is the virus causing chickenpox (varicella) in children. After the primary infection with the virus the individual retains an immunity to new infections, but the agent remains in a dormant form in the body associated with cells of the nerve system. Activation of such dormant/

Table 4.1. Human herpesviruses.

No. 1	**Herpes simplex virus type 1**
No. 2	Herpes simplex virus type 2
No. 3	Varicella-zoster virus
No. 4	Epstein-Barr virus
No. 5	Cytomegalovirus
Nos. 6 & 7	T cell lymphotropic viruses
No. 8	Kaposi's sarcoma-associated virus

latent virus allows it to spread from central nerve ganglia, where it may have been hidden, to the periphery of the body. This spread occurs inside neurons where the virus is inaccessible to the immune system. When it reaches the skin it can multiply and give local lesions, which occur in the region of the skin — the dermatome — in any part of the body that is served by the afflicted nerve. This expression of the infection is called zoster (shingles). The disease is often very painful and the symptoms may last for months. The grandfather with shingles can infect his grandchild, who then develops chickenpox. This is an elegant way for the virus to secure its survival in nature. Today we can prevent the occurrence of chickenpox by immunizing children with a live virus vaccine. Recently this vaccine has been licensed for use in adults too. It is employed to improve the immunity in people of the age of 60 or above. The reason for this vaccination is to compensate for the progressive weakening of the immune system in elderly people. The reduced immunity at higher ages is an important factor in the activation and spread of varicella virus leading to the development of zoster. The weakening immune defence in elderly people is a general problem.

In the 1960s a technician in Werner and Gertrud Henle's virus laboratory at the Children's Hospital in Philadelphia provided a serum to be used as a control in studies of particular tumor cells from African patients associated with a herpes virus called Epstein-Barr virus (EBV). To the surprise of the researchers the serum reacted strongly with antigens in the infected tumor cells. This led to the discovery that the virus present in the tumor cells was the cause of the common disease infectious mononucleosis, which the technician had just recovered from. This is a disease that is most common among adolescents and young adults. It often leads to relatively severe symptoms and there is a long convalescence. Infections with EBV are common in the population, but when they involve people at a young age, there are normally no symptoms. As the immune system continues to develop in the teenage years conditions are set for developing the cumbersome symptoms. Others factors may also contribute. The illness is sometimes referred to as "deep kissing" disease, possibly emphasizing a role of transmission of infected cells rather than of virus particles. In the symptomatic patient a war develops between the main actors of the immune system. B cells infected by the virus are attacked by the cytotoxic (CD-8 positive) T cells mobilized by the host immune response. This is just one of many examples of the fact that our finely tuned immune system can sometimes contribute to disease instead of preventing it.

Human cytomegalovirus (HCMV), yet another herpesvirus (Table 4.1), generally causes a harmless infection involving the salivary glands. Its name derives from the fact that it may cause the presence in these glands of abnormally large cells containing accumulated virus products, *inclusions*. Like rubella virus HCMV can be harmful when transmitted from the pregnant mother to her foetus. Besides being of importance for congenital infections, HCMV may cause serious challenges in connection with immunosuppression in transplant patients as we shall see. The virus has a capacity to persist because it has evolved a particular mechanism to interfere with MHC class I presentation of viral antigens. We will meet further examples of persistent herpesviruses in the discussion of AIDS below.

One more form of persistent infection is the one caused by hepatitis B virus, discussed previously (Ref. 7, Chapter 2). It is appropriate to ask how a virus that releases infectious particles exclusively into the circulating blood, can spread under natural conditions. After all blood transfusions are a modern invention depending upon knowledge about the blood groups as described in Chapter 2. The answer is that originally the dominating source of transmissions of this chronic infection was from mother to child during pregnancy or at the time of delivery, so called *vertical* rather than horizontal transmission. A similar situation of transmission is seen in cases of HIV infections with the predominant spread of virus at delivery. It is now possible to prevent such vertical infections of newborns, in the case of hepatitis B by vaccination and in the case of HIV by treatment with antiviral drugs. Let us now discuss the situation in HIV-AIDS, because, as the name implies, it represents the most spectacular example of virus-induced immunosuppression and its consequences.

In the early 1980s a complex and fatal disease started to afflict male homosexuals in San Francisco. Their whole immune system seemed to have collapsed; parasites like *Pneumocystis carinii* caused pneumonis; cytomegalovirus caused inflammation of the bowel; Kaposi's sarcoma, later shown to be caused by human herpesvirus type 8 (see Table 4.1, p. 141), caused major skin lesions. It did not take long before the name GRID — gay-related immune deficiency — was changed to AIDS and the derangement of the whole immune system was demonstrated to be caused by HIV. The two types of this virus as already mentioned represent a special form of human retroviruses, the lentiviruses. They have a unique capacity to interfere with functions of the immune system. Their preferred target cell was found to be activated CD4 cells.

Before further discussing the disease-causing mechanisms of HIV a few comments on the general nature of retroviruses should be given. These viruses have a uniquely long association with different forms of life and HIV is only one of a huge number of members in this group. One unique character of these kinds of viruses is that their genetic material is RNA, but that they function like DNA viruses. They have an enzyme that can transcribe their RNA "backwards" into DNA. This enzyme is called reverse transcriptase and its discovery was the basis for the 1975 Nobel Prize in physiology or medicine to David Baltimore and Howard Temin. They shared this prize with Dulbecco, Tonegawa's post-doctoral mentor, with the prize motivation "for their discoveries concerning the interaction between tumour viruses and the genetic material of the cell". It is characteristic of these viruses that they can shuttle in and out of the genome of cells. This shuttling presumably has played a major role in evolution through billions of years and the genome of us humans reveals many signs of this. A major fraction of it is represented by more or less complete — vestigial and "rusty" — retroviral genes. There have been many attempts to demonstrate a possible importance of these *endogenous* retroviruses for disease, but so far no clear evidence for a role in causing illness has been found.

There are in principle three central mechanisms that viruses may use to dominate their multicellular host with the potential final outcome of death. All these mechanisms can be illustrated by the categorically persistent infections of man by HIV, which therefore will be used as an example. Before discussing these mechanisms it should be noted that both HIV-1 and HIV-2 cause harmless persistent infections in their natural hosts, the chimpanzees and the sooty mangabey monkeys. A balanced relationship, benefiting both the host and the virus, has evolved. It is not known why these animals do not develop disease, but hopefully with time some insights into the critical mechanisms might be gained. This could give access to new means for managing the HIV infection in man.

The mechanisms of importance for the progressive HIV disease process in man are: (a) antigen instability, (b) integration of the virus genetic material in cells in a quiescent state undetectable by the immune system and in particular (c) suppression of immune function(s). The origin of the antigenic instability is the high mutation rates of viral genomes. Changing the antigenic properties of immunodominant virus components allows a virus to escape the immune response mobilized by the host. This phenomenon, in another context, provides an explanation for the recurrence of influenza epidemics due to the antigenic drift and shift allowing repeated acute infections as already introduced in Chapter 1 and mentioned again above. However, fortunately, most viruses causing diseases in man, in spite of the relative imprecision of replication of their genomes, are relatively antigenically stable. Thus there are, for example, only three types of poliovirus, one type of measles virus and so on. We should be grateful for this because if this had not been the case we would not have been so successful in developing vaccines that protect against these illnesses, and also many other viral diseases.

By way of contrast, attempts to develop a vaccine against HIV have failed so far and there are many reasons for this. One reason is that the integration of virus genetic material into host cell DNA facilitates the stealthy behavior by the virus. It should be emphasized again that in their latent persistent state in cells, viruses may totally avoid immune clearance for extensive periods of time. A particular problem with HIV infections is the capacity of the virus to selectively attack and destroy the helper and regulatory T cells, the CD4 cells. In an irony of fate the virus uses the CD4 immunoglobulin receptor as a part of its means of specifically entering this kind of cell. This has major consequences. In untreated patients there is a progressive destruction of the CD4 cells. This facilitates the persistence of this virus and it also paves the way for development of many other viral and bacterial infections as well as the appearance of certain kinds of tumors already referred to above. The level of CD4 cells in the blood is used as guidance on when to introduce antiviral treatment of patients. Although proper use of antivirals has become a very efficient means of suppressing the replication of HIV, the treatment never leads to a complete clearance of the virus from the body. The intimate relationship with the white blood cells allows the virus to stay for life. A single exception to this rule is a German patient who seems to have lost all traces of the virus in connection with a bone marrow transplantation.

In order for the CD4 cells to allow virus replication they need to be stimulated. There are increasingly more refined studies of how stimulation or suppression of CD4 cells is regulated. The complexity of the signalling and the role of cell-to-cell contacts involving different subpopulations of cells is being progressively unravelled. Perhaps it would be possible to suppress in a durable fashion the stimulation of CD4 cells and hence block the replication of HIV in them by some kind of immunoprophylaxis. This would mean a new approach to immunoprotection not dependent on production of specific antibodies or immune T cells. But let us leave this speculation and return to the classical vaccines. The achievements made possible by their use have been astounding as already discussed (Ref. 7, Chapter 4) and there is more to come. In some cases we are aiming at eradicating selected diseases and the viruses that cause them.

The Eradication of a Virus Disease and a Virus Species

There are three conditions that need to be met to make eradication of a virus infection possible. These are (a) that the virus is antigenically stable and that there exists a vaccine that can effectively prevent the infection, (b) that the virus cannot cause persistent infections — although this need not be an absolute criterion — and (c) that there is no animal reservoir from which the virus can be reintroduced into the human population. Several virus infections in man fulfil these criteria. The eradication of smallpox from our world in October 1977, in a program managed by WHO, was a triumph for humanity. A plague that had purged human civilizations for thousands of years was no more. During the 20th century alone many millions of individuals had died of this disease. General vaccination could cease. If a Nobel Prize in physiology or medicine was allowed to be given to an organization — as in the case of the Peace Prize — the WHO might have been recognized for this unprecedented achievement. However one would have had to define what the discovery was.

The last natural case of smallpox occurred in Ali Maow Maalin, a hospital cook in Somalia who had attended a child with the disease. He survived the infection. Sadly there was to be one more human case. It was a female medical photographer who became infected in September 1978 when working at the anatomy department of the University of Birmingham. The virus causing this laboratory infection originated in a microbiology department on the floor below. The head of the latter department, Professor Hendry Bedson, committed suicide following this event.

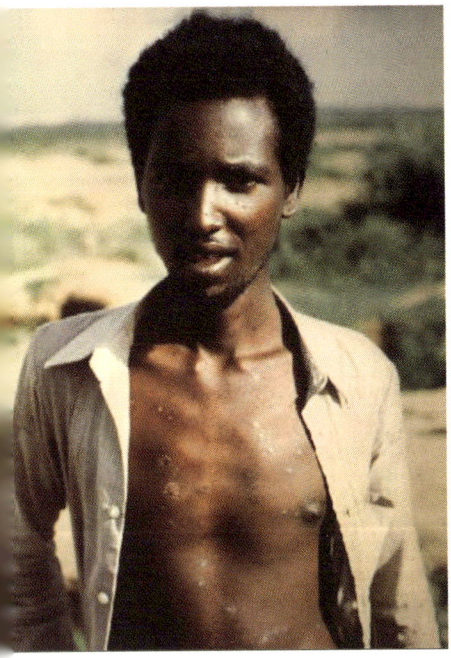

Ali Maow Maalin, a hospital cook in Somalia, who was the last individual to contract smallpox through natural transmission. [Credit: CDC Public Health Image Library.]

Although little spoken of there is one more virus disease that has been globally eradicated. This is rinderpest (from a German word for cattle-plague), a highly infectious disease in cattle and related wild species of ungulates, caused by a virus closely related to measles. It would in fact be more appropriate to say that measles virus is related to rinderpest virus, since it most likely was the spread of the latter virus to man that allowed establishment of the highly contagious measles virus in humans. The successful eradication was the result of initiatives by the United Nations Food and Agricultural Organization and the World Organization for Animal Health. The program was launched in 1994 and it was coordinated from the Institute for Animal Health at Pirbright, Surrey. The leading personality in this project was Walter Plowright. He was the father of the vaccine employed and a central figure throughout the campaign for eradication. When we were studying the relationship between measles, canine distemper and rinderpest viruses, Plowright kindly provided us with sera from animals infected by rinderpest virus. However, it was absolutely forbidden for us to work with this virus in Sweden. The formal declaration of the successful eradiation was made in June 2011. One may wonder which viral disease will be the third one to be fully wiped out from the earth?

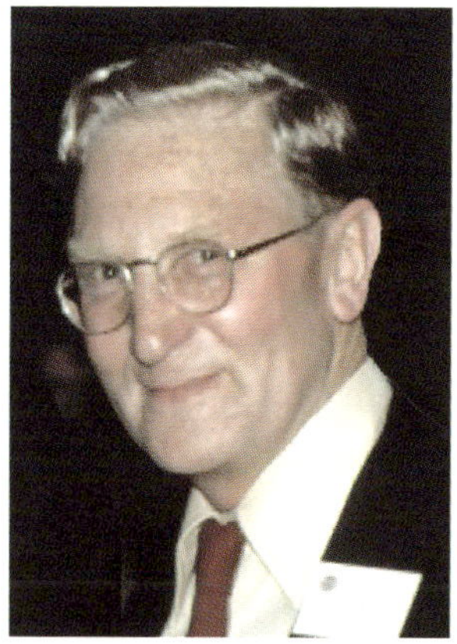

Walter Plowright (1923–2010), who played a central role in the global eradication of rinderpest. [From Ref. 15.]

The success in eradicating smallpox inspired WHO to attempt the eradication of other virus diseases. Poliomyelitis was chosen as the next target. Again the early phase of the program gave excellent results as described previously (Ref. 7, Chapter 5). In a little over ten years after 1989 when the program was started the number of countries with continuous infections with the virus — endemic polio — was reduced from 125 to 4 (see figure below). The major

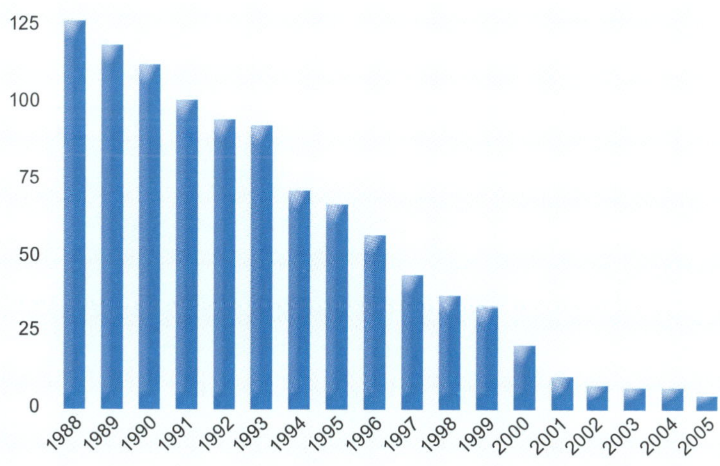

The reduction of countries with endemic polio after WHO in 1988 had initiated a program for eradication of the disease.

parts of our world — the Americas, Europe, East Asia and Australia have been declared to be free of polio, meaning that no case has been registered for more than two years. Regrettably it has not been possible to conclude the program of eradication during the last ten years and still in 2013 there have been flare-ups of polio in Pakistan, Afghanistan and Nigeria. India for a long time belonged among the nations that still had endemic polio, but that has changed. This large country with a population exceeding a billion people has now been declared free of polio, an impressive achievement. The intensity of the campaign is presently being increased in the remaining three infected countries, but regrettably social unrest and cultural conflicts have so far blocked a final successful eradication.

In parallel there is also an unofficial program to eliminate measles. This disease may in fact be easier to get a grip on than polio since essentially all infections are associated with clear symptoms, whereas the absolute majority of all polio infections are symptomless. In spite of access to an effective vaccine since the 1960s, the number of children dying of measles in our world for many years stayed at about one million. Between 2000 and 2011 there was a major improvement. The number of measles cases has been reduced by 65% and the estimated deaths caused by the disease were reduced by 71%, from 542,000 to 158,000. Regrettably the coverage of vaccination has diminished in some of the industrialized countries during later years. This may to some extent be due to disinformation not infrequently accepted by the well-educated sections of society. Because of the high level of contagiousness of the virus it can spread from one unvaccinated to another possibly unvaccinated individual if the total coverage of vaccination is lower than 90%. If the value is higher than this figure the likelihood that a chain of infections between non-immunes can be established is so low that no epidemic will arise. There is so-called *herd immunity*. In parallel with the campaign to eliminate measles, WHO is also pushing for the elimination of rubella. In the latter case the aim primarily is to prevent the occurrence of damage by congenital infections. This campaign too is developing well.

The statement that only acute virus infections can be eradicated needs to be qualified. It is possible to discuss approaches to eradication also of human viruses causing certain kinds of persistent infections. One example is varicella/zoster virus infections. If it becomes possible to let the mild live vaccine virus substitute globally for the wild virus infection, the circulation of the virus will be extensively reduced or even eliminated. There will also be a consequential marked reduction of the eventual number of zoster infections in the vaccinated individuals. A supplementary immunization of adults may further reduce the occurrence of such infections which may eventually lead to the final eradication of the virus. Another special form of persistence of viruses is seen in individuals infected with the agent causing hepatitis B. As was mentioned the natural chain of transmission is predominantly from mother to child at the term of gestation and at delivery, a transmission that can be prevented by vaccination. Thus also in this case it might be feasible to interrupt the continued existence of the virus.

It is worth noting that at a time when there are extensive discussions about means to preserve biodiversity by saving as many species as possible, we are simultaneously, for anthropocentric reasons, searching for possibilities to actively eradicate selected species of viruses. If we are successful in such endeavors it will be possible, as in the case of smallpox, to cease vaccinating against the eradicated virus. This would mean enormous progress, but it would also put a demand on us to build a world on trust and not on mistrust. Theoretically some of the agents we will eradicate could be considered for use as bioterrorism agents. One approach to managing this threat would be to destroy all existing laboratory virus of the kind eradicated, but not even that may provide a guarantee against unethical behavior. The reason is that with the advance of technology it is now possible to create infectious viruses in the test tube, as already demonstrated for the agents causing polio and influenza. In theory it would be possible to synthesize the genomes of even more complex viruses, since scientists have managed to synthesize nucleic acids containing as many as one million base pairs. This was demonstrated by the high fidelity recreation of the whole genome of a small form of bacterium[8]. It is to be expected that this field of the writing of the books of life will continue to expand in the coming years.

It is to be hoped that the deeper an insight we get into the detailed functions of the immune system the more successful we will become in interfering with and preventing acute as well as persistent infectious diseases. One of the deadliest virus epidemics in modern times was the 1917–1918 Spanish flu. It has been estimated that more than 50 million people died from this disease. Many of the victims were younger men in their prime and they succumbed to a rapidly developing disease in what was later described as a cytokine "storm". A deeper insight into signalling in the immune system may help in counteracting such an event. As has already been mentioned another gain in deepening our understanding of the immune system is the possibility of interfering in situations when it makes mistakes in distinguishing self and non-self. There are a number of medically important autoimmune diseases in need of more effective treatment. Distinguishing self and non-self naturally leads us to the final Nobel Prizes to be discussed in this chapter, the 1990 prize recognizing the medical importance of organ and cell transplantation and the prize given two years earlier for the development of drugs allowing such transplantations.

The Developments in Tissue Transplantations in Humans

One of the major arguments for awarding the prize to Burnet and Medawar was that the understanding of the rejection of transplanted tissues as an immunological reaction should pave the way for future transplantation of organs between humans. This is certainly true, but the argument needed to be qualified. In Medawar's own words:

> Thus the ultimate importance of the discovery of tolerance turned out to be not practical, but moral. It put new heart into the many biologists and surgeons who were working to make it possible to graft, for example, kidneys from one person to another — a procedure already shown to be both genetically and physiologically possible by the brilliantly successful transplantation of a kidney from a patient's identical twin donor, at the Peter Bent Brigham Hospital in Boston.

What Burnet's and Medawar's prize illustrated was that if a match between the MHC antigens of a donor and a recipient of a transplant could be met, at least reasonably well, and in addition drugs to achieve a graded immune suppression could be developed, it might be possible to transplant organs between humans. This is exactly what happened. The successes in transplanting organs between humans were recognized by the Nobel Prize in physiology or medicine in 1990 to Joseph E. Murray and E. Donnall Thomas. The citation for their prize was "for their discoveries concerning organ and cell transplantation in the treatment of human disease". This prize represented a very attractive meeting point between theoretical and practical medicine. Both the awardees had a solid background in clinical medicine and in experimental science.

I had many interesting encounters with these two prize recipients during their visit to Stockholm. Chairing the Nobel Assembly is a one year responsibility and in 1990 it was my turn. Therefore it was my duty to manage the proceedings of the assembly in its meetings that led to its decision for the

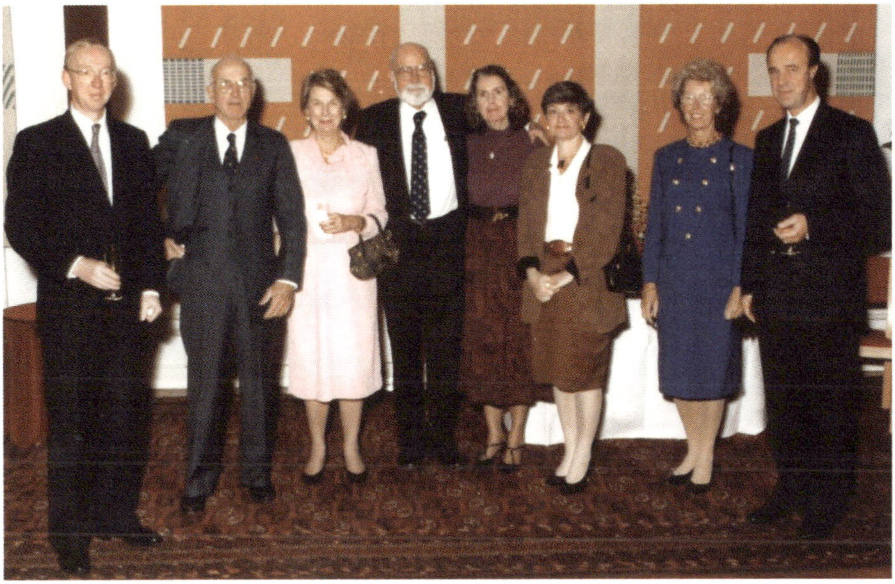

Reception for the 1990 laureates at the Karolinska Institute. *From left*: Bengt Samuelsson, Nobel laureate and Vice-Chancellor, Dr and Mrs Murray, Dr and Mrs Thomas, Mrs Samuelsson, the author and his wife.

prize. Being chairman of the Assembly also gave me the right to take part in the meetings of the Nobel Committee that particular year. Finally, together with the President of the Karolinska Institute at the time, Bengt Samuelsson, who had received a shared Nobel prize in physiology or medicine eight years earlier, I had the pleasure to host the two Laureates at the reception arranged by the Institute after their Nobel lectures.

Transplantation of Solid Organs

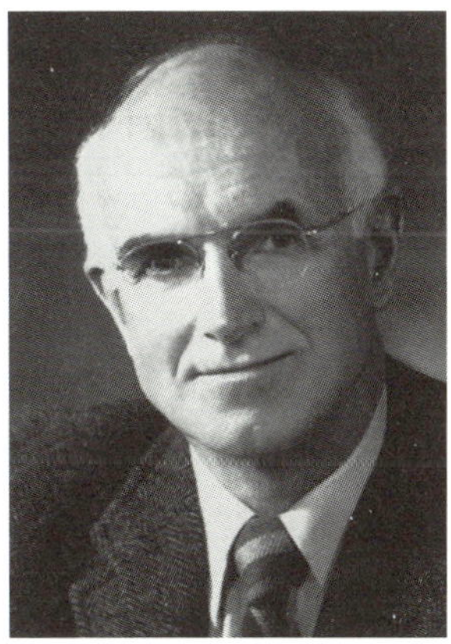

Joseph E. Murray (1919–2012), recipient of the shared 1990 Nobel Prize in physiology or medicine. [From *Les Prix Nobel en 1990.*]

Murray grew up in a family that stressed the importance of taking advantage of educational opportunities and that also emphasized the need for service to others. He decided to be a surgeon inspired by the family doctor. He found his four years of studies at Harvard Medical School to be very enriching. It was during his military experience at Valley Forge General Hospital in Pennsylvania that Murray developed an interest in the biology of tissue and organ transplantation. There were many patients with burns in the ward for plastic surgery that he served. He learnt that the degree of genetic relationship between the donor and recipient might be a factor influencing the survival of temporary skin allografts. Skin grafting between identical twins had been made successfully for the first time in 1937.

Conditions for future successful transplantations of kidneys emerged at the Peter Bent Brigham Hospital in the late 1940s and Murray became the leading figure in these developments[9]. The first great success by the group came in 1954 when a kidney was transplanted between two identical twins as mentioned in the citation by Medawar. A few years later certain immune suppressive drugs were being tested in dogs with results indicating that they might facilitate transplantation between non-identical individuals. On the advice of Medawar one of the researchers involved in these studies, Roy Calne from London, went to Boston to work with Murray.

In the late 1950s another important step was taken. A scientist thought that the immature lymphocytes observed in connection with an activated immune response looked like leukemic cells. He therefore tested the effect of 6-mercaptopurine (6-MP) on the activation of an antibody response. As already mentioned briefly it was found that blocking of cell division interrupted the mobilization of an antibody response. This observation led to the development of the first immunosuppressive drugs allowing successful organ transplantations in man. The first idea was to use 6-MP, since this drug had been found by Calne to prolong the survival of an allotransplanted kidney in dogs. Further discussion came to involve George H. Hitchings and Elion, briefly mentioned above, at Burroughs and Wellcome, whom Calne had introduced to Murray. These dedicated scientists, who were later to receive a shared Nobel Prize two years prior to Murray, had become enthusiastic collaborators and the discussions of the teams eventually led to that another compound, azathioprine (Imuran), being tested instead. The latter serves as a pro-drug and is metabolized to 6-MP in the body, a process that reduces its toxicity. It was the use of Imuran that supplemented with other drugs, that set the stage for successful organ transplantations in man beginning 1962. But the drug also had other beneficial effects. It could be utilized to treat autoimmune diseases, like rheumatoid arthritis.

There are two phases after transplantation that need to be managed by immune suppression. The first one is immediately after the surgical procedure when it is critical to ensure that the organ can survive in the new environment.

Once this has been successfully achieved it is possible to reduce the intensity of the immune suppression treatment to a level combining the long-time survival of the transplant with a minimal of side effects from the drugs used. In 1961 the first attempt was made to transplant a kidney in a patient treated by azathioprine. There were problems with toxicity and the patient eventually died. Within a few years the dose of the drug could be properly adjusted and already in 1965 the survival rates of kidneys transplanted from living related donors had reached 80% and from cadavers 65%. In order to dampen the risk for an early rejection of a transplanted organ a temporary supplementary treatment with corticosteroids was introduced. The identification and early clinical use of this group of hormones was recognized by a Nobel Prize in physiology or medicine in 1950 (Chapter 6, Ref. 7). In further developments also anti-lymphocyte serum and later specific monoclonal antibodies, like for example one that reacts with the cellular receptor for one of the interleukins, were also tried to reduce the risk of early organ rejection. With time progressively improved immunosuppressive drugs have been developed.

Following the successful transplantation of kidneys, attempts were also made to transplant other organs like the liver and the heart. As techniques developed there were also successes in these procedures. Transplantation has become a standard medical procedure and the most urgent present problem is shortage of organs. The possibility of moving from heterotransplantation to transplantation of organs from animals, *xenotransplantation*, is being seriously considered. One circumstance holding this back is consideration of the risks that endogenous animal viruses, like retroviruses, would be transmitted to man. This seems very unlikely, but improved documentation is needed to evaluate the potential threat from such foreign viruses.

Murray's brief autobiography presented at the time of his Nobel Prize[10] gives a picture of a scientist with many interests outside his professional engagements. He seems to have been a very likable person and the development of his life was markedly enriched by a happy marriage and a large family. We will return to his choices of lifestyle in the last chapter in a discussion of this matter in a larger context. Murray had a long life dying in 2012 at the age of 93 years.

Transplantation of Bone Marrow

Thomas, the second person recognized by the Nobel Prize for discoveries connected with transplantation, was a pioneer in transfer of bone marrow.

His decision to choose a medical career emanated from his father who was a general practitioner. Like Murray, Thomas got his training at Harvard Medical School and during his internship he spent a year at Peter Bent Brigham Hospital where the two of them met. Early in the course of his studies he became interested in bone marrow and leukaemia and during a few years at MIT he studied factors stimulating the growth of bone marrow cells. Very little progress was made in this research and it would take a considerable time before this field consolidated. His work on bone marrow transplantation continued in a more clinical environment and was first developed at the Columbia University-affiliated Mary Imogene Hospital in Cooperstown, N.Y. During this time, in 1959, the first successful transplantations were made between identical twins. The recipients of the transplant were given heavy doses of irradiation to destroy their own bone marrow. This treatment by definition was lethal but intravenous injection of bone marrow from their twin allowed the patients to survive. A certain step forward had been made but it was apparent that many challenges remained to manage in the continued work. In 1963 Thomas moved to Seattle where a new team to work on different aspects of bone marrow transplantation was established. This team later (1975) moved to the Fred Hutchinson Cancer Center where excellent resources for the forthcoming work were made available.

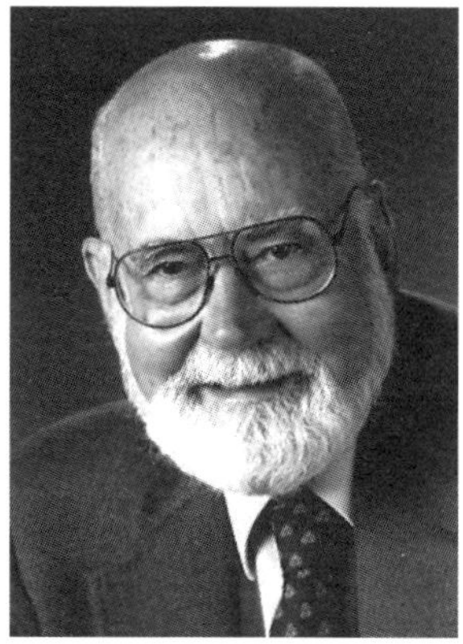

E. Donnall Thomas (1920–2012), recipient of the shared 1990 Nobel Prize in physiology or medicine. [From *Les Prix Nobel en 1990*.]

Developments in the field have led to the term bone marrow transplantation being exchanged for *hematopoietic stem cell transplantation (HSCT)*, since it has been found that there are different alternative sources of donor cells. Besides the bone marrow one can also use peripheral blood stem cells and in the case of newborns also umbilical blood cells. Today it is most common to use peripheral blood stem cells. HSTC is a risky procedure and is therefore used selectively and almost only in life-threatening diseases. One distinguishes between *autologous* grafts, using previously collected and frozen cells from the patient himself, and *allogenic* grafts. Somewhat more than half of the latter come from family donors and the rest from unrelated, but optimally matched donors. About 90% of HSCTs are on the indication of lymphoproliferative disorders and leukaemias. The indications in the remaining cases are disabling auto-immune diseases and particular kinds of cardiovascular disease.

Bone marrow transplantation poses a particular challenge since it involves the kind of tissue that is heavily engaged in various immune reactions[11]. The first step in the treatment is to abrogate the pre-existing bone marrow. This is presently done by radiotherapy and chemotherapy. In the cases of allogenic transplantations a central problem to manage is the previously mentioned graft versus host reaction. In order to reduce the magnitude of this, effective procedures allowing the best possible matching of donor and recipient tissues needed to be developed. The introduction of Dausset's tissue typing technique was indispensable for the selection of the best matches. Furthermore it was critical to develop a properly adjusted level of immune suppression and as mentioned, progressively improved drugs became available. One more challenge was to control possibly activated quiescent persistent virus infections. There were many failures during the 1960s and only after some ten years of trials did it become possible to develop the right conditions for optimal takes of the grafts. It was Thomas and his collaborators who pioneered these developments. The first successful bone marrow transplantation in humans on a non-cancer patient was made in 1968 at the University of Minnesota by Good, already introduced in Chapter 3. Organ and bone marrow transplantations have become routine clinical interventions, but in the latter case the unavailability of matching donors can sometimes be a continuing problem.

A Committed Female Scientist

The successes of organ and cell transplantation have very much been dependent on the development of drugs that allow a properly adjusted immune suppression both during the immediate post-operational period and for the long-term survival of the transplanted organ. Availability of drugs to manage activated virus infections is also of great importance. Elion and Hitchings have been pioneers in both these fields. The significance of their contributions was recognized by the 1988 Nobel Prize in physiology or medicine. The motivation for this prize, which was shared with James W. Black, was "for their discovery of the important principles of drug treatment". As was mentioned Elion and Hitchings established an important collaboration with Murray's team at Peter Bent Brigham hospital.

In a recent book *Drive and Curiosity* by Istvan Hargittai[12], one chapter on Elion has the title *Pushed by personal tragedy. Lifesavers*. It describes how she developed into a devoted chemist in the pharmaceutical industry where

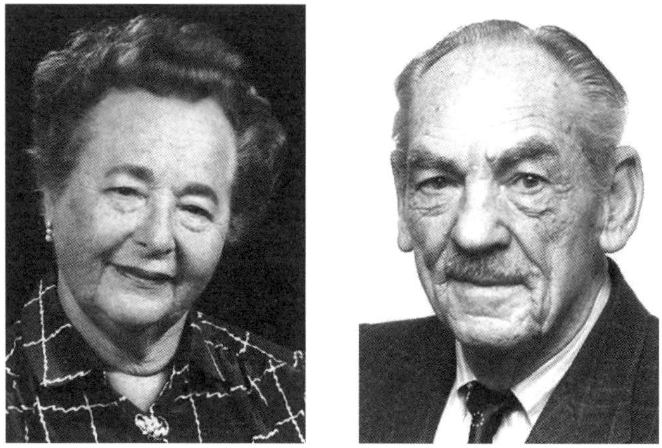

Gertrude B. Elion (1918–1999) and George H. Hitchings (1905–1998), recipients of the shared 1988 Nobel Prize in physiology or medicine. [From *Les Prix Nobel en 1988.*]

she became heavily engaged in her work. She had many odds against her as she got her education in the 1930s due to being both Jewish and a female. The family had limited means since her father, an immigrant of Lithuanian origin, who was a dentist, had lost all his investments during the depression. When she was 15 years old her beloved grandfather died of cancer. This experience motivated Elion to aim at a career in the health sector. She went to the (free) Hunter College aiming to major in science and, in particular, chemistry. Her years of further education were a continuous struggle. Saving money from various teaching jobs enabled her to enter New York University. In her graduate chemistry class she was the only woman. Doing research work at night and over weekends she got her Master of Science in chemistry in 1941. After having tried a number of jobs, Elion was hired as assistance to George Hitchings at the Wellcome Research Laboratories in Tuckahoe, New York. She was given free rein and their collaboration developed in a very fruitful way. Her increasing degree of independence did not detract from this — quite the opposite — and their joint pursuit came to last for some 40 years. In order to complete her studies Elion wanted to get a PhD and to manage this she started night school at the Brooklyn Polytechnic Institute. She was soon informed that she needed to change to full-time studies to get her degree. This she decided not to do since she did not want to interrupt her productive collaboration with Hitchings. Similar to a number of other Nobel laureates, like for example Medawar in Chapter 2, she had to manage without a formal academic higher degree.

It was Hitching's original idea to develop chemical knowledge about the building blocks of nucleic acids. One may wonder why he selected this group of chemicals in the early 1940s for their studies. At that time no one had a premonition about the central role in turnover of the genetic material that they were demonstrated to have in later studies (Ref. 7, Chapter 7). According to Elion[13], "Hitchings theorized that, since all cells required nucleic acids, it might be possible to stop the growth of rapidly dividing cells (e.g. bacteria, tumors, protozoa) with antagonists of the nucleic acid bases." However the chemical knowledge about the building blocks of nucleic acids, the purines and pyrimidines, and their metabolism was rather rudimentary at the time and the important discovery in Avery's laboratory at Rockefeller Institute in 1944, as yet had essentially no impact. Still, the later development of the field showed that the selected targets were very fortunate.

Some of the purine analogues synthesized were tested for their anti-tumor activity at the Sloan-Kettering Institute in New York in the early 1950s. One compound was particularly promising. It was the already mentioned 6-MP. This was the first drug that could induce complete remission in children with leukaemia. It was the beginning of the successful treatment of this disease. With time further effective drugs were discovered allowing combination therapy with excellent results. Today almost all children with this formerly always lethal disease can be cured. The further studies of 6-MP led to the development of Imuran, which provided the conditions for the early successful kidney transplantations and came to serve the same important role in the early cases of bone marrow transplantation.

In her biographical presentation in *Les Prix Nobel*[14], Elion presented herself in a very humble way. She stated simply "Over the years, my work became both my vocation and avocation. Since I enjoyed it so much, I never felt a great need to go outside for relaxation." Having stated this she acknowledged that she did in fact love travelling and to use her camera, and also to listen to music, not the least opera. As concerned family relationships she noted tersely "Although I never married, my brother fortunately did, and I have had the pleasure of watching his three sons and daughter grow up. Several of them now have children of their own. We have a close-knit family, although often separated by distance, and have shared each other's happiness, sorrows and aspirations."

Complications of Medically Induced Immune Suppression

A final word in the context of tissue transplantation concerns the consequences of a general suppression of the immune system in an individual. Releasing the physiological control provided by this system can have two consequences. One is that dormant viruses in our body may become activated and the other that emerging abnormally dividing cells get improved possibilities for expansion. Sometimes, as we shall see, the two effects may be intertwined. As presented above we normally carry, in a silent form, a number of viruses with a capacity to persist in our body. Among these in particular the different herpesviruses and papilloma viruses can cause complications.

Since the late 1940s Elion and Hitchings had been interested in antiviral drugs but it took time until a compound with a capacity to block virus replication without accompanying toxicity could be found. In the 1970s Elion's group discovered that an analogue of guanine, acycloguanosine, later called acyclovir was highly effective in blocking the replication of herpes viruses. This was very useful in the management of activated virus infections in transplanted patients although the effect on different viruses of this kind varied. The best effect was achieved on the replication of herpes simplex types 1 and 2 and varicella-zoster viruses, but there was almost no effect on cytomegalovirus. Acyclovir and other related antivirals have become indispensible in the management of viruses activated by the intense early immune suppression in patients receiving organ or bone marrow transplantations.

The appreciation of a connection between an infection with a certain virus and a later development of cancers underlined a potentially dangerous indirect effect of immune suppressive treatments. The activation of a dormant virus might lead to a harmless infection but this potentially later could lead to the evolution of cancer cells. In his Nobel lecture[15] zur Hausen cited a study of the relative frequency of many different forms of cancers in a large group of kidney transplanted patients followed for a long time. Some forms of cancer do not show any increased frequency of occurrence, and in a few cases it appears as if the immune suppression, for unknown reasons, even decreases the emergence of certain forms of tumors. However there are other cancers which show a distinct increase after immune suppression. The major increase, about 200-fold, involved a tumor originating in connective tissue, Kaposi's sarcoma. Unsurprisingly this was the dominating cancer form seen in the early full-blown cases of AIDS as already mentioned. This form of cancer was recognized as early as 1872 by a Hungarian dermatologist working at the University of Vienna. The tumor was easily recognized by its papular cutaneous lesions but the tumor cells could also spread throughout the body. The critical role of immune control in this type of tumor was recognized in a conspicuous way in the first epidemic of AIDS in the early 1980s. Later it was demonstrated to be due to an activation of a previously unknown herpes virus that came to be labelled type 8 (see Table 4.1). Other forms of cancers too, in particular those involving the lips, the vulva, the penis show a distinct increase in patients subjected to immunosuppression. It remains to determine if this is also due to activation of (papilloma?) virus infections, possibly involving as yet undetected forms of viruses or some other phenomenon that may favor the replication of certain tumorigenic cells.

It is impressive how the challenges to transplantations have been met by the development of various forms of balanced interventions. An important new form of medical treatment has become available adding years of high quality life to many severely ill patients. All together modern transplantation of organs is an excellent illustration of the cross-fertilization of basic science and clinical medicine successfully giving major benefits to patients who previously could not be helped. This is indeed life-giving medicine.

A Management of Bereavement

In the early 1990s I got to know Marcus Storch and his wife Gunilla. He has a background as a civil engineer and is a very influential industrialist in Sweden. In 1991 the family's only son, the teenaged Tobias, died of aplastic anaemia. This disease is caused by a complete abrogation of the functions of the bone marrow. The only chance for survival was bone marrow transplantation. However no donor that matched Tobias' tissue characteristics was found and he tragically succumbed to his disease. As a way to manage the bottomless sorrow and sublimate their grief the Storch family established the Tobias Foundation and I am proud of having been a member of the board of this Foundation since its inception. Considerable resources have been accumulated within the Foundation by money given by the family and a number of external donors. These financial resources have been used to establish a rich bone marrow register in Sweden, listing potential donors whose cell characteristics have been determined. This national register interacts with corresponding registers in other countries around the world. Their global interaction makes it possible to find a matching donor even for individuals with very unique tissue characteristics. The resources of the foundation have also been used to give important support to research focussing on haematopoietic stem cells and for donations of personal chairs in this field at the Karolinska institute and at other universities. Marcus Storch has been the Chairman of the Board of the Nobel Foundation since 2005 and together with his wife, was the host of the Nobel banquet at the Stockholm City Hall on December 10. He brought this important function to a conclusion in 2012.

Chapter 5

Transgressing Borders in Science and Scenes of Life

INVISIBLE LIGHT
A VALUABLE SHADOW
SECRETS UNLOCKED

In 1944 George de Hevesy received the 1943 Nobel Prize in chemistry "for his work on the use of isotopes as tracers in the study of chemical processes". The Nobel committee at the Royal Swedish Academy of Sciences had already recommended in 1940 that he should receive the prize, but the recognition of his pioneering science was delayed because of the ongoing Second World War. When the prize was eventually awarded the war still had not ended and only a small private ceremony was arranged for de Hevesy at the Academy. He had a background as a physicist, who came to receive a Nobel Prize in chemistry for the development of techniques with extensive applications in the life sciences. Thus he pioneered a multidisciplinary approach to science — reflecting its indivisible nature — but he did not only transgress borders in his science. He also did this frequently in his private life, because of repeated confrontations with new political realities in the Europe of the first half of the 20th century. For various periods of his life he lived in Budapest, Freiburg, Zürich, Karlsruhe, Manchester, Wien, again in Budapest, Copenhagen, again in Freiburg, again in Copenhagen and finally Stockholm. It was during his stay with Ernest Rutherford in Manchester in 1912 that he got to know Niels Bohr. Their friendship came to have a decisive influence on de Hevesy's joint development as an individual and as a scientist. It was in Bohr's institute in Copenhagen that de Hevesy made his major discoveries and it was in Denmark that he also met his future wife.

The Assimilated Jew and the Budding Scientist

De Hevesy's life has been described by his collaborator during his second sojourn with Bohr, Hilde Levi[1] and a more recent, detailed and less subjective presentation has been given by Siegfried Niese[2]. George Marx[3] has also included de Hevesy among the twenty remarkable scientists of Hungarian origin that enigmatically have been referred to as the Martians. This strange denomination probably has its origin in a myth that developed at the Los Alamos laboratory during the Second World War. Some of the most influential scientists at the laboratory, like Theodore von Kármán, John von Neumann and Leo Szilard had had their upbringing within a few city blocks in Budapest. It was Szilard who suggested that "The Martian spaceship landed indeed in Budapest around 1900, then departed, and due to overweight had to leave the less talented Martians behind." It is questionable if de Hevesy really was on the spaceship, since the stranded passengers referred to were all born between 1890 and 1910. De Hevesy was born as early as 1885, but like the true Martians his upbringing was in central Budapest. His background was exceptional, but he never mentioned this even to his closest family.

Both his parents belonged to Jewish families who during the 19th century had risen in society and accumulated considerable wealth. His maternal grandfather was one of the biggest landowners in Hungary and in 1863 was the first non-converted Jew to become a Magyar nobleman. In 1895 his father's family was ennobled too and changed its name from Bischitz to Bisicz de Heves, with time modified to Hevesi de Heves and eventually de Hevesy. In the following, Hevesy will be used without the added *de* or the Germanized *von*. George, sometimes Georg according to the German tradition, was to be one of the eight children of Louis de Hevesy, Court Counsellor, and his wife Eugénie, née Baroness Schosberger. He was the youngest of the first born five boys. All of the boys were brought up in a stern monastic Catholic atmosphere at the Piarist Order at Budapest with emphasis on knowledge in the broad sense, including Latin as well as natural sciences. They went on to have successful careers in different fields. George went his own way and decided to become a scientist.

There are two different principal patterns of cultural development among European Jews. One cultural pattern is to carefully nurse the Jewish traditions in the Diaspora as a means of survival, but the alternative has been to assimilate into society, even to the extent of denying one's Jewish origins. Examples of extensive assimilation can be found in the Austro-Hungarian Empire during the latter half of the nineteenth century[4,5]. The golden age of the Hungarian

Jews during this century is an excellent case in point. At the beginning of the century the percentage of Jews in the Hungarian Kingdom was only about 1.5%, but a century later it had increased to 5%. Most of these lived in the cities and Budapest had as many as 21%. During the century they had become an important factor in the industrial development of the country. They came to have a decisive influence on the development of the financial sector and also the intellectual professions. In 1900 about 50% of all physicians and lawyers were Jewish and the corresponding figure for engineers, scientists in general and authors was 30%. In general these Jews had abandoned Judaism and pursued the Magyar gentry's lifestyle. It was an advance by denial. The Hevesy family is an excellent illustration of this and George himself was a typical example of a refined bourgeois gentleman. Still, behind the surface of cultivation there remained the traits that through centuries had facilitated the societal advance of people with his ethnic background — the ambition, the energy and the maximal exploitation of intellectual resources, developed in challenging dialectics, to reach the defined goals. The emphasis was on becoming and not only on being.

Hevesy started his academic studies in Budapest but soon moved to Berlin and then to Freiburg im Breisgau, where the climate suited his fragile health better. This city retained a Habsburg atmosphere and had been a part of Austria until 1902. There he advanced his studies in physics and chemistry. In 1908 at the age of 23, Hevesy presented his thesis on the interaction of metallic sodium with molten sodium hydroxide under the supervision of George Meyer. He received his *venia legendi* and became "Privatdozent" in December 1912. To further his academic training he continued to Zürich to work at the famous Eidgenössische Technische Hochschule (ETH) with Richard Lorentz in the chemistry department, headed by Richard Willstätter, the forthcoming 1915 Nobel Prize recipient in chemistry. The motivation for his prize, awarded during the early part of the First World War, was "for his research on plant pigments, especially chlorophyll". During Hevesy's time in his department he met Albert Einstein for the first time and Hevesy had a

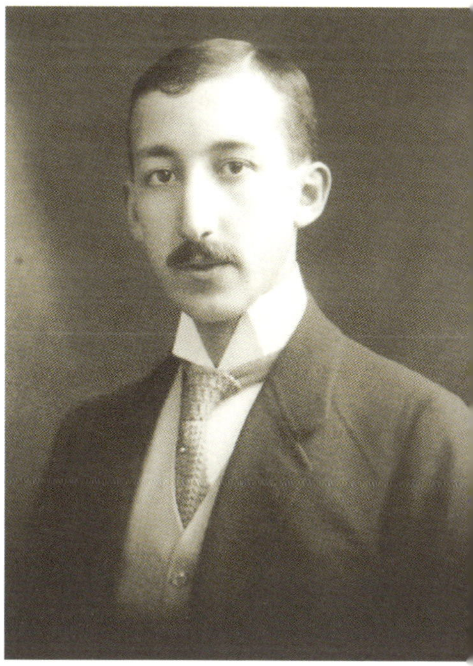

Hevesy in Manchester in 1912. [From Ref. 2.]

unique opportunity, as one of a few, to attend an inaugural lecture given by him at the occasion of his appointment as an associate professor at ETH. Hevesy then moved on to work with Fritz Haber (p. 171) in Karlsruhe, whose interests he deemed to be closer to his own. Haber was later (in 1919) to receive the 1918 Nobel Prize in chemistry "for the synthesis of ammonia from its elements". This was an enormously important achievement because of its application to agriculture — it truly was "to the benefit of mankind" — but the prize was also highly controversial because of Haber's other engagements. He had become listed by the Allied Powers as a war criminal. Hjalmar Branting, who was to become the first social democratic prime minister of Sweden and to receive a shared Nobel Peace Prize in 1921, was very critical of the choice made by the Royal Swedish Academy of Sciences.

Haber was an extreme example of an assimilated Jew. In his patriotic fervor he had instigated the use of chlorine gas which he himself had developed into the form of a weapon. It was employed on many fronts of the war with devastating consequences. This initiative led his wife, herself a qualified chemist, to commit suicide in their garden in 1915 by means of his service pistol. In 1946 their son, who had moved to the US. also committed suicide out of shame over his father's chemical warfare work. At that time it had also become known that the Nazis had developed Zyklon B from Zyklon A, by a refinement of Haber's original work. The B substance, representing a more lethal variant, was the one used to exterminate Jews in the gas chambers at Auschwitz-Birkenau and other camps. Another of Haber's sons, from a second marriage, became a respected historian publishing a book — *The Poisonous Cloud* — about chemical warfare in the First World War. A particular expression of Haber's patriotism was his failed attempts to extract gold from sea water to pay the heavy German war debt after the First World War. The concentration was too low. Possibly there was a romantic underpinning of the imaginative project. Richard Wagner's Ring cycle, *Das Rheingold*, comes to mind.

In the early 1930s when Haber witnessed his fellow Jewish scientists being dismissed from their academic positions he eventually saw the truth of excessive human evil. Realizing that he could not escape the eventual vilification of his own heritage, he finally left for England in 1933, where Rutherford refused to shake his hand. Haber died in Switzerland in 1934 on his way to the Sieff Institute that in 1949 became the Weizmann Institute in the newly re-established Israel, invited by Chaim Weizmann himself. Haber's library remains at the institute.

Rutherford's Laboratory

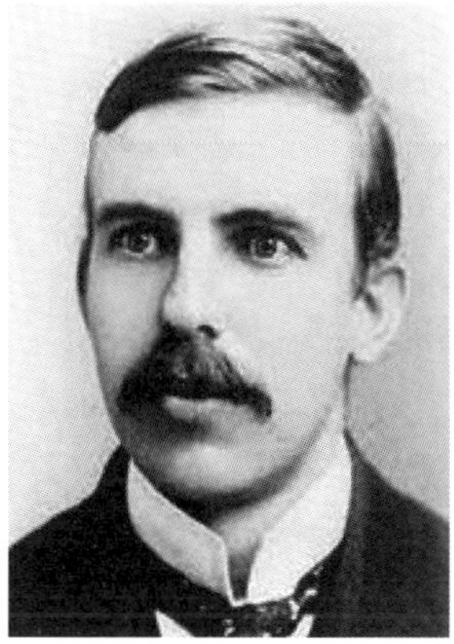

Ernest Rutherford (1871–1937), recipient of the Nobel Prize in chemistry in 1908. [From *Les Prix Nobel en 1908*.]

Hevesy's time with Haber was not as productive as he had hoped for. He wanted in particular to study the effect of oxidation of liquid Na-K alloys by electron emission and in order to learn this he moved after three months to Manchester to work in Rutherford's laboratory. It should be mentioned that Hevesy at the time was financially independent. He was admitted as a research student paying his own fee and with full access to the laboratory facilities. His arrival in Manchester was delayed, since, because of his fragile health, he wanted to avoid the harsh winter there. Rutherford had been awarded the 1908 Nobel Prize in chemistry "for his investigation into the disintegration of the elements, and the chemistry of radioactive substances" and his prestigious laboratory provided a fertile soil for the development of Hevesy's scientific mind. In 1911 he conceived his original idea to use isotopes as indicators to follow the fate of different compounds in various processes in nature. The story has been told innumerable times, including by Hevesy himself in his autobiographical notes and his Nobel lecture[6,7], of how Rutherford said to him "My boy if you are worth your salt you will separate the radium-D (a lead isotope) from all that nuisance of lead". At the time it was known that radium, from Lat. *radius*, a ray (the spoke of a wheel), was a unique radioactive substance. Radium had been identified by Marie and Pierre Curie more than a decade earlier and it was this discovery which led to their shared Nobel Prize in physics in 1903.

After many attempts Hevesy had to conclude that it was impossible to separate lead and radium-D. He then turned the problem around and proposed that the addition of small amounts of a radioactive substance to a compound from which it was inseparable might be a sensitive way of tracing its processing under various given conditions. He was to return to this concept repeatedly during his long and productive scientific career and it came to provide the basis for his most important contributions in science, the ones that earned him a Nobel Prize. Because of his new preoccupations he lost interest in the problems he had originally planned to attack in Haber's laboratory and he therefore never returned to Karlsruhe.

The Rutherford laboratory provided an exceptional breeding environment for young budding scientists and Hevesy made many contacts that were to have a major influence on his future development. His acquaintance with Niels Bohr who came to Manchester in 1912, was to be of the utmost importance. The two scientists developed a rich friendship that lasted throughout their lives. Bohr was fundamentally a shy person and in their interactions this could be given balance by "the young Hungarian aristocrat". This longstanding interaction and mutual admiration can be seen from their rich correspondence. They were born in the same year and came to have their early maturation as scientists in the same creative environment of atomic physics. It was in Bohr's future Institute that Hevesy made his major discoveries.

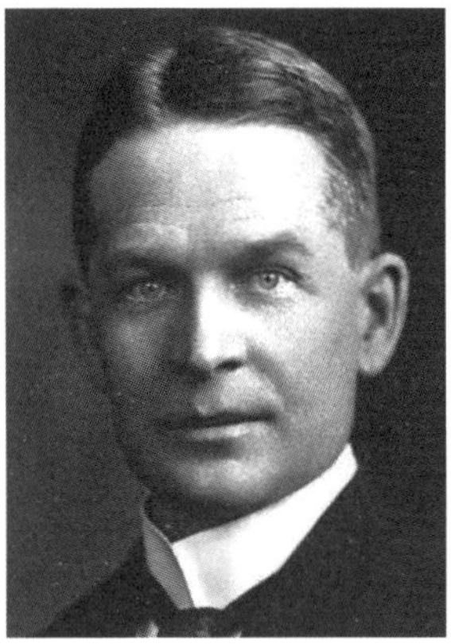

Frederick Soddy (1877–1956), recipient of the 1921 Nobel Prize in chemistry awarded in 1922. [From *Les Prix Nobel en 1921*.]

The atomic nucleus had been discovered and an increasingly clearer picture of the nature and origin of ionizing radiation started to emerge. The term "isotope" had not as yet been coined, but it was understood that substances could behave chemically in an identical way although they had distinct atomic masses. Only a year later the term was introduced by Frederick Soddy, who in 1922 was to receive the reserved 1921 Nobel Prize in chemistry "for his contributions to our knowledge of the chemistry of radioactive substances, and his investigations into the origin and nature of isotopes". The prize in chemistry for 1922 was awarded to Francis W. Aston "for his discovery, by means of his mass spectrograph, of isotopes, in a large number of non-radioactive elements, and for his enunciation of the whole-number rule". The term has its origin in *iso-* meaning the same and Gr. *topos* place. The isotopes of an element occupy the same place in the periodic table. The isotope concept had in fact originally been formulated but not named in Uppsala by Daniel Strömholm and The (Theodore) Svedberg (p. 180). Like many other scientists at the time they were engaged in studying the chemical properties of radioactive substances. Due to lack of follow-up experiments the priority of the discovery was lost to Soddy, who, however, cited their critical 1909 publication in the field in his Nobel lecture[8].

Other relevant topics in the early Manchester days concerned the emission of radiation of different kinds and the modification of products potentially leading to a change of their position in the periodic table. Hevesy was intensely involved in experiments to resolve these kinds of issues. These different topics were the subject of rich discussions between himself and Bohr and came to inspire the latter in his thinking about the nature of the atom. Eventually this conjecturing led to Bohr's model of atoms with multiple layers of electron shells filled to varying degrees with these charged particles. It took time for his model to be accepted by the scientific community but in 1913 it started to make an impact. Hevesy met Einstein in Vienna in September that year and asked him what he thought of Rutherford–Bohr's model. At first he gave only some reserved praise but when he was told about the most recent results he said "This is an enormous achievement. The theory of Bohr must then be right."[9] The pattern of the periodic table became more and more developed and ambitions to make it complete became a central interest of both Bohr and Hevesy as will be discussed below.

Through the experience of working in Rutherford's prestigious Manchester laboratory, Hevesy gained considerably in self-confidence presumably reflecting his privileged upbringing, his superior intellect and his command of experimental science. It is said that he was quick to judge both his own performance and that of other scientists. His own commitments were very demanding and as a result he wore himself out. To recuperate he took a break and returned to Hungary to rest in a nursing home and to enjoy a vacation together with his family. During this intermission he also visited the Radium Institute in Vienna headed by Stefan Meyer, where he discovered that the problem of separating radium D from stable lead, independently, was also being pursued by Fritz A. Paneth and collaborators.

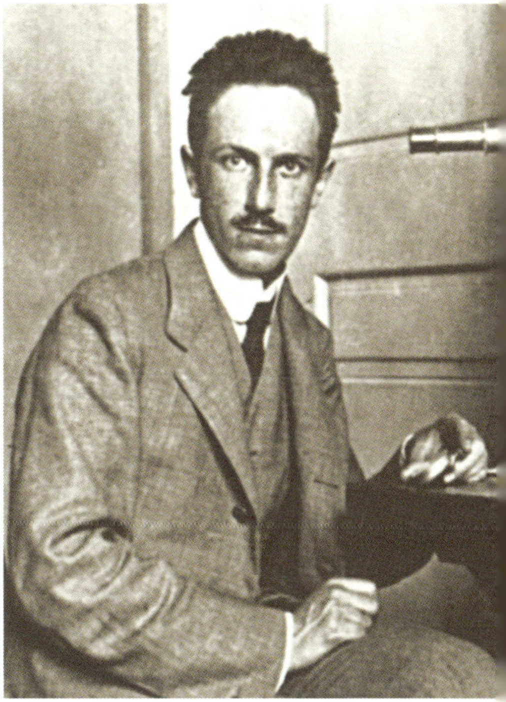

Friedrich (Fritz) A. Paneth (1887–1958). [From Ref. 1.]

In 1912 he made extensive experiments to evaluate the usefulness of radioactive isotopes as indicators of the natural processing of their stable homologues. The foundation was laid for his very successful return to this field some 20 years later — his finest hours crowned by the Nobel Prize. Before that many impressive contributions were to be made. Late the same year he returned to Hungary to formalize his rights to teach at the university by obtaining his "Habilitation" and on the way there he again visited the institute in Vienna and learned more about Paneth's work on the indicator technique. This led to the establishment of a friendship and a long-standing collaboration, both of which developed in a very productive way. They came to publish a number of articles together (cf. Ref. 10). The two scientists complemented each other in an excellent way — Hevesy being the energetic driving force and Paneth the painstaking worker ensuring that the experiments were conducted in a focused and correct way. The important thing to Hevesy was to choose important problems to study, to push through experiments and to publish rapidly to make the discovery known and then if necessary follow up with detailed measurements. Claiming priority is important in scientific endeavors, as in many other competitive human interactions. The friendship established between the two scientists lasted throughout life and can be followed in their frequent correspondence. Paneth became one of the rare people with whom Hevesy was willing to share his innermost thoughts. Stimulated by his personal contacts with Friedrich Nietzsche and Sigmund Freud, he also made a good partner for discussion of philosophical problems.

The Turmoil of the First World War

For shorter periods of time Hevesy attempted to develop his science in Budapest, to work in Vienna with Paneth and to learn X-ray spectroscopy from one of Rutherford's more promising pupils, Henry G. J. Moseley, who had established himself in Oxford. During 1912–1913 Hevesy managed a laboratory at the College of Veterinary Medicine in Budapest. The outbreak of the First World War on July 28, 1914 created havoc in international collaborations and Moseley was tragically killed in the battle of Gallipoli. As a Hungarian citizen, Hevesy had to serve in the army but he was soon found to be seriously unfit for this. He was therefore ordered to perform special tasks, which he could combine with certain scientific activities at the Budapest University of Sciences. He managed to continue his collaboration with Paneth at a distance and a number of joint papers were published. Times became hard and the academic work was interrupted by the special tasks Hevesy had been allocated. He had a particular insight into the technique of using electrolytic separation of copper and other metals from bronze alloys. This technique he developed first at a factory in Nagyteteny-Diosd, south of Budapest and later at the copper works in Beszterczebanya, a small town then in the far north of Hungary. One of his tasks was to supervise the melting of old church bells taken from the Balkan countries to produce copper for military use. Prior to the melting of the bells they were smashed to pieces by Russian prisoners of war. Hevesy disliked his wartime responsibilities intensively, but tried to rationalize them to ensure that he got time to pursue his science.

He was able frequently to return to Budapest where intellectual exchange with a number of qualified Hungarian scientists provided important stimuli during the harsh conditions caused by shortage of food and energy. In order to take advantage of all the non-productive time Hevesy proposed to Paneth that they should write a joint book about radioactivity. Hevesy accelerated his engagement in the project but Paneth for various reasons, including the contentious part of his nature, was slower to join in. It would take several years before the book finally was published[11], but before that a lot of things had happened. When the war finally ended Hevesy was able at last to return to Budapest from his isolated temporary posting in the northern part of the country. The maps of central Europe were redrawn; the region of Beszterczebanya was occupied by the Czech republic and Hungary and Austria were separated and became republics.

In Budapest he was able to take up a position at the university, holding a department chair at the Second Experimental Physics Institute. He employed a number of qualified scientists, including the talented chemist Michael Polanyi. Later Polanyi moved, first to Berlin and then he eventually settled in Manchester, England. Later in life he became involved in the philosophy of science and wrote books focusing on two themes in particular. These were tacit knowledge and the hermeneutics of suspicion. He used the term "tacit" to describe implied or silently acquiescent insights going beyond textbook knowledge, a particular quality guiding successful scientists. The second theme was his stated opinion that philosophers who argued that the primary driving force of scientists was to gain power and/or financial profit were wrong. He even argued that this interpretation was a way of poisoning the well of scientific discovery. One needs only to review the discoveries recognized by Nobel prizes to appreciate that Polanyi was right on this point. Michael Polanyi's son John also became a famous chemist. He developed his science in Canada and shared the 1986 Nobel Prize in Chemistry.

In November 1918 the republic of Hungary was established and the liberal politician Graf Karolyi became leader of the country. The famous aerodynamic technologist Theodore von Kármán became minister of culture and Hevesy was appointed professor in physical chemistry at the Budapest University

Gustav Buschböck. Very soon there was additional political turmoil. The Communist pro-Russian Béla Kun, a friend of Lenin, took over power after another revolution. In spite of this change it was possible for von Kármán and Hevesy to continue with their plans to improve conditions at the University. However this did not last long because the allied powers did not like the Communist regime in Hungary. In the early summer Romanian troops invaded the country and Kun had to flee. Admiral Horthy returned to power and the "white terror" followed and in its trail overt anti-Semitism emerged. Von Kármán had to return to a professorship in Aachen which he had temporarily left and in 1934 he eventually left for his final homeland, the United States, where he made a spectacular career. There developed a mounting threat to Hevesy's position at the university and also to his financial resources, originating in his family's wealth and properties. He had to resign from his academic position but attempted temporarily to continue some experimentation at the College of Veterinary Medicine, where he had worked before. Eventually he felt forced to leave Budapest. In desperation, he finally called upon his particular friend Bohr, who quickly read his signals.

Bohr's reputation was growing rapidly and in 1920 a new institute was to be opened for his expanding activities. During a visit by Hevesy to Copenhagen in 1919 it had been decided that he should return to join the new institute in 1920. Eventually Bohr managed to secure a scholarship from the Rask-Örsted Foundation established by Danish law in October 1919 "for the support of Danish science in connection with international research". This Foundation came to support Hevesy for a stay of six years in total with Bohr. Before Hevesy's departure from Budapest the situation went from bad to worse as an epidemic of anti-Semitism grew and flourished. It can be seen from his correspondence with Paneth that Hevesy worried a lot about the future. He was grateful for the opportunity to work next to Bohr — "this unique human being" — but what were the possibilities for a long term development of his scientific talents considering the language, financial, and also climatic difficulties in Denmark?

The First Stay with Bohr — The Hafnium Years

It was a relief to Hevesy to be able to leave the tumultuous and increasingly hostile atmosphere of Budapest and in April 1920 he set out for Copenhagen. He traveled via Berlin to meet up with Bohr, who had been invited to give a lecture in that city on his atomic theory. The lecture was received with exceptional

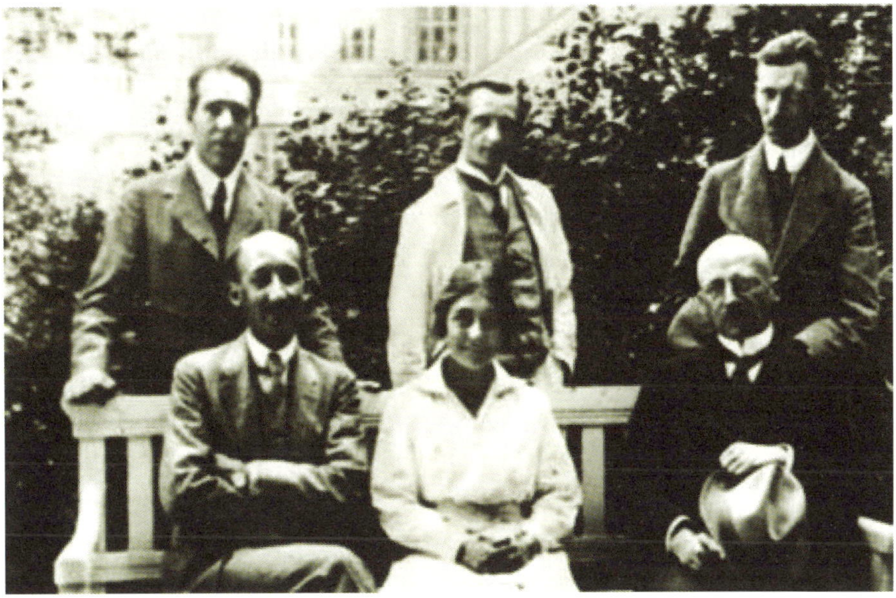

Group photo at the Bohr Institute in the early 1920s. Front row: Hevesy, Mrs A. Delbanco and Haber; back row: Bohr, E. Güntelberg, and Johannes N. Brönsted. [From Ref. 1.]

enthusiasm and the two scientists arrived in high spirits in Copenhagen. This state of mind did not last long for Hevesy. The completion of Bohr's new building was delayed and it would take about a year before it finally opened. In the meantime Hevesy had tried to manage his listlessness and depression by finishing off the writing of several articles and working on the joint book with Paneth, who at the time had moved to Hamburg. For considerable periods Hevesy had problems with insomnia, which he himself explained as due to restlessness. On Bohr's advice he spent some time at a convalescent home called Montebello in North Zealand, but the only form of leisure, besides walks in nature, that he knew of was reading of scientific material. Nevertheless some experimental work was in fact performed together with Johannes N. Brönsted and colleagues at Copenhagen Technical University. Brönsted was a highly respected chemist and a particular authority on catalysis and acid-base theory. Brönsted and Hevesy together applied fractional distillation to separate isotopes, in particular of mercury and chlorine.

Bohr's institute eventually opened in March 1921 and it was promptly filled by a number of visiting scientists besides talented Danish students[9]. Hereby began what for a number of decades became the Mecca for advanced studies in theoretical physics. No other place has been the host of more already recognized or forthcoming Nobel laureates in physics than the Bohr Institute in Copenhagen. When the new building opened Hevesy's situation was stabilized. The problem whose solution in particular challenged him derived from Bohr's now famous theory that the atomic nucleus was surrounded by layers of shells, each of which could only contain a fixed number of electrons. It was postulated that the properties of elements were determined by the mass and charge of the nucleus and the degree to which the outermost shell was filled with electrons. This model made it possible to explain the fixed properties of elements at regular intervals moving from lighter to heavier entities. Hence a theoretical background could be provided to the well-established periodic table originally developed by the Russian scientist Dimitri I. Mendeleev.

Mendeleev's periodic table was developed by use of the 63 elements known at the time. The predictive value of the table became apparent within a few years of its presentation in the early 1860s when new elements were discovered that fitted into the empty gaps identified by Mendeleev. In 1879 Lars Nilson at Uppsala University discovered an element named scandium that fitted into a space in between calcium and titanium and some years later Clemens Winkler at Freiburg University identified a semi-metal named germanium which filled a gap between silicon and tin. The important discovery of the periodic table could have been recognized by a Nobel Prize in chemistry in 1906, had it not been for a single member of the committee, Peter Klason. He managed single-handedly to swing the opinion of the Academy away from Mendeleev to choose Henry Moissan for the prize "in recognition of the great services rendered by him in his investigation and isolation of the element fluorine, and the adoption in the service of science of the electric furnace called after him". Mendeleev died the following year, as did Moissan, and the mistake could never be corrected. The background to this major omission by the Academy was recently described in a book[12].

According to Bohr's atomic model it was the electrons located in the outermost shell that determined the chemical properties of an element and elements with shared properties formed the groups 1–18 in the periodic table. When these rules were applied it was found that six elements, numbers 43, 61, 72, 75, 85, 87, remained to be identified among the potentially naturally existing 92 elements of the periodic table recognized at that time. In the case of element 72, a French group headed by Georges Urbain argued that they had already identified this as a member of the rare earth elements. This group of elements includes 17 members of group 3 in the periodic table; number 21 scandium, number 39 yttrium and numbers 57–71, referred to as the lanthanides from the first member in the group, lanthanum. As a curiosity it can be mentioned that the first rare earth element was discovered by the Swedish Lieutenant Carl Axel Arrhenius in 1787 in minerals from a quarry at the village of Ytterby and since then a number of elements in the group have been identified by Swedish chemists and metallurgists, as is evident from their names; scandium, yttrium, terbium, holmium (from Stockholm, Lat. Holmia), erbium, ytterbium and thulium. The number of rare earth elements remained unclear for a long time. It was first when Moseley managed to deduce, from the X-ray spectra he had generated, that the precise number of lanthanides should be 15 and that in this group element 61 remained to be identified. Moseley's data together with Bohr's atomic model allowed the prediction that element 72 should not be a member of group 3 of the periodic table, as proposed by Urbain, but instead of group 4, which includes titanium and zirconium. As a result of this insight the Copenhagen group decided to isolate element 72.

The most important technique to characterize new compounds was the X-ray spectroscopy originally developed by Charles G. Barkla and by Moseley. In 1918 Barkla himself, in the absence of Moseley, because of his untimely death, alone received the 1917 Nobel Prize in physics "for his discovery of the characteristic Röntgen radiation of the elements". The spectroscopic technique was further developed by K. Manne Siegbahn of Lund in Sweden, who also received a Nobel Prize in physics. His prize was for 1924, awarded in 1925 and the motivation was "for his discoveries and research in the field of X-ray spectroscopy". In order to have access to the most advanced form of the technique at the institute Bohr invited a researcher from Holland, Dirk Coster, who had received his training with Siegbahn. He arrived in September 1922. This allowed for an attempt to discover the unidentified element.

Coster's familiarity with advanced X-ray spectroscopy and the special interest in geochemistry that Hevesy had developed during the summer were important factors favoring the pursuit. Following Bohr's predictions zirconium minerals were used as suspected host structures for the missing element. The Geological Museum of Copenhagen provided zirconium minerals from Norway and Greenland. Another important source of minerals was the Swiss-born geochemist Victor M. Goldschmidt. Hevesy had made his acquaintance already during his student years in Freiburg and in the 1920s he held a professorship in Oslo. The samples of alvite from Norway that he provided turned out to be very rich in the element they were searching for. The first step in the study was to develop chemical methods that could enrich the unknown element from this material. This was Hevesy's responsibility and he was lucky in the approach taken. He started by dissolving in hydrogen fluoride as much of each piece of zirconium material as he had available and then concentrating the unknown element by crystallizing it in the form of double fluorides. It was found that compound 72 had become so enriched that the 6–7 spectral lines already postulated by Moseley could be identified and agreement with Bohr's theory could be secured. This triumphal discovery was rapidly published in a series of papers (cf. Refs. 13 and 14).

During this time period, in 1922, Bohr was awarded the Nobel Prize in physics "for his services in the investigation of the structure of atoms and of the radiation emanating from them". At the time close to the prize ceremony on December 10 the critical data on element 72 were still being collected, but after the banquet at the Grand Hotel, Hevesy managed to reach Bohr by phone and tell him that he and Coster now were certain they had discovered element 72. Hereafter Hevesy took the night train to Stockholm and managed to be present at Bohr's Nobel lecture the following day on "The structure of the atom"[15]. This was his first visit to what would become his final homeland. Towards the end of his talk Bohr announced the finding of the new element and the special significance of the discovery for the new atomic theory, a climactic closure exciting the audience.

Hevesy's and Coster's findings were not well received by all parts of the scientific community. Completely irrational national chauvinistic considerations and questions of academic specialization came into play. New elements should be discovered by chemists and not by physicists intruding on their turf. The French group led by Urbain persisted in claiming that they had already identified the element, which they called celtium (Ct). They insisted that their discovery was supported by X-ray data obtained by a fellow Frenchman Alexandre Dauvillier. It took a long time before it was generally acknowledged that the French data were incorrect and the name hafnium (Hf) derived from the Latinized form of the name of the city of Copenhagen became the one finally accepted. Remarkably French scientists still today write Ct instead of Hf when the periodic table is presented in French scientific textbooks.

The Copenhagen group had been divided during discussions about the naming of the new element, with Coster and Bohr's collaborator Hendrik Kramers arguing for hafnium and Bohr himself and Hevesy instead preferring danium. Hevesy published some thirty publications about hafnium. He naturally had some hopes that the newly discovered element might have some particular use in technical applications. It came as a disappointment when, at the time, no such applications could be identified. If he had survived beyond the 1970s he would have learned about a number of important uses. It has been discovered that the hafnium-tantalum carbide $HfTa_4C_5$ has the highest melting point ever identified in a material. But hafnium has been found to have other useful properties too. It absorbs neutrons with a high degree of efficiency and is therefore used as a moderator in control rods for nuclear power plants. More recently it has been found to be of importance for the development of the semiconductor industry. Thin films of hafnium oxide have superior insulating properties and thus less electron leakage than films conventionally made of silicon dioxide in the design of miniaturized integrated circuits.

Table 5.1. The last six naturally occurring elements to be discovered.

Element	Symbol	Time of discovery	Discoverer(s)	Character
Hafnium	^{72}Hf	1922	D. Coster G. Hevesy	Stable
Rhenium	^{75}Re	1925	O. Berg W. Noddack I. Tacke	Stable
Technetium	^{43}Tc	1936	C. Perrier E. Segrè	Unstable
Francium	^{87}Fr	1939	M. Perey	Unstable
Astatine	^{85}At	1940	D. R. Corson K. R. Mackenzie E. Segrè	Unstable
Prometium	^{61}Pm	1945	Oak Ridge Laboratory team	Unstable

Hafnium was one of the last stable isotope elements to be discovered in Nature (Table 5.1). Inspired by the discovery of hafnium three of Hevesy's Freiburg colleagues, Walter Noddack and Ida Tacke together with Otto Berg, identified element number 75, rhenium, three years later. At the same time they announced the discovery of the missing element 43 — there was an empty position in between molybdenum (element 42) and ruthenium (element 44) — for which they suggested the name masurium. The "discovery", which Hevesy regarded with some amusement, was however soon disqualified and it was not until 1936 that Emilio Segrè and Carlo Perrier showed that the element technetium — it received this name because it had to be artificially made — was radioactive with a half life of 4.2 million years of its most long-lived isotope. Consequently, if originally present in the Earth's crust, it would since long have

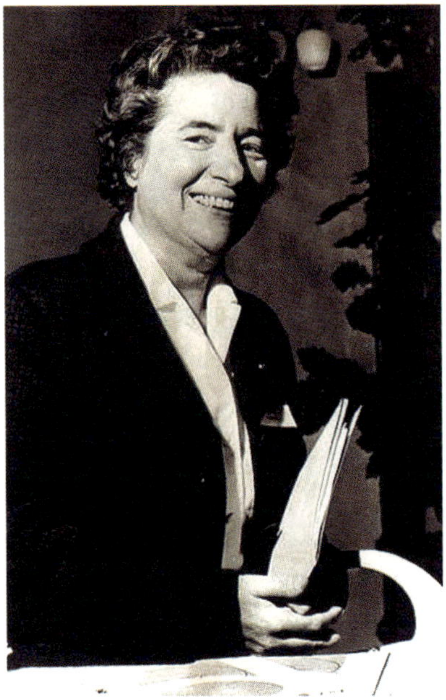

Marguerite Perey (1909–1975). Discoverer of the element francium and th first woman to be elected to the French Academy of Sciences.

disappeared except in minute quantities as an unstable decay product of uranium. As mentioned there were also other missing elements, like number 87, to search for. Hevesy and also Otto Hahn in Berlin attempted to identify this element in the mid 1920s, but failed. It would take until 1939 before Marguerite Perey eventually managed to find it as a radioactive decay product in uranium ores. It became the last among the naturally occurring 92 elements to be discovered in nature and it is the second rarest of all of them because of its instability.

Perey had a background as a test-tube washer in Marie Curie's laboratory but rose to become a famous scientist. She was the first woman to become a member of the French Academy of Sciences in 1962, a recognition that had eluded both Madame Curie and also her daughter Irene Joliot-Curie. The original name for the element was catium, but when the name had to be finally settled in 1947 it was for circumstantial reasons changed to francium, Perey's second choice for a name. Perhaps this provided some consolation for the fact that the discovery and the name celtium proposed by Urbain were never internationally accepted. Perey was nominated repeatedly for a Nobel Prize for her identification of francium, the first time in 1952. Her contribution was reviewed by the committee, which in its summary concluded:

> Marguerite Perey's supplementation of the periodic system by the heavy and radioactive alkali metal 87 francium and her studies of the properties of this element undoubtedly are worth being recognized but it does not have an importance which would motivate it to be recognized by a Nobel Prize.

She was nominated again in 1958 and 1961 and it is possible that she was also proposed after 1962, but this cannot be identified at the time of writing, because of the 50 years secrecy rule. The 1961 nomination had a nice formulation, which however did not make the committee swing into action. It read (freely translated from French):

> … Mrs Marguerite Perey (who is nominated) for her discovery of element 87, named francium, is in fact seriously ill, a victim (of exposure) to radioactivity. To recognize her contribution would be a universal act of humanity and a Christian act of charity."

Like Marie Curie, Perey had been heavily exposed to radioactive material in the early phase of her career, at the time an unknown occupational hazard. However, even though she was apparently seriously ill already in 1961, she survived until 1975 when she died of the radiation-induced cancer she had developed. In the later years of her life she received a number of honors, sealed in 1974 by the Commandeur de l'Ordre National du Mérite.

After the discovery of francium there remained only two elements to be identified. They had to be artificially produced. In 1940 Dale R. Corson, Kenneth R. MacKenzie and Segrè managed to produce element 85 which came to be called astatine. Later it was found that this labile element, produced as a result of the decay of heavier elements, did in fact occur in nature but only in exceedingly small amounts. It is the least abundant among the non-transuranium elements in the Earth's crust. In 1945 the last empty slot in the periodic table was filled in. Element 61, named promethium, was synthesized at the Oak Ridge National Laboratory in the US. This element has no stable isotope.

In 1953 Segrè was nominated for the first time for his discovery of technetium and astatine. His contributions were reviewed by Arne F. Westgren, a professor of physical chemistry and long term chairman of the Nobel committee and also Permanent Secretary of the Royal Swedish Academy of Sciences, who we will meet again in this chapter and also repeatedly in Chapters 7 and 8. Based on his review the committee concluded:

> … his contributions to filling in the last empty spaces in the periodic system without doubt are very large but they are still not sufficient to become recognized by a Nobel Prize in chemistry. If Segrè were to receive such recognition it would be appropriate by the same token for Mrs Marguerite Perey, who was proposed last year for her discovery of the element 87 (francium) and by Marinsky, Glendenin and Coryell for their synthesis of the element 61 (promethium) to also receive a prize. The fact that so many researchers in later years have contributed with great success to the completion of the periodic system demonstrates that the difficulties that they have had to surmount have not been

> overwhelmingly large. Disregarding McMillan's and Seaborg's discovery within the chemistry of the transuranian elements, which two years ago received their well deserved recognition (the 1953 Nobel Prize in chemistry recognized Edwin M. Mattison and Glenn T. Seaborg from the USA "for their discoveries in the chemistry of the transuranum elements", my remark) one can note that the developments seen during the later years within the field of radioactive elements and synthesis of them are to be regarded as having been possible to anticipate and as not too surprising consequences of the rapid development of techniques within nuclear research. The discovery of technetium and astatine has their origin in Lawrence's construction of the cyclotron. Hence the committee cannot find support for Segrè's candidature.

Besides the prize to Mattison and Seaborg it is only during the first decade of awarding Nobel Prizes that the identification of new elements has been recognized. A particular example is the prize in chemistry in 1904 to William Ramsay. His addition of a whole group of gaseous elements which completed the periodic system by the addition of group 18 was considered highly worthy of a prize. This also applied to Marie Curie's studies of radium and polonium awarded with a prize in chemistry in 1911, her second Nobel Prize. It was much more debatable if the above-mentioned chemistry prize in 1906 to Moissan, recognizing his investigations and isolation of the element fluorine, had been a fair choice.

The discovery of hafnium made Hevesy a famous scientist. He received several invitations to lecture in different parts of Europe, including participating in the famous yearly Solvay meetings of physicists in Belgium. As might have been expected, there were speculations at the time about the possibility that the discovery of element 72 would be recognized by a Nobel Prize.

The Deliberations by the Nobel Committee on the Discovery of Hafnium

Hevesy was proposed for the first time for a Nobel Prize in chemistry in 1924. Three separate nominations were submitted by researchers in Dresden and they cite the discovery of hafnium. A similar joint nomination was also given by two additional researchers from Dresden, but this nomination also included Coster. Henrik G. Söderbaum, a member of the Nobel committee, made a five pages long evaluation. He first noted that the nominations in an exceptional manner fulfilled the criterion in Nobel's will by the fact that the discovery was published the previous year. He then concluded that the identification of a new element, named hafnium, closely related to zirconium, was important but that it was dependent on the availability of the improved technique for measuring the emission of X-rays originally developed by Barkla and Moseley, further improved by Siegbahn, and also on Bohr's theory about the structure of the atoms, already recognized by a prize in physics. For these reasons the discovery was not considered to be of sufficient magnitude to be recognized by a prize. By contrast the studies by Georges Urbain and Auer von Welsbach to find new elements among the rare earth metals were viewed as being more demanding. Still these discoveries had not been considered worthy of a prize in previous evaluations. Söderbaum also discussed the claims by the French group led by Urbain that they had already discovered element 72 in their work on rare earth metals and named it "celtium". He concluded that the claims were incorrect and that the Copenhagen group had priority both in the discovery and the naming. The review ended as follows:

> Departing from the fundamental premises that Nobel Prizes should be reserved for research contributions of more fundamental nature, the discovery of hafnium, although fully confirmed, could hardly be seriously considered for a prize this year, even when consideration is taken to how beautiful and meritorious it must be considered to be and what a justifiable sensation it has caused.

It would take three more years before the discovery of hafnium was again recommended for a prize. One nomination from M. Le Blanc from Leipzig proposed de Hevesy and Coster, whereas another from J. Perrin in Paris recommended Urbain and Hevesy. There was also a separate nomination of Urbain. The committee did not make a new evaluation but a reference was made to previous reviews of Urbain made by Söderbaum in 1923 and 1926 and his above-mentioned 1924 review of Hevesy and Coster. The committee concluded that nothing new had been added which at the time would motivate it to recommend the discovery of element 72 for a prize. In 1929, after another two years, there were five nominations from scientists in Berlin. One of them was from Paneth, who had now moved to this city. All of them included both Hevesy and Coster and in one case also, as a third candidate, Bohr. One of the nominators was Otto Hahn (p. 217), who was later to be awarded the Nobel

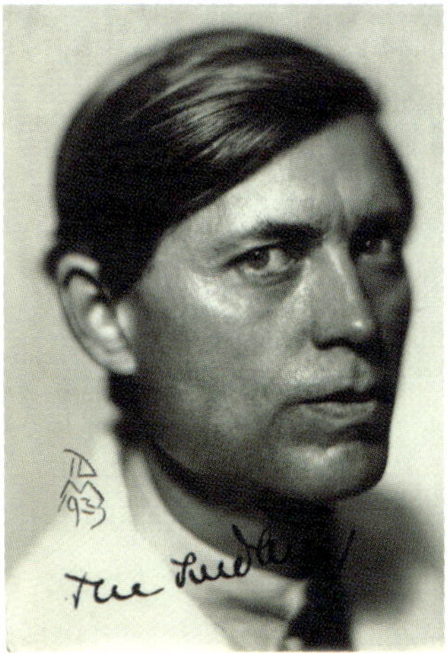
The (Theodor) Svedberg (1884–1971), recipient of the Nobel Prize in chemistry in 1926.

Prize in chemistry for 1944 "for his discovery of the fission of heavy nuclei", received in 1945. Hahn's nomination did not only mention the discovery of hafnium, but also Hevesy's and Paneth's work on radioactive indicators. This was the first time that the use of radioactive indicators was proposed. A new evaluator was the recipient of the 1926 Nobel Prize in chemistry Theodor (The) Svedberg. Although he was rewarded "for his work on disperse systems" he was especially well familiarized with isotope work, as already mentioned. Because Svedberg was to become heavily involved in evaluating Hevesy's science a brief digression presenting his background will be made.

Svedberg was born in 1884 and he defended his PhD in chemistry at Uppsala University in 1908 and was appointed professor of physical chemistry in 1912. In 1913 he was elected a very young member of the Royal Swedish Academy of Sciences in the class of physics. In 1933 he was moved to the class for chemistry. His rapidly rising star also led to nominations for a Nobel Prize in chemistry. In 1926 Svedberg was elected a member of the Nobel committee for chemistry, a responsibility he was to carry for decades to come (Chapter 7). The year 1926 became very special in the annals of the Nobel Prize for physics and chemistry as has been discussed by Friedman[16]. The first problem confronting Svedberg as a member of the committee was that he himself had been nominated for a prize. The 1920 Nobel laureate Walter H. Nernst had proposed, as his second alternative, Jean B. Perrin and Svedberg for the prize. This was solved by the committee in the following way. After the list of nominated candidates in the beginning of its annual report the committee stated:

> The deliberations by the committee, in the first place, have focused on the alternative nomination by W. Nernst for a joint prize between J. Perrin and Mr T. Svedberg. In this context it (the committee) expressed the unanimous opinion that this proposal in its present form was not of such a kind that it could be used by the committee as a proposal of its own. Thus it would be possible for Svedberg to participate in the treatment of the remaining proposals (of candidates).

Svedberg reviewed the candidate Richard A. Zsigmondy, whom he himself had proposed. The committee was so impressed by Svedberg's analysis that it decided to recommend Zsigmondy for the reserved 1925 Nobel Prize in chemistry and to reserve the 1926 prize for the coming year. However this was not to the taste of the academy members when they met on November 11 to decide on the prize. There was a revolt initiated by the academy member Carl Benedicks, a physicist who was Director of the Metallographic Institute in Stockholm. He pointed out that it was 25 years after the first Nobel Prizes had been awarded and that therefore it would not be appropriate to withhold the 1926 prize in physics. He managed to make the members of the academy override the committee of physics and select his own favorite Jean B. Perrin, who had since long been written off by the committee. And once he got started he also scooped the committee of chemistry by getting a majority for awarding the 1926 prize in chemistry to his countryman Svedberg. These events explain how Svedberg could receive his Nobel Prize "for his work on disperse systems" the same year that he had become a member of the Nobel committee of chemistry.

Let us now return to Svedberg's evaluation of Hevesy. It was brief and covered two pages, with half of the text discussing Hevesy's work on isotopes. It mentioned some important achievements but it concluded succinctly that "The contributions that de Hevesy has made to our knowledge of separation of isotopes are not of such importance that they deserve to be awarded by a Nobel Prize". Svedberg was somewhat more positive than the previous evaluators to the discovery of hafnium as a candidate for a Nobel Prize. He noted the previous decisions by the committee not to put the hafnium discovery forward for a prize, but he emphasized that the discovery of this element had come to play a particularly important role in further developments. Hafnium had been used as a touchstone of deepening understanding of structural conditions providing a basis for the periodic system. He argued that: "The discovery of hafnium therefore seems to exceed, with a wide margin, the importance of discoveries of other elements made recently (masurium, rhenium, illinium). The proposal to reward this discovery by a joint prize to de Hevesy and Coster in this year seems to be better motivated than before." In spite of this upgrading of the discovery, the final conclusion was still that the magnitude of the discovery did not reach the level required for a prize. Regarding Bohr's possible inclusion among the prize recipients it was noted that he already had received a prize.

The last time that the discovery of hafnium was discussed by the Nobel committee was in 1933 when Hevesy and Coster had been nominated by

K. L. Wagner, Prague. This year the committee, as evidenced by the archival materials, had had a general discussion about the importance of discoveries of new elements for the prize. It gave the foundation for the highly selective attitude already discussed above. The conclusion of the committee was that only true pioneers should be recognized and that Hevesy and Coster did not belong among them. The prize money was reserved this year.

The Age of the Earth and the Rare Earth Elements

One can distinguish three phases of intensified creativity in Hevesy's career. The first one (1923–1928) was the intense focusing on the characterization of element 72, as already discussed, and the second one, which concerned cosmochemistry and geochemistry, overlapped with and connected to the previous phase and lasted until about 1936. Thereafter he became completely absorbed by the problems of using isotopes for studies of biological phenomena, an engagement that kept him fully occupied until his death in 1966.

Hevesy's interest in what today is generally referred to as earth and space science derived naturally from his curiosity about how the presence of elements in the universe might be deduced from their radioactivity and nuclear stability[17]. Charles Darwin in his 1859 book *The Origin of Species* had assumed, on the basis of geological evidence, that the earth was some 300 million years old. He reduced this "guestimate" after being impressed by authoritative statements by the Irish-Scottish mathematician-physicist Lord Kelvin, born William Thomson. Based on the assumption that the heat from the sun originated in gravitational contraction and that the Earth had cooled from a molten state, he had calculated the cooling of its crust by thermal radiation to have taken only 20 million years. In his first paper on the age of the earth, in 1923[18], Hevesy, in a confirmatory statement, commented on the potential importance of radioactive decay and hydrogen fusion as sources of energy emanating from the sun. These sources were not known to Kelvin and invalidated his age estimate as being far too small. As an alternative method for geological and cosmic age determination Hevesy discussed a possible use of the immutable decay of radioactive elements. Isotopes introduced at a single specific time could serve as a clock with the degree of decay providing a measure of time. This was not a new idea. It had already been proposed by Rutherford and Bertram Boltwood. The question was which element to use and how to ensure that an accurate estimation of the radioactive decay could be

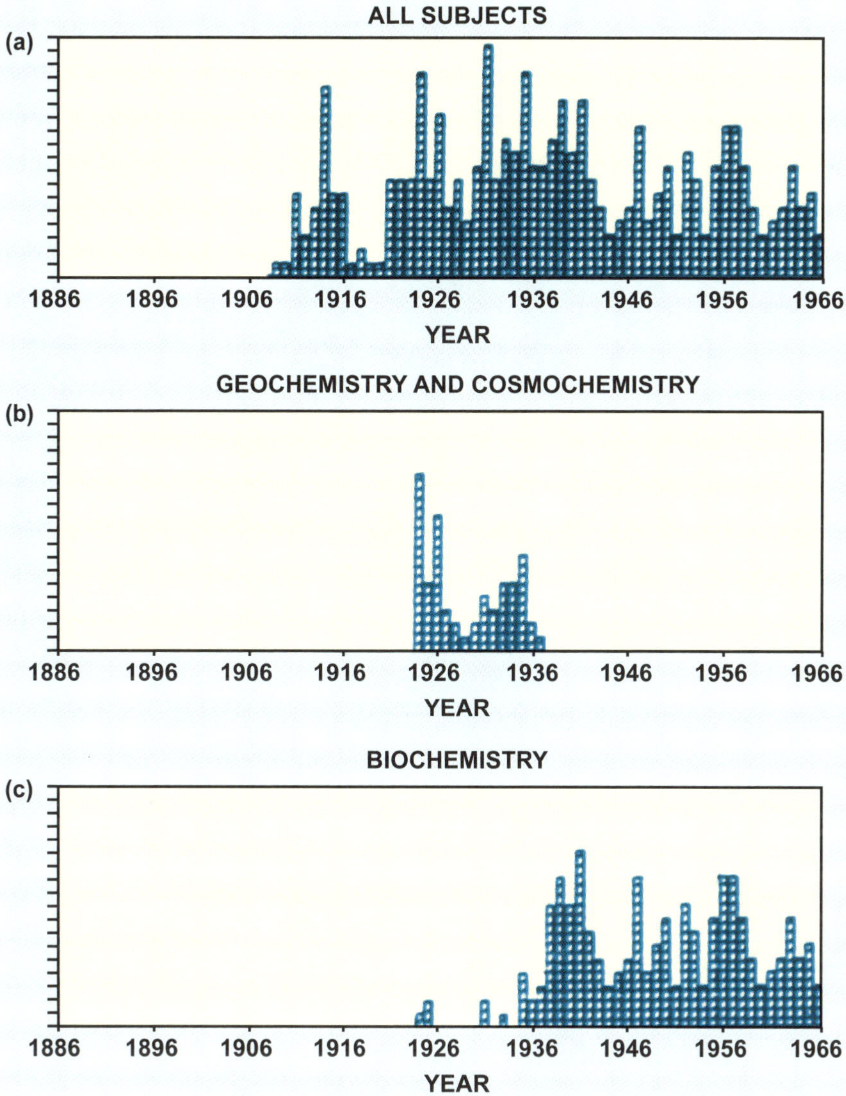

Hevesy's different research interests summarized into a graph of his publications over time. His particular focus on hafnium and geochemistry and cosmochemistry in general and his all-consuming engagement in the use of isotopes in biochemical studies from the mid-1930s have been illustrated separately. [Figure modified from Ref. 17.]

made. He discussed the possible use of the ratio of uranium/lead and thorium/lead to determine the age of crystallized minerals. Taking into consideration that the minerals would have pre-existed in a molten form he calculated a figure of 6000–7000 million years, but pointed out that this value would be lowered if additional lead isotopes were to be found.

Hevesy did not pursue these early speculations and experiments, most probably because he became absorbed by his studies of hafnium. However, it is evident from his further publications on this theme[19,20] that he retained an interest in the problem. He extended the search for other naturally radioactive elements of potential use for geochronological purposes. When he eventually came to make the experiments he had shifted his focus from lead to other isotopes, which he decided at the time would offer better opportunities for studies of nuclear structure and systematics. Zirconium and hafnium as well as the related elements titanium, niobium and tantalum, the latter two being members of the neighboring group 5 in the periodic table, were included in the studies but their main focus was the rare earth elements. The reason for this choice was a well-known problem that Hevesy wanted to avoid. This was that different intermediate daughter elements, e.g. in the uranium-thorium-lead-helium chains, end up in or pass through different groups in the periodic table and therefore are subjected to different geochemical fractionation processes. In contrast any purported radioactive elements well within the lanthanide series, undergoing single step decay, would form daughter elements remaining in this series and therefore have closely similar chemical properties, protected against selective export. In view of this chemical coherence, Hevesy systematically searched the entire lanthanide series of elements for traces of activity, except for thulium, presumably because of lack of a suitable sample. Only in one single element — in all four samples that he had of element 62, samarium — did he find activity, so he could establish that it was due to alpha particle (=helium 4) emission, indicating the samarium was decaying to an isotope of element 60, neodymium with four fewer mass units than the parent samarium isotope. It was important to ascertain that none of the observed alpha emission was contributed by the preceding element 61 which at the time had not been identified. Much later element 61 was demonstrated to be a short-lived nuclide called promethium, as mentioned above (Table 5.1, p. 175).

For this and other studies Hevesy needed access to as many of the rare earth elements as possible. For some years back he had had contacts with the above-mentioned renowned geochemist Goldschmidt and the private scientist Carl Auer von Welsbach. The latter Austrian nobleman, a Baron and scholar, carried out frontier-breaking research in his castle in Kärnten, Austria. Among other things he was the first to identify element 59, praseodymium, and number 60, neodymium. He generously shared his envied collection of natural rare earth compounds with Hevesy. The majority of these samples were found by Hevesy to contain radioactive impurities from uranium and thorium series elements, leading to erroneous claims by other workers, and Hevesy had to expend a lot of effort on purification to guarantee the reliability of his data. In the end it was only samarium that could be identified as a naturally radioactive surviving species among the rare earth elements. The low activity of the samarium was compromising the accuracy of the measurements if carried out by the current methods and Hevesy ascribed his success to the new counting techniques developed by his friend Hans Geiger at Rutherford's institute. Based on the half-life deduced for the radioactive samarium Hevesy estimated 3×10^9 years as a possible age for the Earth[20], which is not too far from the current estimate discussed below.

Other scientists were also pursuing the problem of radioactivity among the earth elements. One of them was Willard F. Libby, who used 57 lanthanum and 60 neodymium in his studies. However, it was politely pointed out by Hevesy that the activities recorded were most likely due to contamination by nuclides of the uranium and thorium series. These constructive comments were of certain concern to Libby, at the time a young scientist. Much later, in 1960, he was to receive the Nobel Prize in Chemistry "for his method to use carbon-14 for age determination in archeology, geology, geophysics and other branches of science". In time Libby came to reconcile himself to the criticism of his early work by Hevesy, not least since Hevesy came to precede him by 16 years as a chemistry Nobel Prize recipient. Over a number of years the two of them had close professional contacts, but their principal use of radioisotopes developed in different directions. Libby used radiocarbon as a clock in studies of materials from earlier settled human civilizations, which is discussed further at the end of this chapter.

To return to the question of the age of the Earth it would take some 40 years before scientists would again pick up on the application of the decay of radioactive samarium for the purpose of its determination. It was the Austrian physicist Günther Lugmair working at the University of California San Diego who refined the mass spectrometric method and led to the actual applicability of Hevesy's samarium method. Data of high precision could now be obtained and meaningful data in the four billion years plus range were now estimated. The final value of the age of selected meteorites and indirectly of Earth has been estimated to be 4.55 billion years, with 1% marginal error.

Years of Interlude in Freiburg

Hevesy let himself be fully absorbed by his work and there was little time for social interactions. He remained a bachelor until reaching mature age. In the summer of 1923 Hevesy visited, for the third time, the convalescent home of Montebello, close to the city of Elsinore. There he met his future wife. Her name was Pia Riis. She was visiting Montebello as a companion to one of her aunts. Pia had been born in Argentina and her father was a Danish ship owner. When she was eight years old she had lost both her parents and thereafter she and her sister were cared for by their father's sister, their aunt Dagmar, in Denmark. Pia had had her professional training as a nurse in London and she returned to this city after her encounter with Hevesy at Montebello. However, the mutual attraction remained and she soon returned to Denmark. In early 1924 they became engaged and were married soon thereafter. George was 39 years old and she was 22. They had a rich joint life until his death.

Based on his fame as a scientist Hevesy in the mid-1920s could negotiate conditions for affiliations with different universities. In 1925, after much vacillating, he accepted a chair of physical chemistry in Freiburg, returning to an environment he knew from his early years of study and succeeding his mentor, Meyer. This came to be his first and last stable academic employment. His young wife liked the life in Freiburg and when they moved their first child, a daughter Jenny, had already been born in 1926. The family grew rapidly and a son Georg was born in 1928 and another daughter Ingrid, three years later. Quality of life was good and Hevesy had more time for his family. He also liked the surroundings. Although not at all athletic he was an outdoor person enjoying long walks in the countryside and, when conditions permitted, cross-country skiing. When his mother died in Budapest in 1931 he said that Freiburg changed from being 75% to 100% his home. At the time it would seem that his life had entered a smoother phase and in 1932 he became a Baden citizen (his citizenship was rescinded in 1941 by the Nazi regime). However, by the early 1930s clouds were again starting to appear on the political horizon.

Hevesy's work changed both in structure and pace. He needed to catch up with himself after the six intense years in Copenhagen. The focus was on managing the department also including the teaching for which he was responsible. The scientific engagements calmed down temporarily, but he remained a highly prolific researcher and author. As a well-known scientist he was invited to give lectures and participate in congresses. This travelling also took him out of Europe to South Africa, where, together with Rutherford, he was proud to receive an honorary doctorate. After 1929 he came to receive 12 more honorary doctorates in different parts of the world throughout his long life. In fact two of them were awarded after the Second World War by both the technical (1949) and the medical faculty (1959) at Freiburg University.

He also travelled to the US where he established contact with the Rockefeller Foundation which had a very positive view on his work. He was appointed Baker lecturer at Cornell University, Ithaca, in 1930. Further travel took him to California and from there to Japan, a country he came to like very much. In Pasadena he again met Einstein. Hevesy also took time to have his hair cut. The barber, who was from Konstanz, on the Bodensee, told him about a secret wish of his, namely to cut Einstein's hair. When Hevesy told Einstein about this particular wish he said "Since he was not able to achieve anything on your head (Hevesy had sparse hair) he wanted to go wild on mine!"

However, at home his situation continued to worsen and he eventually had to acknowledge by contacts with his selected friends that the situation in the Third Reich might evolve into a threat also to himself and his family. Although seeing himself as a Hungarian aristocrat with a conservative political orientation it dawned on him that he could not possibly present the "Aryan" descent required to remain a full professor at a German university. He was in fact classified as 100% Jewish in 1933 by the political authorities, something he kept strictly to himself. Not even to his children would he acknowledge his and hence also their ethnic background. His lack of a stable home environment was further amplified and it was during a vacation in Denmark in 1933 that he decided to return to his invaluable friend in science, Bohr. The alternative was to go to England and work with Rutherford, but his wife's Danish origin had a large bearing on his final decision. He took another year in Freiburg to settle his responsibilities to his students and to his colleagues but in July 1934 he asked to be allowed to resign and moved with his wife and the three children to Denmark. By force of circumstances it was time once again to turn a page.

One year earlier the Rockefeller Foundation had created a new program, the International Education Board (IEB). The purpose of IEB was to support European refugee scholars. It became a very important initiative which aided some 300 scholars before it ended at the cessation of the Second World War. Bohr had close contacts with the Foundation and eventually he obtained a sizable grant, $40,000, which allowed him to employ several high caliber visiting scientists in his Institute. One of them was Hevesy. It could be added that since 1932 the program of the Foundation was headed by Warren Weaver. He came to hold this post for twenty years and, during this time, showing a great foresight, he reoriented the focus of the Foundation towards experimental molecular biology. This suited the shift in Hevesy's scientific endeavors at the time excellently.

Return to Copenhagen — The Indicator Method Comes of Age

Originally Hevesy called his isotope marker technique the *indicator* method. It was not until after the Second World War that a new term, *tracer*, started to be used. This modern term will be used occasionally as an alternative in the following. The potential of the indicator method had remained in Hevesy's mind throughout his career ever since he formulated the concept in 1912–13. It was originally applied to studies of metals and alloys, but in 1922, at the time when he was intensively engaged in the hafnium work, he also did his first experiments in life sciences systems. He tried to follow the dissemination of labeled lead in bean seedlings. An uneven distribution of the labeled material in the plant was found. Similar experiments were made with radium D and thorium B, both of which are lead isotopes. However, the toxicity of the naturally occurring compounds, all of them salts of lead or bismuth together with their lack of natural metabolic roles, limited further studies. Sometime later dermatologists interested in replacing arsenic by bismuth in syphilis therapy stimulated Hevesy to perform indicator studies of the uptake, distribution and excretion of labeled bismuth in rats. The results of this study, published in 1924, represent the first data on the study of animal metabolism by use of tracers. However, it was developments in nuclear physics in the early 1930s that truly made the concept take off.

In 1932 Harold Urey discovered the heavy hydrogen isotope deuterium. The importance of this finding was quickly recognized by the committee for the

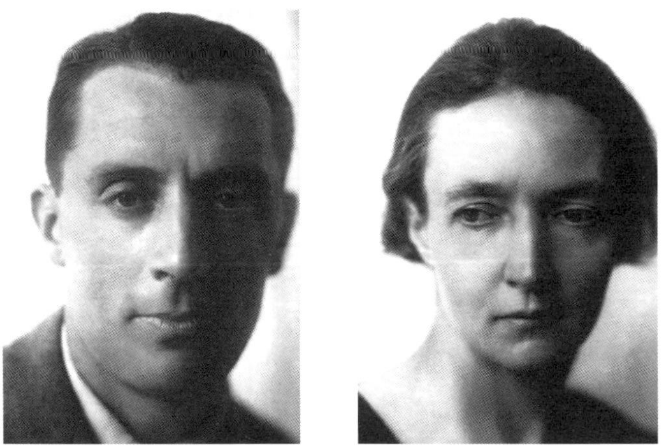

Frédérick Joliot (1900–1958) and Irene Joliot-Curie (1897–1956), recipients of the 1935 Nobel Prize in chemistry. [From *Les Prix Nobel en 1935.*]

Nobel Prize in chemistry and in 1934 the discovery was recognized by a prize. The prize motivation succinctly read "for his discovery of heavy hydrogen". Hevesy, who had known Urey since the earlier Copenhagen days, was quickly provided with some dilute heavy water. He immediately used this to study the turnover and total volume of body fluids in organisms using both fish and himself as study objects. He used the straightforward dilution technique comparing the dose of the inoculums and the concentration of isotope after mixing with the total body fluid[21]. But even more attractive isotopes were soon to become available.

The new field of induced isotopes was opened up by Frederic and Irène Joliot-Curie. They found that bombardment of aluminum by alpha particles led to the formation of radioactive material that after decay for a short time returned to its original stable aluminum state. Again the discovery was quickly recognized by a Nobel Prize in chemistry. They were given the award in 1935 "in recognition of their synthesis of new radioactive elements". Hevesy got to know them during a visit in 1938 to Paris, a city where many years earlier he had also become acquainted with Irene's mother. In the same year that the Joliot-Curies received their prize, the Nobel Prize in physics recognized James Chadwick "for his discovery of the neutron". This newly discovered elementary particle was used by Enrico Fermi and collaborators to bombard a number of light elements. It now became clear that essentially any element in the periodic table could be transformed into an unstable element, which after varying times returned to its original state. The rate of decay (half-life) of the isotopes varied.

When Hevesy resumed experimental work in Copenhagen in 1935 the possibilities for his work had changed dramatically because of the induced isotopes that had now become available. Another very powerful phase of development of his science started (p. 183). His biographer Hilde Levi contributed markedly to the buildup of the equipment needed for measuring radioactivity. She herself was the last Jewish PhD student of Max von Laue, the elder statesman of physics, who received a Nobel Prize in 1914 "for his discovery of the diffraction of X-rays by crystals". She was allowed to present her thesis in spite of the emerging threat of the Third Reich. This was permitted only on condition that she afterwards left the country. The first collaborative efforts in Bohr's institute by Hevesy and Levi concerned studies of rare earth elements, the former's favorite toys. By use of induced radioactivity they could trace the admixing of one element in a sample also containing other compounds. One example was the determination of the percentage of dysprosium in an yttrium sample. This technique came to be of more general use later and was referred to as neutron activation analysis. They were to publish four articles together on these topics. The focus of their joint efforts hereafter changed drastically.

Since Levi came to be one important biographer describing Hevesy's life it may be worth taking a closer look at their relationship. They never became close and Levi remained in the position of a qualified technician in Hevesy's laboratory. She was never a guest in Hevesy's otherwise open and often social home. At Christmas time it was a task of his son Georg to take a tram carrying a box of chocolate to Levi, who shared an apartment with Bohr's secretary Sophie Hellman. In return he received a box of homemade marmalade candy. Levi was proud of her Jewish heritage, but such recognition did not foster a common ground for interaction with Hevesy. Very surprisingly Levi did not even know that he was Jewish. It was made clear to her first when she took the initiative to write his biography after he had died. It was the oldest daughter Jenny who told her this secret which Jenny herself had never discussed with her father. Levi must have seen this as some kind of betrayal, but it may just reflect the conditions of extreme assimilation of a person with a Jewish background basing his existence on complete denial.

In the mid-1930s Hevesy had a relatively poor insight into the fields of biology and medicine. However at the mature age of 50 he completely shifted the focus of his science towards these fields and in time he became more and more acquainted with their particulars. In fact about 200 articles that were still to be added to his very long list of publications, (see figure on p. 183) almost all focused on problems in these disciplines. Parenthetically it can be mentioned that Hevesy published articles in five different languages, German, English, French, Danish and Swedish. In his spoken language this polyglot is said not to have been a purist. This may however not be a completely true statement. With one exception he was very careful to keep the languages separate. The exception was the two Scandinavian languages Danish and Swedish. When he eventually settled in Sweden he decided to continue to use his Danish and in the end he came to use a mixture of the two Scandinavian languages for practical purposes.

The transformation of his professional orientation towards biology was markedly facilitated by the relationships he developed with a good friend of Bohr, Ole Chievitz, the head surgeon at the Finsen Hospital, and August Krogh, a visionary Nobel laureate who in 1920 had received the prize in physiology or medicine "for his discovery of capillary motor regulating mechanisms" as described previously[22]. Both of them fully appreciated the potential usefulness

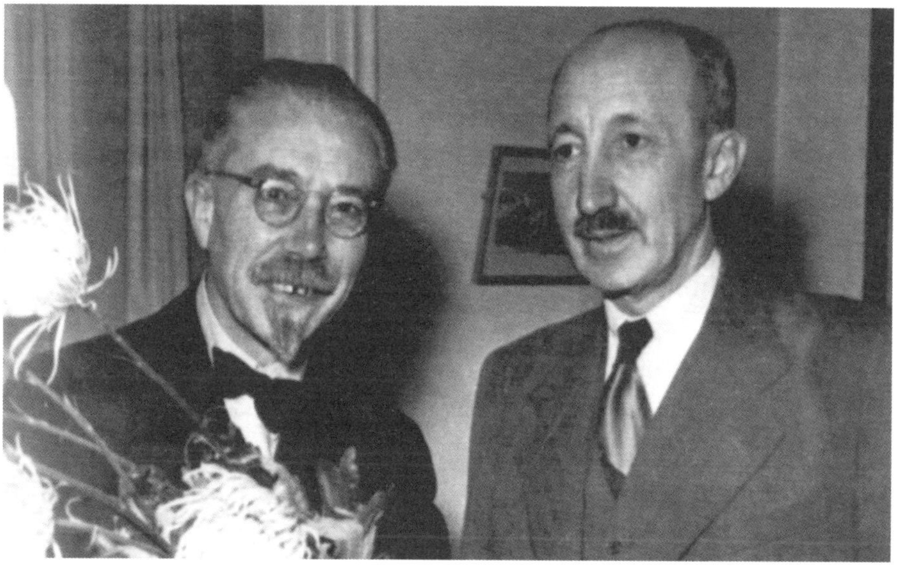

S. August S. Krogh (1874–1949), recipient of the 1920 Nobel Prize in physiology or medicine together with Hevesy in the 1930s. [From the Hevesy family collection.]

of the tracer method and one of Hevesy's first publications in the field, in which heavy water was used, was together with Krogh[21]. But, as mentioned, even better tracers progressively became available.

Hevesy decided to use radioactive phosphorus for biological experiments. It had the attractive properties of emitting readily identifiable beta radiation (electrons) and the rate of decay was14 days. He used this isotope in very imaginative experiments to examine the interaction between phosphorus and bone tissue. The results were spectacular and revolutionary. In a letter to the editor of Nature submitted in September 1935[23] de Hevesy stated: "The results strongly support the view that the formation of bones is a dynamic process, the bones continuously taking up phosphorous atoms which are partly or wholly lost again and are replaced by other phosphorus atoms." Who would have thought that there would be such a turnover of bone tissues? These were indeed heterodox interpretations. The first author on the Nature communication was Chicvitz. He arranged for the conditions required for execution of the animal experiments. It was by means of this kind of experiment that the indicator method moved from being a tool for biochemists to being one of indispensable value to biologists. The outreach of Bohr's Institute for Physics was indeed impressive. Hevesy had developed scientific collaborations all over town and transported his isotope containers wrapped in newspaper during his travel on streetcars.

The isotope *par excellence* that Hevesy used in his expanding biological experiments came to be ^{32}P, but with time progressively many more, very useful isotopes became available. These were ^{15}N, ^{14}C, ^{24}Na, ^{42}K, ^{72}Zn and ^{59}Fe. Later in life he summarized his efforts in using the tracer (indicator) methods in two volumes[24] and under Life Sciences he lists: Skeleton — Phosphatides — Permeability — Labelled Blood Corpuscles. The theme phosphatides illustrates his talent for intuitively choosing a field of emerging importance. He studied nucleic acid turnover long before it had been clarified that these are the information carrying molecules in all forms of life. Together with Hans von Euler, professor of chemistry at the University of Stockholm, he investigated the metabolism of the nucleic acids in a special line of sarcoma tumor cells and they published more than ten articles in this field. We will meet von Euler again later in this chapter. Similar studies were also performed in collaboration with Einar Hammarsten at the Karolinska institute, a very influential scientist in the field of nucleic acid research frequently referred to in my previous book[22]. It was found that the nucleic acid turnover was high in the spleen and the intestinal mucosa of the rat. The permeability studies — the movement of ions and molecules across membranes — were also pioneering. Before the access to isotopes it had not been possible to perform the kind of crucial experiments that he did with his qualified Danish collaborators Krogh and Hans H. Ussing.

In the beginning it was difficult to get access to sufficient radioactive compounds. A charming story describes how Bohr on his 50th birthday was presented with 100,000 Danish crowns to buy radium, which could be used for the generation of radioactive materials. Another development was the construction of accelerators which eventually became indispensable for production of isotopes with markedly improved specific activity. Support from the Rockefeller Foundation in 1935 allowed the building in Copenhagen of one of the first cyclotrons in Europe. Before access was gained to this accelerator, isotopes were obtained from the Berkeley laboratory in California managed by Ernest O. Lawrence. He was to become the 1939 Nobel Prize recipient in physics "for the invention and development of the cyclotron and for results obtained with it, especially with regard to artificial elements". ^{32}P was sent from Berkeley by (surface) mail! The successful applications of induced isotopes followed over many years with studies of renewal and exchange processes in many different animals, in different organs, in normal and cancerous tissues, etc. A completely new field of science had become available. It was harvest time for the advances of Hevesy's research endeavors. It was time for a Nobel Prize.

The Evaluation of the Indicator Method by the Nobel Committee

The first time that Hevesy's engagement in separation and use of isotopes was mentioned in a nomination for a Nobel Prize in chemistry was in 1929, as already referred to above. The evaluator Svedberg did not consider that the advances made until that time justified recognition by a prize. A nomination by Arthur Hantzsch from Dresden in 1934 proposed the discovery of hafnium by Hevesy and Costner one more time, but the main emphasis of the nomination concerned radiochemical studies. However, the proposal concerned the early indicator studies undertaken prior to the involvement in studies of biological phenomena. The committee referred to previous evaluations and did not consider these contributions for a prize. The following year Hevesy was proposed by H. Mark from Vienna again for his work on radioactive indicators, but now the nomination for the first time mentioned the new applications to physiological and biological chemistry. The committee let Svedberg make a new evaluation. He gave a state of the art analysis and emphasized the advances made in studies of the radioactivity of samarium, the isotope of future use to estimate the events in the most distant part of the history of Earth. Svedberg's conclusion was "The publications discussed above concerning the radioactivity of samarium seem to me to be from a general point of view the most important that de Hevesy has produced." Still he concluded that altogether the studies did not have sufficient importance to justify discussion of a Nobel Prize. The committee concurred with this opinion.

In 1936 there were three nominations of Hevesy. One was by the prize recipients the previous year Frederick Joliot and Irene Joliot-Curie and it included Urbain. The nomination focused on the rare earth metals and stated that the two nominees had encountered the elements samarium and neodyme which show a weak spontaneous radioactivity — "On y rencontre des elements, samarium, neodyme, qui montrent une faible radioactivité spontanée." This is in fact a misunderstanding. It was Hevesy who discovered the alpha activity in samarium, which his systematic search of the lanthanide series showed to be the only member of the series to have a natural radioactive isotope. Urbain had made other important observations in his studies of the rare earth elements. One more nomination for both Urbain and Hevesy was made by another French Nobel laureate, the prize recipient in physics in 1926, Jean Perrin. He made it clear that both the nominees had made important contributions to the understanding of the properties of a range of rare earth elements, but interestingly, in spite of being a Frenchman, he gave Hevesy alone the credit for the final identification of element 72, hafnium. Finally there was one nomination by A. von Eiselsberg in Vienna for Hevesy alone. The committee referred to earlier evaluations and did not take any action.

Three years later the scene had changed dramatically. There were three nominations. One came from Bohr and this was the first time that he had made a nomination for a chemistry prize. He emphasized the revolutionary consequences of using induced isotopes for studies of living organisms. The second proposal came from Tibor Széki and Julius Gróh in Budapest. In their nomination they reviewed the whole history of the development of the concept of using a radioactive compound to trace a homologous element and discussed the relative merits of Hevesy's and Paneth's contributions. In the end they proposed Hevesy alone as a candidate. The third nomination was by Soddy and he recommended both Hevesy and Paneth as candidates but still emphasized the significance of the use of the recently introduced induced radioisotopes. The committee asked Svedberg to make another evaluation.

In a very thorough presentation of the development of the field he noted that the idea of using indicators was introduced in 1913 jointly by Hevesy and Paneth. He then pointed out that of the two Hevesy had followed up the field more effectively by his work on radioactive indicators, already discussed earlier in the reviews in 1929, 1934 and 1935, and on radioactive elements with a low atomic weight also reviewed earlier in 1934 and 1935. Throughout these years his contributions were concluded not to be prize-worthy, but the recent access to artificial radioactive isotopes representing essentially all elements implied a revolutionary change of possibilities.

Hevesy had pioneered the foray into new applications involving biology and medicine. Already before the access to the new forms of isotopes he had tried in 1924 to examine the uptake and accumulation of bismuth and lead in animals and plants with some interesting results. The problem, as mentioned above, was the toxicity of the short-lived and hence highly active isotopes decaying by emission of destructive energy particles. Svedberg then noted the impressive and dramatically new data obtained by use of radioactive phosphorous and other isotopes in collaboration with Chievitz and Krogh. He saw a major potential in future applications of the technique. Finally he commented on the use of heavy inactive isotopes of H, O and N with the early important results also published by Hevesy. Svedberg's concluding paragraph was laudatory but contained a reservation that is difficult to understand. It reads:

> To follow the fate of atoms in chemical reactions and biological processes by use of labeling must be considered to be one of the most important methodological innovations for studies of chemical kinetics during recent times. From this perspective this advance, in its totality, is worthy being recognized by a Nobel Prize. The question of whether de Hevesy's and Paneth's work on radioactive indicators can also be viewed to be of fundamental importance for the use of inactive isotopes is more difficult to answer. At least there is no reference in the nominations given for such an importance of de Hevesy's and Paneth's investigations.

The committee agreed with Svedberg and did not recommend a prize.

The Shadow of the Second World War

1940 turned out to be a decisive year. Three nominations were given for a prize to Hevesy. One was from Aston in Cambridge, the 1922 laureate in chemistry mentioned above. Although his nomination briefly mentioned the identification of hafnium its main emphasis was on the indicator method. The other two proposals came from members of the committee, Svedberg and Wilhelm Palmaer. One wonders why supplementary in-house nominations had to be submitted by 40% of the committee members. Further, the uncertainty from the previous year as to whether the indicator method should include both radioactive isotopes and non-radioactive isotopes is said in the summarizing text to have been addressed in all three nominations submitted, but in fact it is only the one from Palmaer which addressed this specifically. Be that as it may, the committee was now wholeheartedly supportive of a prize to Hevesy. This is anchored in a comprehensive review — of his own nomination — by Svedberg. He gave a detailed historical and comparative up-to-date analysis of the whole field covering 14 pages and added a reference list including 70 publications by Hevesy. Svedberg's conclusions were echoed on four pages out of the 12 in the summarizing report by the committee. It appropriately concluded that Hevesy has opened a new field of science of immense importance. The motivation given by the committee was "for his work on the use of isotopes as indicators in the study of chemical processes". Paneth was not discussed as a serious candidate for a prize although he had independently formulated the idea of the indicator method and experimentally documented its use in parallel with Hevesy in the early studies. However, it was noted in the follow-up of the original idea that

Hevesy had an obvious lead. He had made the most original contributions of applications of the indicator method to inorganic systems and he was the sole initiator of its use in a wide range of biological systems.

However, the story did not end here as it should. Hevesy did not receive his Nobel Prize in 1940 because, as already mentioned, due to the Second World War, no prizes in chemistry were awarded in 1940 to 1943. The committees continued their work throughout the war years although the number of nominations dwindled. In 1941 it was concluded that Hahn was a strong candidate to a Prize in chemistry, second only to Hevesy, who in this year had been nominated by Urey. The following year Hevesy was proposed in a comprehensive nomination by his collaborator Krogh and the committee noted that the proposed candidate retained his position as number one. In 1943 Hevesy was nominated by Luigi Rolla from Genoa University. Due to the fact that three years had passed since the previous evaluation of Hevesy the committee asked Svedberg to undertake yet another evaluation. He elaborated over 12 pages, with an added list of 16 publications by Hevesy, on the impressive developments of the applications of tracer technique and the clear lead in the field retained by Hevesy and collaborators. A multitude of radioactive and heavy isotopes had come into use as markers; ^{32}P, ^{24}Na, ^{42}K, ^{15}N, radioactive chlorine and fluorine and heavy water. He concluded that over the last three years the usefulness and importance of the tracer method had become further documented. The technique had now become adopted by many other researchers — "Qualitatively, however, the studies by de Hevesy and collaborators still remain in the frontline". The committee reiterated a major part of the assessments made in Svedberg's evaluation in its annual overview and repeated that among the candidates, Hevesy retained his leading position. In 1943 Hevesy was also nominated for a prize in physics. It was submitted by a fellow countryman from Budapest, R. Ortvay and highlighted four contributions; separation of mercury isotopes, purification and identification of hafnium, demonstration of the radioactivity of samarium and the development of the method for use of radioactive isotopes in solving problems of chemical, physical and biological nature. The Nobel committee of physics referred to the thorough evaluations already made by the committee of chemistry and did not make any independent evaluation of the proposal.

In 1944 the number of nominated candidates for a prize in Chemistry was still low, 26, and in this year Hevesy was nominated by Goldschmidt and by Luigi Mazza from the University of Genoa. The committee was very meticulous and asked Svedberg to make yet another update of Hevesy's contributions to the field, assessing the news of the preceding year. Svedberg first took notice of the increasing number of useful isotopes for biological work, like the access to tritium — ^{3}H— and radioactive carbon — the short-lived ^{11}C and the long-lived ^{14}C — created by scientists in Berkeley. As a digression it can be mentioned that the ^{14}C isotope, which is exceptionally useful for biological studies, was discovered in 1940 by Martin Kamen and Sam Ruben when they bombarded graphite in the cyclotron. Kamen had a difficult life and was fired from Berkeley in 1945 accused of having leaked weapon secrets to Russia. The validity of this accusation was never substantiated and after many years he was again able to obtain a passport and return to academic life.

Svedberg reported that Hevesy's contributions during the year included determination of the half-life of erythrocytes using ^{32}P and further studies of the metabolism of nucleic acids in normal and cancerous cells also using this isotope. The latter work, as already mentioned, was carried out in collaboration with von Euler, one of the five members of the committee. The committee repeated Svedberg's remarks in its summary and stated "de Hevesy's indicator method has been found to be a great tool to research chemical and physiological sequences of events and has year by year been demonstrated to be of increasing importance". It then discussed Hahn's contributions and the evaluations made of this branch of chemistry and recommended that the reserved Nobel Prize in chemistry for 1943 should be given to Hevesy and the one for 1944 to Hahn.

The eventual decision by the Royal Swedish Academy of Sciences became to award Hevesy the reserved 1943 prize in chemistry, but to reserve the 1944 prize for the coming year. Hahn was awarded this reserved prize in 1945, but could not collect his prize until 1946. His prize motivation was "for his discovery of the fission of heavy nuclei". Hevesy, however, had settled with his family in Sweden in 1944 and worked at Stockholm University and therefore was available to receive his prize. The other prize recipients in the fields of natural sciences in 1944 were in the United States and a ceremony was arranged in New York under the auspices of the American–Scandinavian Foundation (Ref. 22, p. 175) and greetings were transmitted by radio between Sweden and the USA. There was also a prize awarded in literature. The recipient was a Dane Johannes V. Jensen, but he could not come to Stockholm and therefore received his insignia the following year. However, he was greeted over the radio and the person giving the laudation commented that the Swedish prize could be seen as "a support to its suffering brother country".

A Final Home Country

The shifting focus of Hevesy's science after he had settled in Copenhagen for the second time in 1935 led, as already mentioned, to a very productive period. The different kinds of radioactive isotopes that could be applied in the experiments increased and their suitability for such a use improved markedly. Hevesy's range of collaborators expanded as did his involvement in various central biological and medical problems. He seemed not to miss his precious experience from Freiburg of managing a large institution and controlling considerable resources.

Interestingly it was revealed[1] that Hevesy might not have been a skilled experimenter. This is illustrated also by a cartoon made by none other than Brönsted. It is not clear what Hevesy would have thought about this caricature. His biographer Levi has said that he never laughed in front of people but that he always had a polite smile on his face. However this may reflect the fact that she only saw him in formal professional settings, since, as we have mentioned they did not have more personal contacts. His close relations describe a much larger emotional register. I myself recognize a trait for genial contacts over many years with his eldest daughter Jenny, who was the wife of the renowned origin-of-life geochemist Gustaf Arrhenius at the Scripps Institute of Oceanography in La Jolla. My wife and I, on a number of occasions, have had the privilege to be dinner guests at the charming Arrhenius home on the upper mesa in La Jolla with a grand view of the southern California coast and the Pacific. There were always interesting guests representing science and academia, like Manfred Eigen, Albert Eschenmoser, Richard Lerner, Leslie Orgel, Jack Dunitz, Philip Sandblom to mention just a few. Jenny was the perfect hostess, always very positive, in

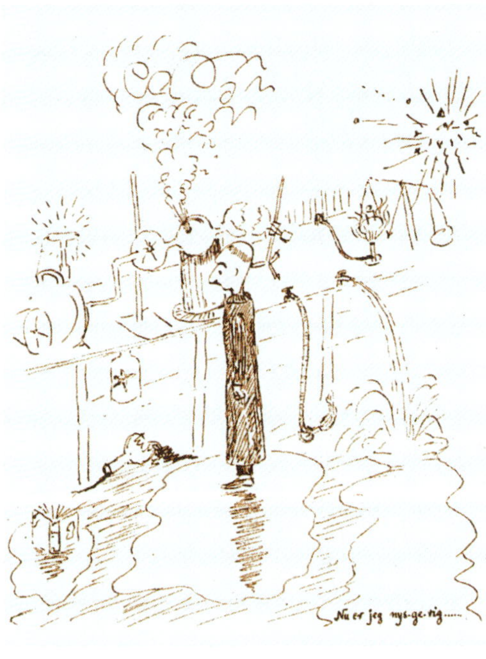

Brönsted's interpretation of Hevesy's limitations as an experimenter. The small text at the bottom reads "Now I'm curious". [From Anders Lundgren, courtesy of the Brönsted family.]

a pleasant and non-committal way, in her remarks on people or subjects of discussion. However, talking to Jenny's closest family has revealed that she could be strongly opinionated and could aggressively stand up for her views. But one wonders how her father could emotionally unload all the turbulence he frequently had to internalize during his eventful life. The picture generally presented is the one of a cultivated, correct, courteous, gentle and distracted professor forgetting one overshoe outside his office. This could mean either that he was in his office and still had one overshoe on or that he had left forgetting one of them. Still this picture cannot be complete. His letters showed that he was a man of deep involvements in human affairs too. He naturally had deep emotional concerns about the turbulent political affairs of Europe and did enjoy subjecting them to philosophical discussions. He also had his own sense of humor, often sarcastic, but still not unkind.

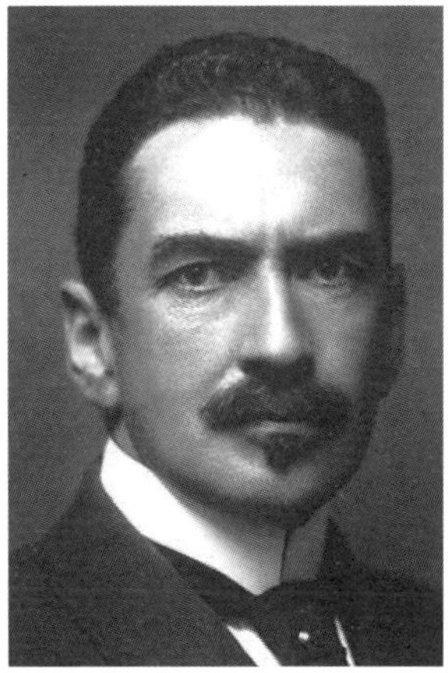

Hans K. A. S. von Euler-Chelpin (1873–1964), recipient of the shared 1929 Nobel Prize in chemistry. [From *Les Prix Nobel en 1929*.]

Maybe the presence of a perpetual smile in some cases is a way of keeping people at a distance improving one's focus on the problem at hand, but this does not seem to be the appropriate description of Hevesy's attitude. His son-in-law Gustaf has given the following description of Hevesy "I have often seen George laughing heartily in the company of colleagues and friends. In the multitude of ceremonial situations he always maintained a diplomatic and ceremonial demeanor but when relaxed he often sank into a pensive and absent state, sometimes morose when he thought of life's adversities." It is not surprising to note that in a way Hevesy's method way of managing crises, like the impending threat of another World War, was simply to submerge himself in his work. But he also demonstrated repeatedly that he could take action when an emergency situation required this. Levi has emphasized that he was an energetic and inspiring promoter of new ideas and that he expected as much from his co-workers as from himself, which meant a lot.

There were parts of his personality that he kept closely to himself or at most shared with a few selected friends. Thus, surprisingly, he did not comment on the progressively worsening political situation in Europe. The fact that he had Jewish ancestry that had forced him to leave Freiburg, although formally voluntarily, obviously came to be of increasing importance when the

Nazis annexed Denmark in April 1940. Even after this event he continued to be very productive in his science. There are however certain private letters, for example to Urey, that demonstrated that at the time he was in despair. He tried, unsuccessfully, prior to his move to Sweden, to find ways to travel to the US. This turned out not to be possible since transports both by boat and by the trans-Siberian railway were blocked.

At the time of the German invasion Hevesy helped Bohr to resolve a very unusual situation. During the 1930s the mounting oppression of Germany's Jewish scientists led to two Nobel laureates in physics, the above-mentioned von Laue and also James Franck, who together with Gustav L. Hertz had been awarded half of the 1926 prize "for their discovery of the laws governing the impact of an electron upon an atom", smuggling out and depositing their Nobel gold medals in Bohr's institute. It should be clarified that von Laue was not Jewish, but he was not well regarded by the regime in Germany. He actively obstructed the removal of scientists with a Jewish ethnic background from university appointments in Germany and as president of the German Physics Society he had a considerable influence. The fact that Levi could finish her PhD thesis is only one example. Bohr's own Nobel medal had already been put up for auction to assist in the war effort, but he was concerned about the two concealed medals belonging to his two physicist friends. If they were found they might compromise their owners, since their names were engraved on them and it was illegal to take gold out of Germany. Bohr discussed this situation with Hevesy, who proposed that they should simply bury the medals. However, they did not feel confident about doing this and instead Hevesy dissolved the medals, by the only means possible, in *aqua regia* — one part nitric acid and three parts hydrochloric acid. The German occupants searched Bohr's Institute and stole some possessions, including the Bohr family silver that for some reason was kept there, but they were not impressed by two bottles of green liquid on a shelf. When the war was over the gold was recovered and new medals were minted by the Nobel Foundation and returned to the two physicist laureates.

Until 1943 daily life in Denmark was not drastically altered by the German invasion. But then everything changed and resident Jews came under immediate threat. Thousands of them fled over the Öresund to Sweden, very often under dramatic conditions. Bohr, half-Jewish by birth and an ardent opponent of the Nazi regime, was brought by emergency efforts to Sweden in 1943 and then flown to England. A few weeks later Hevesy also left and although he might have used his Hungarian passport and simply boarded a train for Stockholm in Copenhagen, it is not clear if this is what he did. His son and son-in law have been looking for Hevesy's passport to settle the matter, but as yet have not been able to find it. The possibility that he was taken illegally by a Danish fishing boat to the Swedish coast at night remains a possibility. Many months later his collaborator Krogh did flee by the latter route. He was wanted by the German occupiers because he, like Bohr, had been very outspoken in his criticism of the Nazi occupation and he was assumed to be high on the death list of Danish Nazi sympathizers. For almost a year Krogh developed his activities in Sweden mostly at the University of Lund, staying with his daughter.

Some weeks after Hevesy had left Denmark the rest of his family, his wife and now four children — another daughter Pia had been born in 1937 — departed for Sweden and came to settle into what became their final home country. It was a difficult transition, uprooting from their Danish home and finding a new one in Stockholm. After the family had lived temporarily in a place at Saltsjöbaden von Euler helped them out by letting them have an apartment above his laboratory at Stockholm University, right in the center of the city, at Sandåsgatan 2. Space in this apartment was somewhat limited and the two older children, Jenny and Georg continued to live in the suburbs visiting the family over weekends. They were nearing the end of their high school *(gymnasium)* studies at the time. Once they had *studentexamen* (high-school leaving-certificate), Jenny travelled to London to work for the Swedish Institute and the BBC and later to study staying with the Paneth family in Durham. Georg started to study medicine at the Karolinska institute. The two youngest daughters Ingrid and Pia were still in their early school years. Hevesy's home was open and friendly and Georg Klein remembers afternoon tea sessions when he and his wife Eva met many other interesting guests, as for example Lise Meitner, a close friend of Hevesy's, who had also settled in Sweden. Over a few years the Kleins also had some scientific collaboration with Hevesy.

Von Euler's involvement was of major importance for Hevesy's assimilation into the Swedish academic environment. They had already had close scientific collaboration for about the last three years and von Euler had invited Hevesy to join him in Stockholm. In 1929 von Euler had shared a Nobel Prize in chemistry with Arthur Harden "for their investigation on the fermentation of sugar and fermentative enzymes". He was a professor at Stockholm University and a member of the Nobel committee at the Royal Swedish Academy of Sciences as mentioned above. Not surprisingly he had a major influence at the University. There is a paradox in this collegial friendship, reflecting a frequently cited special feature of Hevesy's personality, namely the capacity to manage to keep an emotionally watertight separation between work and politics in his dealings with people. Von Euler was openly pro-German and even wrote "Heil Hitler" in his letters.

Hevesy, once more, and for the last time, transplanted himself into a new scientific environment which he seems to have enjoyed. However he was never appointed formally to a tenured post at the University of Stockholm. Throughout the remainder of his career he had to rely on support from various grant-awarding authorities, including various foundations. The remaining family resources in Hungary were lost after the Communist takeover. As can be seen from his publications he continued to be scientifically productive even towards the latter part of his life. He collaborated a good deal with other scientists at Stockholm University, but also at the Karolinska Institute. At the latter institute he researched the metabolism of nucleic acids together with Hammarsten, as already mentioned above. He also studied nucleic acid metabolism together with Swedish colleagues at the department of pharmacology. The synthesis and breakdown of haemoproteins was examined in collaboration with the forthcoming recipient of a Nobel Prize in physiology or medicine Hugo Theorell and his collaborators at the medical Nobel Institute for biochemistry. At the department of histology he studied the effect of heavy water on the organism together with Gösta Häggqvist, another professor with Nazi sympathies. He also interacted with clinical departments. Isotopes were tried out for early diagnosis of cervical cancer together with colleagues at Radiumhemmet, the cancer center section at the Karolinska Hospital, and finally he published many papers on the effect of radiation on tissues together with Arne Forsberg at the laboratory for radiophysics at the hospital.

His close early interaction with the Karolinska institute is also obvious from his appointment in 1948, for one year, as an adjunct member of the Nobel committee for physiology or medicine. It should be mentioned that whereas members of the decision-taking body — originally the college of teachers at the Karolinska Institute and presently the Nobel assembly — have to be employees of the institute this does not apply to adjunct members of the Nobel committee. During the late 1970s Peter Perlmann, a professor of immunology at Stockholm University, was an adjunct member of the Nobel committee at the Karolinska Institute, as mentioned in Chapter 3. Hevesy's engagement in the Nobel committee was only for a single year and the reason that it had made him an adjunct member was a proposal by Theorell for a prize to Chester H. Werkman and Harland G. Wood, State College of Agriculture, Ames, Ohio, for their discovery of the CO_2 assimilation also of heterotrophic organisms, a finding of great significance for the understanding of the role of intermediary metabolism. Hevesy reviewed their work over 10 pages and concluded that they might be considered for a prize. The reason that he was selected to carry out this analysis was that the work that developed during 1935–1940 in its later part was heavily dependent on the carbon isotopes that had become available at the time. The committee concluded that Werkman and Wood were worthy of a prize. The following year they were nominated again, but this time together with Hans A. Krebs. Hevesy was no longer involved in the work of the committee and in his place Hammarsten made an extensive and full investigation of all three candidates. Eventually Krebs received the 1953 Nobel Prize in physiology or medicine "for his discovery of the citric acid cycle", whereas the other two scientists joined the large group of prize-worthy candidates who never received a prize.

The Nobel Prize

Hevesy's recognition by the award of the Nobel Prize in chemistry in 1944 was a decisive event. For once the monetary part of the prize came in handy, when he and his family settled in their new home country. Also, being a Nobel laureate obviously facilitated his wish to finally change citizenship. His Hungarian passport was eventually exchanged for a Swedish one. One frequently finds citations in the literature that a Nobel laureate of a foreign nationality has the option to become a Swedish citizen. I have not found facts to support this statement, but of course it markedly improves a person's credentials if he is a non-Swedish Nobel laureate and applies for Swedish citizenship. As was mentioned earlier, there was no collective prize ceremony in 1944. On the appointed day, December 10, Hevesy's work providing the background for his prize was presented on Swedish radio. The presentation[25] was given by Westgren, already introduced earlier (see also Chapters 7 and 8). Hevesy sent a telegram expressing his thanks for the honor to the Royal Swedish Academy of Sciences. The following day the Academy had one of its formal monthly meetings and a part of that was used to award Hevesy his prize.

Hevesy was a foreign member of the Academy. In 1942 it was recommended by von Euler supported by Westgren and Tiselius, members of the class for chemistry (IV) that he should become a foreign member of that class. A special reference was made to the evaluation of his work by the Nobel Committee for chemistry in 1940 recommending him for a prize. One may ask how Hevesy reacted to this recognition. As was mentioned in Chapter 1, Burnet took his election as a foreign member of the Academy as a signal that he might not after all receive a Nobel Prize. It is hard to conjecture if Hevesy might have had similar thoughts. We have no insight into the inner reflections on this matter by this personally rather reclusive man. If he did think about the matter at least he did not mention it in the private letters to his best friends, like Paneth. In parentheses it should be mentioned that Paneth himself was very disappointed not to be included in Hevesy's Nobel Prize. Gustaf Arrhenius tried to explain to him that the main emphasis of the prize was the application of the indicator method in biology, but Paneth was inconsolable.

Hevesy's number as foreign member of the Academy was 806 but after he had become a Swedish citizen in 1951 a transfer to Swedish membership was formally arranged for him. This did not require any further evaluation of his merits. His number as a Swedish member became 965. Since the Royal Swedish Academy of Sciences was founded in 1739 members have been given consecutive numbers and the personal number is important. The rank of a member of the Academy is determined by the day on which he or she is admitted which is reflected in the personal number. At the present time this is considered in the rare cases when a member is transferred from being a foreign member to becoming a Swedish one. The date at which the scientist became a foreign member is considered and he is given a number corresponding to that. This is arranged, in a typically pragmatic Swedish way, by using the number of the Swedish member admitted immediately before the particular time and adding ½. If that rule would have been followed at the time, Hevesy should have been given the number 894½ instead of the higher number that he received, but perhaps he could live with that.

Because Hevesy was a foreign member of the Academy he had the right to be present at the meeting of the Academy on December 11. He could follow the proceedings held in Swedish since he spoke the related Scandinavian language Danish. After having listened to a number of matters relating to Nobel prizes, including a decision to build a rain shelter at the bus stop close to the Nobel Institute for its personnel, the second to last paragraph of the protocol specified

> After a presentation by the Preses (the chairman) he handed over the Nobel Medallion, the Nobel diploma and a check for the Prize sum to the 1943 Nobel Prize recipient in chemistry Mr Hevesy (members of the

Academy dismiss their titles and are addressed Mr or Mrs, in Swedish Herr or Fru, my remark).

This is the only time that a Nobel Prize has been handed out at the Academy, but there is one more interesting detail and that is that Hevesy received a check representing the monetary award connected to the prize. This is not the way transfer of prize money is arranged today. At present the prize recipients pay a separate visit the day after December 10 to the Nobel Foundation where arrangements are being made for transfer of the prize sum. This is convenient for the laureate, but in fact the arrangement made in connection with the improvised prize ceremony for Hevesy was more appropriate from the point of view of principle. It is the Academy, as one of the prize-awarding institutions, and not the Nobel Foundation, that gives the prizes and the money is a part of the prize. As it is today it cannot be seen from the annual financial report by the Academy that it carries this responsibility. However, the expenses involved in selecting prize recipients and for the virtual Nobel Institute are apparent from the annual reports. When, as a member of the Board of the Nobel Foundation, I proposed that the prize-giving institutions should hand over the check this suggested change of arrangement was not well received.

After the meeting by the Academy a dinner was arranged to honor Hevesy. It took place in the reading room of the library, which at this time was a part of the Academy. The room was decorated with a Swedish flag and a bust of Alfred Nobel. Hevesy as the guest of honor was seated with the Preses, Tore G. E. Lindmark, professor of steam technology at the Royal Institute of Technology in Stockholm, on his left and Westgren, the Permanent Secretary, on his right. Both of his neighbors were dressed in tails as was required when they served in their official Academy functions. This tradition was maintained until the late 1970s. Other members of the Nobel committee present at the table were Svedberg and von Euler. It is worth remembering that this cozy gathering took place at the time when many parts of Europe were in flames and millions of Jews were being murdered in the Holocaust. The developments in Hungary during the last year of the war represent one of the worst atrocities committed by mankind according to Winston Churchill. Hitler's army invaded Hungary on March 19, 1944. A program for the extermination of all Jews was immediately initiated supervised by Adolf Eichmann. Edmund Veesenmayer was able to report to Berlin that during the time period May 14 to July 8, a total of 437,402 Jews had been transported to the concentration camps for extermination. The

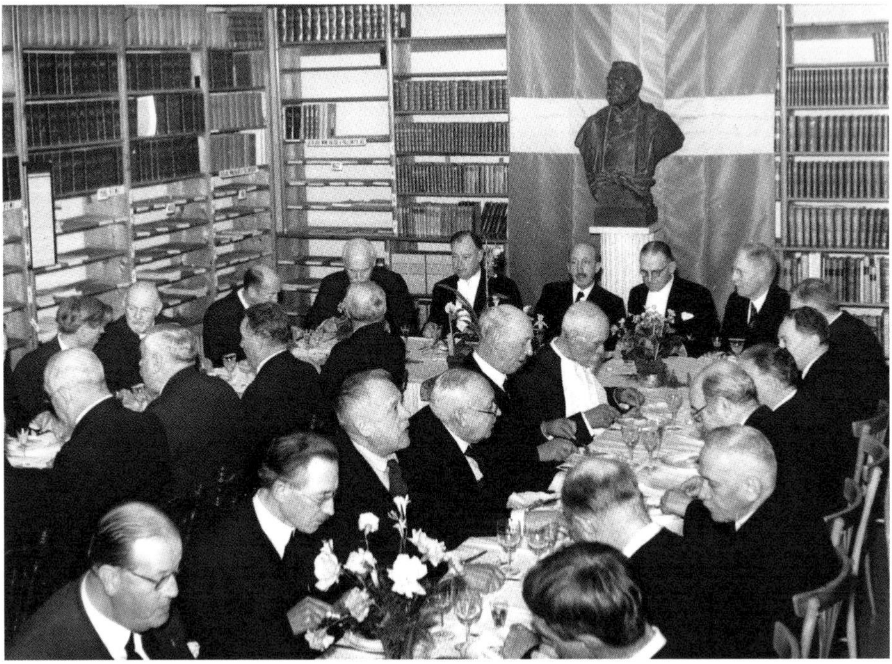

The unique Nobel dinner arranged for Hevesy at the Royal Swedish Academy of Sciences. This is the only occasion when this feast was held at the premises of the academy. Hevesy has the president of the academy Lindmark on his left side and its permanent secretary Westgren on his right side. Both of them are dressed in tails.

overall majority of them came from the rural parts of Hungary. The efficiency of the Germans in carrying out this operation was improved by increasing the number of trains delivering prisoners to the concentration camps beyond what was originally thought to be possible to handle. During the autumn of 1944 several different initiatives were taken to save as many as possible of the remaining 230,000 Jews in the country.

Hevesy's closest family fared comparatively well under the conditions. One brother Edmund (Ödön) was brought to a concentration camp in Germany, but survived. He stayed temporarily in Sweden and then settled in the South Tyrol. One sister Hanna was also brought to a concentration camp, but survived. Late in life she settled in Stockholm. Most other brothers and sisters of this rootless family settled in different parts of the world. The brother Paul (Pal) is of particular interest. He became a diplomat and after various appointments he lived for a longer time in London, but eventually died in Kitzbühel. He was the French teacher of Queen Mary and became a good friend of Charlie Chaplin, who in turn introduced him to many influential statesmen and personalities of the 20th century. He wrote influential books on the economic developments of our world[26] and also an entertaining biography *Eighty Years Around the World*. He was proposed for a Nobel Peace Prize by the British foreign minister Lord Butler. His comment on this nomination was "We have all been normal children from birth except George, my younger brother, who in 1943 received the Nobel Prize in chemistry. How interesting and nice would it not have been to have two recipients of Nobel Prizes in the family."

Characteristically for the times there were only men at the table of this Nobel dinner. The Royal Swedish Academy of Sciences has an interesting history when it comes to the election of female scientists as national and foreign members. The first female member to be elected was Eva Ekeblad, born De la Gardie, in 1748. She contributed some new observations to the annals of the young academy but never participated in a meeting. Thereafter it took another 200 years before another female national member was elected. This was a very special case. In 1945 Lise Meitner had been elected as a foreign member. She had worked close with Otto Hahn in Berlin for about 20 years before, on account of her Jewish background, having to flee Germany in 1938. It has been discussed at length whether she should not have shared the 1944 Nobel Prize in chemistry awarded in 1945 to Hahn[16]. However she was awarded an honor, which was not allotted to Hahn. One of the new unstable large elements meitnerium, 109 Mt, was named after her. In this prestigious recognition she is in good company, given the nearby element, nobelium, 102 No. In 1951, after Meitner had came to live in Sweden, her foreign membership was converted to a Swedish one in 1951. The first time a Swedish female scientist was elected was in 1975. It was an astronomer Aina Elvius. To this can be added that Meitner was not the first foreign female member of the Academy. There had been two predecessors. The first was the Russian scientist Yekaterina Romanovna Dashkova, a remarkable intellectual with wide international contacts, who at a young age assisted Catherine II to become the Empress of Russia. Princess Dashkova was elected to the Academy in 1783. She had close contacts with Benjamin Franklin and became a member also of the American Philosophical Society, founded as early as 1743. The second female foreign member of the Royal Swedish Academy of Sciences was Marie Curie who was elected in 1910. As already mentioned she never became a member of the French Academy of Sciences.

On December 12 Hevesy gave his Nobel lecture[7]. It provided a grand presentation of the development and application of the indicator technique. The lecture took its origin in the Czechoslovak town of Joachimstal. This Bohemian city is the origin of the pitchblende ore that was used by the Curies to isolate radium for the first time and also provided material for Rutherford's studies of radium and its byproducts. Parenthetically it can be mentioned that metals from the same mines have been used for the minting of coins, which were referred to as *thaler* and this designation is the origin of the more commonly used currency term *dollar*. It was the "radio-lead" — Radium D in lead from pitchblende — sent to Rutherford which he asked Hevesy to separate from common, stable lead, an impossible task as he realized after two years of experiments. It was because of this experience that he initiated decennia of pioneering work using the indicator method.

As already described the possibilities in the early phase were very limited because of the access to only a few useful naturally occurring radioactive materials. Some studies of atom exchange in materials like lead and lead compounds were feasible and it also became possible to determine the lead content of rocks with great precision. However, the opportunity to study biological problems initially was very limited. Certain studies of mineral uptake in plants were examined using lead, but the toxicity of its compounds restricted further use. It was the access first to heavy water and later artificially induced isotopes that would "lead" Hevesy on. The whole field of use of radioisotopes came to explode. Hevesy was in the right position and at the right place to spearhead this rapidly expanding field of research. It is to his credit that he could train himself as a physicist studying chemistry into becoming an authoritative biologist. He approached a number of different fundamental questions, for example the formation of the constituents of the hen's egg. In order to study this he employed the highly useful ^{32}P isotope. Many other applications have already been presented above. Hevesy's last years of experimentation were conducted in collaboration with the hematologist Dieter Lockner at the Karolinska Institute. Lockner was a German physician, who was trained in performing experimental work together with Hevesy in his laboratory at the Stockholm University. The data he generated was used in a PhD thesis at the Karolinska Institute.

In Levi's book it is suggested that although Hevesy was pleased to receive the Nobel Prize, he was not wholeheartedly satisfied. This was probably due to the fact that he regretted not having been recognized earlier, in particular for his discovery of hafnium. He was rather outspoken when commenting on his prize as cited[27]. According to this source he had said "The audience believes that the Nobel Prize is the greatest award for a chemist, but this is not so. There are 40 to 50 Nobel laureates in chemistry whereas the Royal Society includes only ten foreign members, of whom only two (de Hevesy and Bohr) have been awarded the Copley Medal." Obviously Hevesy viewed the Swedish Academy as somewhat provincial whereas the British Royal Society was held up as a paragon of intellectual standards. In a comment given later in life to Klein Hevesy mused: "The happiness the Nobel Prize brings to those who get it is like a feather compared to the massive misery of those who expect to get it but don't."

Clearly there was a streak of vanity in his personality and still I wonder what the true description of his reaction to the Nobel Prize he received might have been. He clearly was a very competitive person who aimed at rapid publications to claim priority. He knew his value and understood that he had opened up a completely new field of research. Still he had a wide perspective on the selection of individuals and their achievements as meriting a Nobel Prize. For example he was well versed in the magnitude of contributions like that of Bohr. The identification of a single element by itself had not previously been considered sufficient to be recognized by a Nobel Prize as discussed above. However, it might be argued that the identification of hafnium represented much more than the demonstration of a single new element. The question is how important it was in providing a key to the electronic structure of the atom postulated by Bohr and how critical it was in furthering an understanding of the mysterious series of lanthanide elements. By way of contrast it should be noted that it was *because of* Bohr's model that Hevesy and Coster looked for a zirconium-related element with a deducible X-ray spectroscopic pattern predicted by Moseley. Svedberg did rate the discovery of hafnium higher than the corresponding identification of other previously unrecognized elements, but still he did not hesitate to state clearly that this contribution was not sufficient to be recognized by a Nobel Prize. I judge that Hevesy understood that in order to merit recognition by a Nobel Prize a discovery should include the demonstration of the existence of new principles or methods, in this case allowing the identification of a wider set of unique elements of compounds.

In the case of the introduction of the concept of the indicator technique the situation was different. It was after the fortunate discovery of induced radioactivity by Joliot-Curie that Hevesy was able to take full advantage of the potential for bold conceptual formulations and of his wide knowledge as well as his dynamic fearlessness with regard to embarking on completely new applications. Sometimes a discovery needs a boost and again the famous Louis Pasteur dictum that "luck strikes the prepared mind" can be cited. In the history books Hevesy is referred to as the father of the ever growing field of nuclear medicine — and the humble giant Bohr as its godfather.

It is said that Paneth was very disappointed not to be included in the Nobel Prize to de Hevesy, but as has already been mentioned, the committee concluded that it was the combination of the original discovery of the indicator technique, by both de Hevesy and Paneth, and the critical follow-up of applications of the technique by de Hevesy alone that justified his being the sole recipient of the prize. Paneth was a highly respected chemist and he appears repeatedly in the annals of the Nobel archives. He was nominated with varying motivations for a prize in 1927, 1932, 1935, 1939 — this time together with de Hevesy by Soddy , as discussed above — 1948 (a nomination together with Morris S. Kharach in a joint proposal by six American scientists from Chicago), 1952, and 2–5 nominations in 1953, 1955, 1956 and 1957. It is not unlikely that de Hevesy, being a generous person and a very good friend of Paneth, had stimulated some of his scientific colleagues to nominate Paneth for the prize. The 1948 nomination of Paneth and Kharasch was "for their work on free radicals" and a ten-page review was done by Arne Fredga, a member of the chemistry committee we will meet again in Chapter 7. In the introduction he again reviewed why earlier contributions by Paneth had not led to serious consideration of him as a strong candidate for a Nobel Prize. As concerns the 1948 nominations for the work on free radicals he concluded that Paneth and Kharasch had made separate contributions at different times and that Kharasch's work was still ongoing. Fredga raised the possibility that a combination of the two for a prize in the future might be an alternative but the committee did not endorse this at the time. Throughout the later years the committee referred back to Svedberg´s and Fredga's earlier reviews, but in 1953 Svedberg did an additional investigation focusing solely on Paneth´s geochemical and cosmochemical studies. The committee cited Svedberg's conclusions in its summarizing review. These were: "He (Paneth) has, by use of the gaseous analytical methods developed by the early English school, developed techniques that make it possible to determine noble gases, in particular helium, in very small concentrations with a high degree of accuracy. Using this method it has been possible for him to determine the age of rock materials of low activity and of meteorites — something that has previously not been possible." The committee agreed with the reviewer that these investigations represented a very important contribution, but that they could hardly justify a Nobel Prize in chemistry. So in the end Paneth's important research in different areas was never recognized by a Nobel Prize. He is certainly not alone in that category. There is after all only one prize per year in each discipline awarded to a maximum of three scientists. Only unique discoveries or improvements can be rewarded by a prize in chemistry.

Modern Tracer Techniques in Biology, Medicine and Archaeology

The tracer technique that Hevesy pioneered has developed in many directions and become a pervasive and indispensable tool in biological research. The principal applications are too numerous to be listed and only a few random examples will be given. Tagging of molecules by an isotope has become an indefinitely useful way of determining specificity and turnover of biologically important molecules. Viruses contain as their genetic material either DNA or RNA, but never both at the same time. In the early 1960s it had not yet been defined which kind of nucleic acid measles virus contained. This virus was the focus of my own PhD thesis. In my laboratory we had developed a technique to purify virus particles by equilibrium centrifugation. By use of tritium-labeled uridine — specific for RNA — and tritium-labeled thymidine — specific for DNA — we could show that only the former isotope-labeled nucleotide was present in the fractions containing virus particles[28]. Hence the virus-specific nucleic acid was RNA.

A combination of isotope-labeled antigens and specific antibodies offer excellent possibilities for quantification. This was recognized by the 1977 Nobel Prize in physiology or medicine one half of which was awarded to Rosalyn Yalow "for the development of radioimmunoassays of peptide hormones" (see Table 3, p. 90). Yalow came from a poor Jewish family and had the double handicaps at the time of her studies in the 1940s of both her ethnic background and also of being a woman. She was the only woman among 400 faculty members and graduate students in the engineering faculty at the University of Illinois at Urbana-Champaign. In time she came to be responsible for the development of nuclear physics at the Bronx Veteran Administration Hospital where in 1950 she had a decisive encounter. She met the physician Solomon Berson. They became an inseparable team of researchers for 18 years pioneering the use of radioactive tracers in studies of physiological problems. They elected to use different isotopes of iodine. One isotope ^{131}I had a high energy of emission and since it specifically associated with the thyroid gland it could be used to medically depress the function of that organ. Another isotope ^{125}I emitted less energy and was

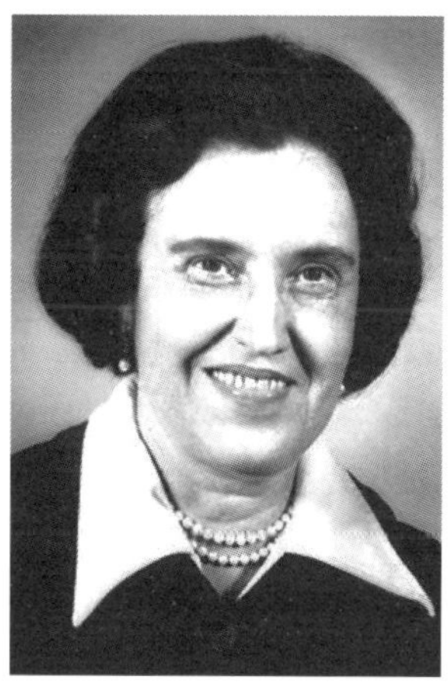

Rosalyn Yalow (1921–2011), recipient of a shared 1977 Nobel Prize in physiology or medicine. [From *Les Prix Nobel en 1977*.]

therefore safer to work with and hence could be employed for experimental purposes. Originally the two scientists used the iodine isotopes for blood volume determination, as Hevesy had done in his original dilution experiments. They also used them for clinical analysis of thyroid diseases and the kinetics of iodine metabolism. Thereafter they expanded their studies to also include diabetes — Yalow's husband Aaron had this disease. These studies allowed an unexpected breakthrough; eventually leading to the shared Nobel Prize awarded to Yalow in 1977. Sadly Berson could not share this prize since he had died five years earlier.

At the time it was believed that patients with diabetes had a shorter half-life of insulin because of the speculated presence of enzymes breaking down the hormone. Yalow and Berson studied three groups of patients; healthy individuals, diabetic subjects treated with insulin and individuals who had received insulin as a shock therapy for schizophrenia. The insulin was purified from pig organs. When insulin labeled by radioactive iodine was injected into these groups of individuals the scientists found to their surprise that the labeled material survived much longer in patients who had previously received injections with the same kind of insulin. Further studies of this phenomenon revealed that this was due to production of antibodies against insulin in the treated patients. It took time for Yalow and Berson to convince the scientific community that there existed antibodies against insulin, since at the time it was not believed that a molecule as small as insulin (about 6,000 Daltons) could induce an antibody response. The original manuscript describing these important findings was rejected by Science and initially by Journal of Clinical Investigation. A modified version of the manuscript was eventually published in the latter journal, but only after the word *antibody* in the title had been exchanged for *immunoglobulin*.

The disappointment at the rejection of their seminal paper stayed with Yalow for many years and in her Nobel lecture[29] she showed a copy of the letter of rejection. However she was not alone in feeling such frustration. The general saying is that attempts to publish discoveries which are later recognized by Nobel Prizes are rejected in about 40 percent of cases. The documentation of the existence of antibodies to insulin allowed the development of a new technique to measure the amount of circulating insulin in a blood sample. The method required access to three ingredients; iodine-labeled insulin, antibodies to insulin and a serum sample containing insulin in a concentration to be analyzed. The reaction between the labeled insulin and the antibodies was interfered with in the presence of *unlabelled* insulin and the degree of this interference under standardized conditions was a measure of the concentration of the latter. This very useful and simple methodology, referred to as the *radioimmunoassay* (*RIA*), was found to be extremely sensitive and could also in principle be applied to measurements of various other kinds of antigens, like different protein hormones. In essence the introduction of this assay revolutionized experimental and clinical studies of endocrinological and many other kinds of diseases. Later on variants of the technique were introduced using a selected enzyme as marker instead of an isotope label, the *enzyme linked immunosorbent assay* (*ELISA*).

With time many further refined forms of immune reactions with isotope-labeled antigens were presented. Employment of monospecific antibodies generated by the hybridoma technology developed by the Nobel Prize recipients Köhler and Milstein, as described in Chapter 3, and antigens separated by electrophoresis gave valuable information. This *radioimmune precipitation assay* (*RIPA*) has been used extensively and in my laboratory we employed it to characterize the different proteins of measles virus and to map the reactivity of sets of monoclonal antibodies unique for each protein[30]. Virus antigens were labeled by growing the virus in the presence of a tagged amino acid, ^{35}S methionine, and the immune complexes formed were selectively isolated by use of protein A from Staphylococci, which has a unique capacity to bind immune complexes. The complexes were hereafter dissociated and the size of the labeled protein antigen determined by electrophoretic separation. Later the same technique was used for studies of the existence and immunological properties of individual components of many other viruses.

Isotopes can also be used to identify the location of particular — natural or foreign — components, specifically labeled by a selected isotope, in cells. The technique is called *autoradiography* and can be applied also to cells examined, not only by the light microscope, but also by the electron microscope. The general principle is to produce a two-dimensional copy — a radiograph — by which it is possible to identify the location of specifically labeled components in a single layer of cells. The radioactivity emitted from the specimen is photographed by some suitable technique. An alternative way to characterize the presence of specific components in cells, not requiring the use of isotopes, is to use *immunofluorescence* by attachment of a fluorescent tag to the reagent, like for example an antibody, providing a specificity of reaction as discussed in Chapter 2.

Recently this approach has become markedly expanded when it was discovered that certain sequences of amino acids in a protein chain can endow it with capacity to fluorescence by itself when activated by ultraviolet light. It was the obsession by a Japanese researcher Osamu Shimura to devote his life to the spontaneous fluorescence of an exotic jellyfish *Aequorea Victoria* that came to open this field of research. Together with two other scientists, Martin Chalfie and Roger Y. Tsien, his finding was awarded a Nobel Prize in chemistry in 2008 "for the discovery and development of the green fluorescent protein, GFP". The advantage of this technique over radiography is that it can be used on living cells and that it can provide a wide range of "tags", representing the whole spectrum of colors in the rainbow, to separately label different cellular components. When applied to brain tissues the technique was referred to as the "brainbow".

All these applications represent further developments of the principle introduced by Hevesy of using isotopes as indicators. However isotopes can also have another principal use. This is to employ them as clocks. Hevesy used isotopes primarily as indicators, but as discussed above he was also interested in applying long-lived radioactive isotopes, like samarium, for measurement of the age of the earth and short-lived isotopes for example phosphorous and iron for measurement of the lifetime of biomolecules. Libby also used isotopes as clocks, taking advantage of their specific half-life. However as described in his Nobel lecture he was interested in a shorter time scale[31]. He used primarily 14-carbon which is generated by the bombardment of the nitrogen by cosmic rays in the outermost part of the atmosphere of the Earth. Carbon is the backbone atom in organic molecules and therefore 14-carbon is built into such molecules during the active life processes. As soon as these life processes cease, as for example at the death of a tree or the harvest of animal or plant material to be used, as for instance, for textiles, no more radioactive carbon is added. The concentration of radioactive material then decreases exponentially with time with a half-life of 5,568 years. The usefulness of this clock could be confirmed in studies of archeological materials collected and dated from before the Common Era (BCE), like brick and wood structures from the first Egyptian Dynasty tombs of the Vizier Hemaka and of King Zet, found at Saqqara (4,900 years before the present time) and the linen wrapping of the Dead Sea Scrolls, the Book

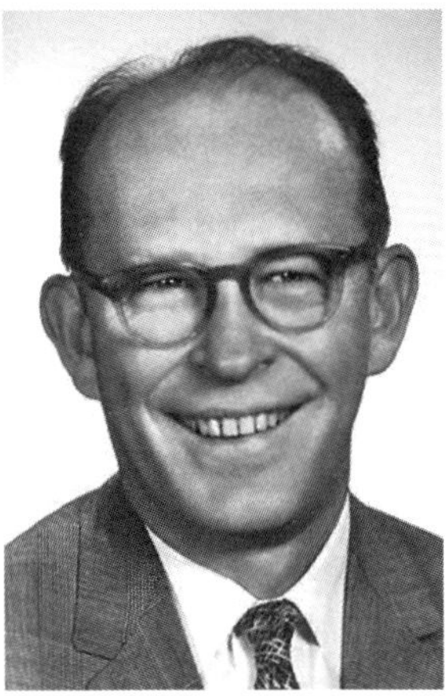

W. Frank Libby (1908–1980), recipient of the 1960 Nobel Prize in chemistry. [From *Les Prix Nobel en 1960.*]

of Isaiah, found in Palestine (slightly more than 2,000 years old). During the 1990s more exact data on the age of the Qumran scrolls have been obtained by accelerator mass spectrometry carbon measurements, an improvement of accuracy of considerable importance in matters of exegetics.

One circumstance that delayed the prize to Libby was a discussion in the committee, initiated by the reviewer, the Nobel laureate Tiselius, of the practical importance of the findings. On this occasion the Nobel committee for the first time used Swedish experts outside its own circle. Wisely it was concluded that human cultures need and are nourished by particular knowledge developed just for its own sake. It is obvious that timelines of and insights into the origin and development of the universe at large and specifically the planet we inhabit as well as our own very short cultural history markedly influence our ways of managing the central existential questions.

Hevesy was interested in the turnover of cells in complex animals and published the first data on the lifetime of red blood cells. He also demonstrated that there was a fast turnover of cells in the bone marrow and in the intestine. It has been a particular challenge to characterize the fate of cells in organs, which originally were believed to have no exchange of cells. Such organs are the brain and the heart. In recent years it has become possible to examine the turnover of cells also in these organs by use of an ingenious technique. In this case it is not possible to use a prospective labeling of cells by adding a suitable isotope labeled compound. Jonas Frisén, a professor of stem cell research at the Karolinska Institute, developed a solution to this problem by skilfully taking advantage of a particular possibility for retrospective age determination of cells. He decided to see if the isotopes released by the open-air testing of nuclear weapons for a few years until 1963 might provide a marker. After the cessation of above-ground tests no more 14-carbon has been released into the air, besides that originating from the natural, continuous cosmic ray production, and therefore its concentration has progressively decreased due to the decay of the isotope. Hence the 14-carbon in the DNA of cells can serve as a marker of their date of birth. However, the application of this approach required major refinements of methods to measure a tiny amount of the isotope in materials. The necessary improvement in accelerator mass spectroscopy measurements became possible by collaborations with physicists. The spectacular results obtained show that there is in fact a certain renewal of cells in the brain, in particular in its central parts. In the case of the heart the startling new findings were that about one percent of the cells of the heart are replaced every year until the age of 25 and that the rate progressively falls towards half a percent at older ages[32]. This means that during a normal life span of an individual, about half of all heart muscle cells are exchanged. These findings amplify the hope for a possible use of stem cells in regenerative medicine applicable to different organs.

Life after the Nobel Prize

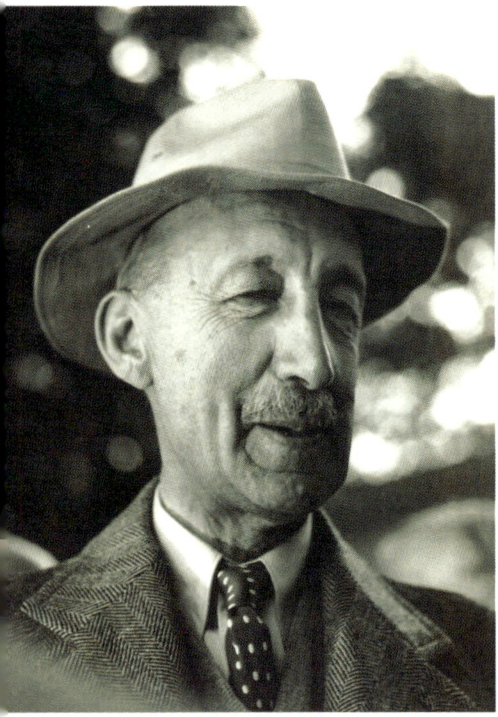

Hevesy at a mature age. [From the Hevesy family collection.]

Hevesy was almost 60 years old when he received his Nobel Prize. There remained still two more decades of his life that allowed him to further develop his curiosity and creativity. Science was the essence of his life. He continued to run a laboratory at Stockholm University and was supported for long periods of time by the Rockefeller Foundation. Even when his involvement in experimental work waned somewhat in later years he continued to be a prolific writer. The field of science he had made accessible for his fellow scientists by the introduction of his tracer technique was essentially limitless. The range of different isotopes available for use progressively increased and methods to detect their radiation also improved. In the field of health care dedicated departments for nuclear medicine were established. The radioisotopes were used both for diagnosis and for treatment of diseases like hyperactivity in the thyroid gland as already referred to. In laboratories studying life sciences tracer techniques were integrated as standard methods and became as indispensable as everyday tools for chemical separations or for morphological characterizations. Various examples of new applications were cited above. Medawar (Chapter 2) drew a parallel between the consequences of the introduction of isotope techniques and those of the development of the microscope.

As a Nobel laureate Hevesy was frequently invited to international conferences. He enjoyed in particular participating in the yearly meetings

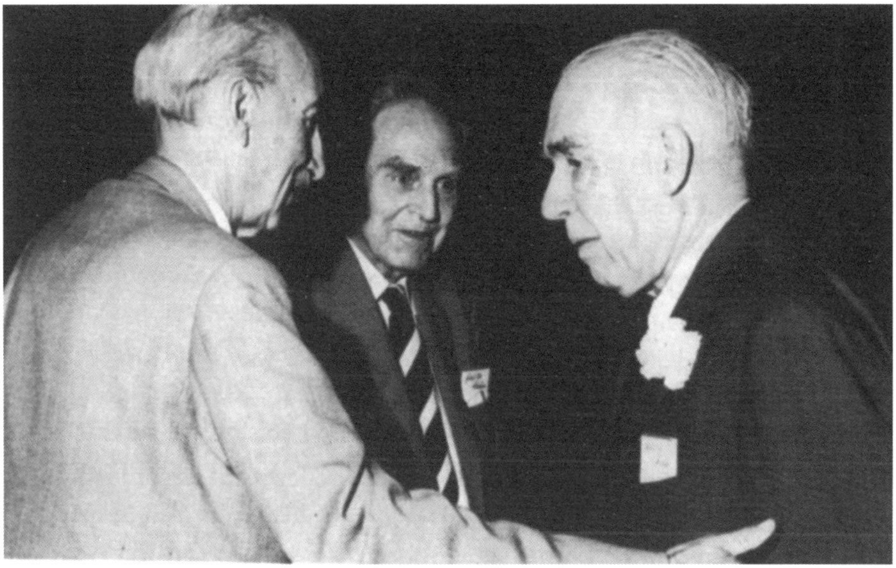

Three statesmen of science Hevesy, Otto Hahn, who received his Nobel Prize in chemistry one year after him, and Bohr meeting at Lindau in 1960. [From Ref. 2.]

by Nobel laureates in Lindau at Lake Constance. This form of meeting has a long tradition by now and has developed to become a globally acknowledged forum for exchange of knowledge between Nobel Laureates and young researchers continuing into the present time. The first Lindau meeting was arranged in 1951 and Count Lennart Bernadotte af Wisborg at Mainau was its host, a responsibility he retained for many decades. Hevesy participated in these meetings between 1952 and 1962 and in 1965, in most cases by giving a lecture on a topic within his field. In 1955 he gave two lectures, one of which was entitled "The way of the atoms through generations" and in that year he also was one of the signatories of the Mainau declaration, an appeal against the use of nuclear weapons.

Hevesy was also recognized by being awarded honorary doctorates, two of which he received from Freiburg University after the end of the Second World War, as mentioned, and also by receiving a number of prizes. Among the latter can be mentioned the Copley medal from the Royal Society in London 1949 and the Atoms for Peace Award which he received at an event at the Rockefeller Institute from the hands of Dag Hammarskjöld in 1959, the Swedish Secretary General of the United Nations at the time. Bohr had received the latter medal the year before Hevesy.

Hevesy had many contacts in the field of science, but there were two individuals who were particularly close to his heart and to whom he made exceptions to his general tendency of not sharing his emotions and personal concerns about life. They were Paneth and Bohr. These friendships came to be very long lasting, since Paneth lived until 1958 and Bohr until 1962. In later years they enjoyed reminiscing about the time that had passed. A year before Bohr's death Hevesy was very proud to receive the Niels Bohr medal at a ceremony in Copenhagen. Hevesy's own health started to deteriorate a year later. He was diagnosed with lung cancer by a clinical friend of his in Freiburg. It can be speculated that this disease could have been due to professional exposure to radium D (^{212}Pb) from its precursor , the gas radon, which might have accumulated in his lung tissues. It should be added that Hevesy was a strict non-smoker. The disease progressively reduced his capacity to work and to engage in scientific meetings. He reserved a good part of his time for his closest family always accompanied by his wife. In La Jolla in California, where their oldest daughter Jenny and three grandchildren lived, he could relax. It even happened that influenced by the local casual dressing traditions he could take a break from his waistcoats and tailor-made suits. In Geneva he could visit their daughter Pia and two other grandchildren and finally at home in Stockholm his son Georg, a physician, with his family and two further grandchildren offered rich contacts. The third child Ingrid had chosen to live in Freiburg, which became particularly important during the last part of Hevesy's life. As the disease advanced he was cared for in this city by his clinical friends there. It was also there that he celebrated his 80th birthday and somewhat less than a year later died on 5 July 1966.

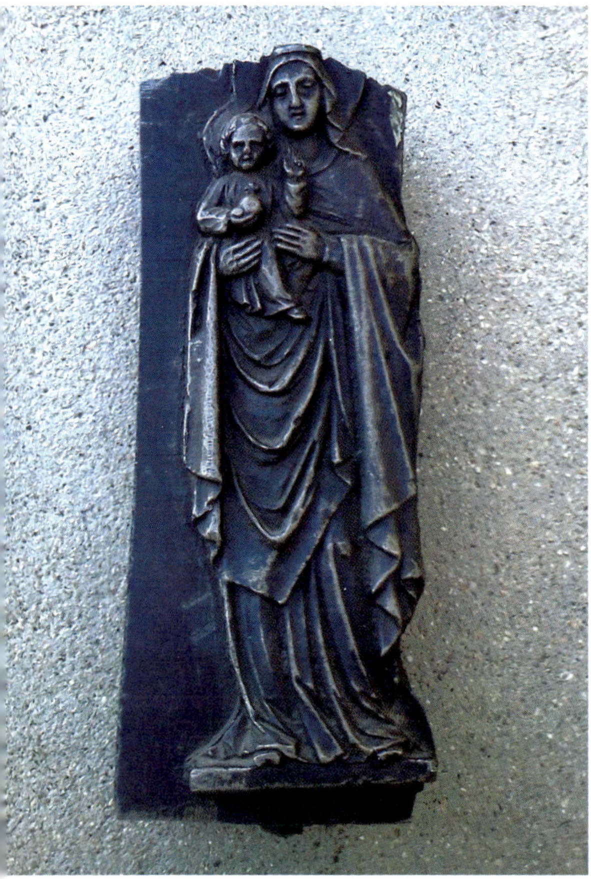

A part of a church bell rescued by Hevesy during the First World War. [From the Hevesy family collection.]

Hevesy was not a religious man in a superstitious sense. He never went to church for personal religious observation. Still he was emotionally firmly attached to some of the ethical concepts of Catholicism, especially its emphasis on humility. He had his upbringing in a Catholic school and he was induced by the diocese in Copenhagen to let his older children have access to extracurricular Catholic instruction. On the occasion of his involvement in copper works in Nagyteteny-Diosd during the First World War he cut out and rescued a part of a church bell showing the Virgin and Child and retained it as an esthetic memory of those bad days. It still remains with his family. In the latter part of his life he became involved with the Pontifical Academy. He showed a particular appreciation of the meetings of this Academy and gave a memorial lecture about Bohr at one of its meetings in June 1963. In spite of the fact that his disease had advanced markedly he managed, with a personal medical carer, two months before his demise to participate in a conference on hematology in Rome, and at his own particular wish to be received once more in an audience by the Pope. He was buried in Freiburg, but in 2001 he and his family's earthly remains, with great civil ceremony supervised by the Hungarian Academy of Science, were moved to a final resting place in his native country in the National Pantheon at the Kerepesi Cemetary in Budapest. The academy also took care of Hevesy's Nobel gold medal, donated by the family.

Chapter 6

Making Sense of Hearing

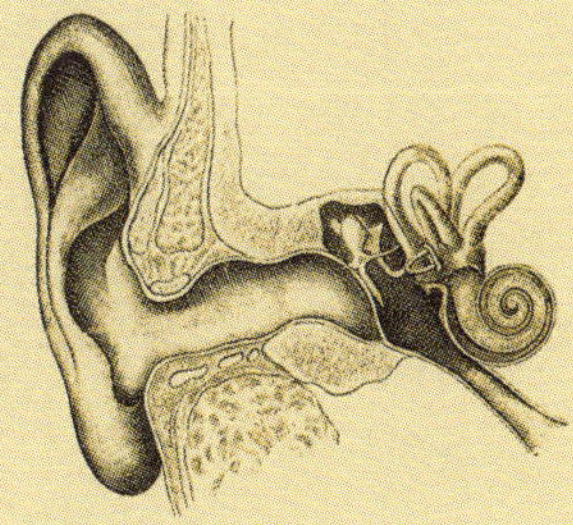

ARTS AND SCIENCES
CREATION – EPIPHANY
REACH BEYOND SENSES

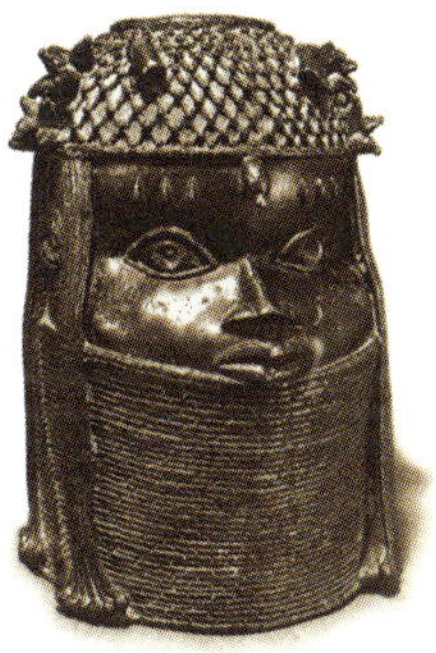

A royal memorial head in bronze from Benin City, Nigeria, in the foyer of the office of the Nobel Committee at the Karolinska Institute. [From Ref. 13.]

In January when I make my yearly foray into the archives of the office of the Nobel Committee at the Karolinska Institute, the first thing I see is a royal memorial head in bronze. This impressive artifact has its origin in Benin City, Nigeria and is 200–300 years old. It represents one piece out of the very rich collection of art that Georg von Békésy accumulated from many ancient cultures during his long life. This collection was bequeathed to the Nobel Foundation upon his death in 1972. It was his way of honoring the organization supporting the prize-giving institution, the Karolinska Institute, which in turn had honored him. In 1961 Békésy had received the Nobel Prize in physiology or medicine "for his discoveries of the physical mechanism of stimulation within the cochlea".

Like Hevesy, whom we met in the previous chapter, Békésy was of Hungarian nobility. His cultivated background encouraged him in the development of his two interests in life, his science and his collections of books and ancient art. He never did clearly distinguish between these pursuits. They were both interpreted by him to have beauty and their creations reflected the skill and ingenuity of their originators. He loved to cite Goethe and one of his favorite quotes was: "If you want to reach the infinite, thoroughly explore every aspect of the finite." His intense involvements in science and the arts allowed him to live a rich life, but he was a solitary person, remained a bachelor and made only a few friends.

There is no complete biography of Békésy but Floyd Ratliff at the Rockefeller University has written about his life both in a biographical memoir published by the U.S. National Academy of Sciences[1] and as an introduction to a catalogue of Békésy's collection of ancient art displayed at the East Asian Museum in Stockholm in 1974[2]. He is also mentioned in Marx's book on Hungarian scientists[3], referred to in the previous chapter .

The Early Years of Studies

Georg von Békésy was born in Budapest half a year before the turn of the previous century into a noble family originating from Debrecen. His father was a diplomat who held posts in different countries, Germany, Turkey and Switzerland. His choice of appointments was directed in part by the consideration that Georg's poor health might be improved by choosing a benevolent climate for the family to live in. In Munich the young Békésy was stimulated by access to a well-endowed museum of the history of science. The technical advances of the time thrilled him. Among other things the first automated telephone appealed to his imagination. But his interest in music, painting and sculpture was also stimulated by the diverse cultural events on offer in the liberal Bavarian environment. The seeds of his lifelong interest in the arts and science were planted early.

When his father was transferred to Constantinople he was exposed to another seductive cultural environment. The beauty of the city — the sunsets on the Bosphorus and striking views of the Sea of Marmara — stayed with him, although the family were to live in Turkey only briefly. The political situation became volatile when the long-lived Ottoman regime was toppled by Kemal Atatürk. A rapid transition to a post for his father in Switzerland implied another major change of cultural environment. Békésy liked the ambiance of Zurich, not least the plentiful access to high quality libraries and many well-endowed museums. He also liked his school, the private Institute Minerva, which applied a uniquely modern mobile class system. His major disciplines were physics and Latin and he did very well in school. Half a year before turning 18 he finished his studies. This allowed him six months to engage in other things before he was allowed to start his theoretical studies at the university.

He chose to study practical mechanics and became an apprentice in a workshop. From the experienced Swiss mechanics he learned the fundamentals of the use of standard tools, like a file, a hacksaw, a drill press, a turning lathe, etc. This experience was to be of great value in his future research, which as we shall see included the examination of the hearing organ *in situ* by careful dissection of the petrous part of the temporal bone and by the design of highly informative mechanical models.

In 1916 Békésy started his studies at the University of Berne. He chose chemistry and after two years he succeeded in gaining his baccalaureate. One particular episode during this time was to further increase his enthusiasm for books and libraries. As has become apparent from the previous chapter it was popular at the time for chemists to try to fill in the gaps that still remained in the periodic table. Békésy thought he had discovered a substance that might be a candidate for one of the gaps and therefore asked his professor what he thought about his findings. He got the abrasive answer, "The library is on the second floor." Once he had searched the books in the library he found that his substance was not new. He took this lesson to heart and the experience strongly accentuated his belief that books, preferably collected in one's own library, are the best "friends" one can have.

For some time Békésy studied music seriously, guided by two famous Swiss pianists. Surprisingly, given that he was to become the world authority on hearing, he never came to love music unconditionally. He found that music stayed with him in an uncontrollable way and he even stated: "… music is different, it occupies the brain and handicaps good logical thinking." He did not have this problem with all the other forms of art, like painting and sculpture. On the contrary, he used visual arts for his inspiration. Over time he developed very personal working habits. During the long days that he put in working on science he took intervals of "resting" which for him meant contemplating a piece of art. He could do this for hours. He also made it a habit to compare similar pieces of art as a way of developing his capacity for judging its quality. To constantly compare and contrast was the basic method that Békésy developed and applied both in his studies of art and of science.

Békésy's studies in Bern also made him familiar with the disciplines of mathematics, astronomy and physics. It remained for him to choose the course of his future researches. This decision was delayed since Békésy was drafted into the Hungarian army at the beginning of the First World War, but due to his fragile health he was not sent to the front line. After the war his idealism and patriotism encouraged him to become involved with the University of Budapest.

He selected experimental optics for his doctoral studies and received his PhD in Physics in 1923. At that time the country was in disarray, as described in the previous chapter, but thanks to material and emotional support from his mother he was able to move on. The only laboratory he could find that was still equipped to keep up its work was the research laboratory of the Hungarian Post and Telegraph. Although formally no position was available he was accepted at this laboratory and even received a small salary. Very soon Békésy became involved in problems of communication engineering. Hungary was at the crossroads of international telecommunications, but there were recurrent problems. When communications were delayed or blocked one tested the international line by closing the circuit in another city. Hereafter pure tones in the form of defined voltage were introduced into the loop in Budapest and then recorded as they returned to the city some 15–20 minutes later. This was a very unreliable and impractical method, so Békésy took a completely new approach. He had noticed that there were "clicks" when phones were connected and disconnected. He chose to use such "clicks" as a test signal. This was an ingenious invention and a line could now be checked in about one second. Information about this new invention was never published. In his Nobel lecture[4] he compared this approach to what a violinist did when he determined the tuning of his instrument by plucking a string — pizzicato — instead of using his bow, which is much more time-consuming. It was the click method that guided Békésy into his future research on the mechanisms of hearing.

The Inner Ear Is So Beautiful that I Must Study It

Because of his important contributions to the laboratory of the Hungarian Post and Telegraph, Békésy was given a relatively free hand to expand his research projects. Using the click method it was possible to determine that the telephone receiver was the weakest part of the communication system. Thus it needed to be improved, but first it was important to determine its sensitivity relative to that of the ear. Unsurprisingly it was found that the eardrum was a markedly superior instrument. This observation led Békésy to focus his research on the mechanisms of hearing, a preoccupation that was to stay with him throughout his life. He made many discoveries in this work that focused on almost all aspects of hearing associated with the structures of the outer and inner ear. These can only be analyzed in the proper context and in order to understand this it is necessary to briefly describe the knowledge of the mechanisms of hearing at the time.

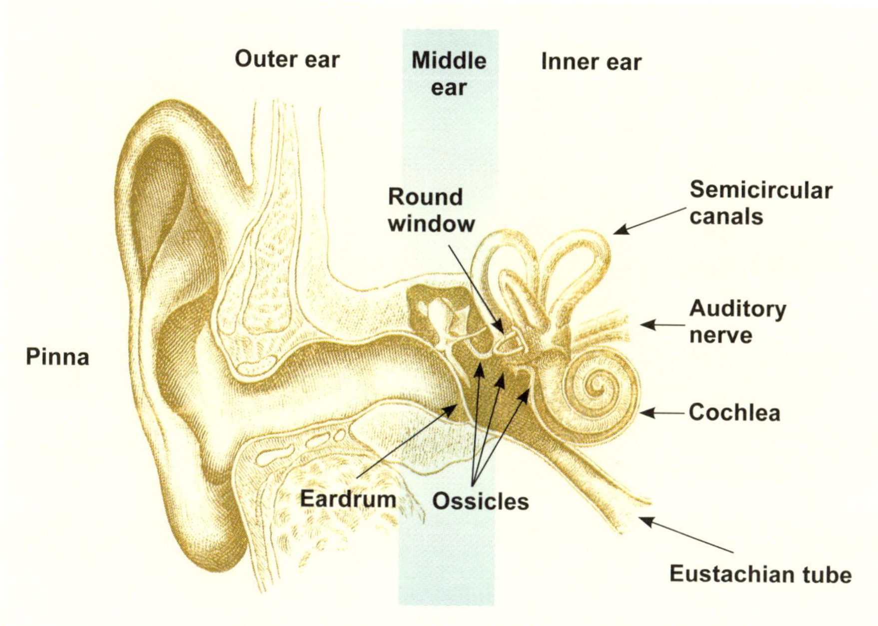

Schematic drawing of the hearing organs.

Hearing is one of the five major senses as defined by Aristotle and like touch it requires sensitivity to the movement of molecules outside the organism. There are three steps in hearing. The sound waves are transmitted by air into the body via the outer ear and its channel to the eardrum. The vibrations of the eardrum are then transmitted mechanically via three bones — the hammer, the anvil and the stirrup bones — to the membrane covering the oval window. This window connects to the inner ear, which has two distinct parts with different functions. One of these is the bone-enclosed helical shell of hearing, the *cochlea*, which at its other end has one more membrane-covered opening, the round window. Like the shell of a snail the cochlea is a three-dimensional spiral with a diminishing diameter towards its apex. It encompasses 2¾ turns. The hollow space is divided by two membranes — the Reissner and basilar membranes — into three channels — *scala vestibuli*, *media* and *tympani*. The middle scala, where the hearing organ is located, is thus enclosed by membranes. The 35-millimeter long basilar membrane carries hair cells which are connected to nerve endings. The cells are sensitive to spatial-temporal patterns of vibrations transmitted by the fluid in the helical structure. The stimulation of the hair cells is executed by contact with a third membrane, the tectorial membrane, which is set in motion by vibrations transmitted by the enclosed fluid. Paradoxically the basilar membrane widens the larger the distance from

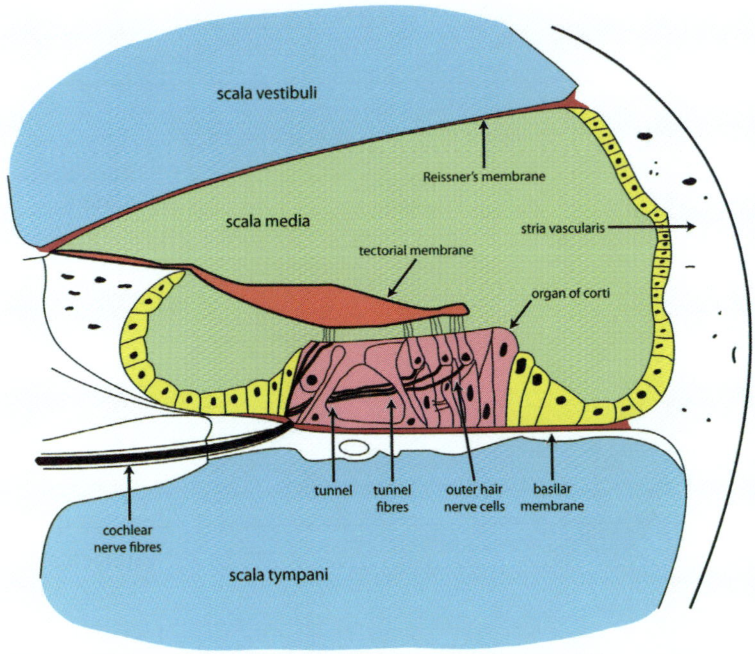

A schematic presentation of a cross-section of the cochlea with the three channels. The organ of Corti is located in the middle channel.

the oval window (see figure on p. 242). The maximum span of the membrane is at the top of the three-dimensional spiral.

The hair cells can activate firing of selected cells in the auditory nerve and this firing transmits information about the sound to the brain. There are 15,000 to 20,000 auditory nerve-cell receptors. The complex structure of the hair cells and the nerve cells is referred to as the organ of Corti, a name deriving from the 19th century Italian anatomist Alfonso Corti, who was the first to describe its structure. Activation of the hair cells can also occur by movement of the fluid caused by sound transmitted directly by the bone surrounding the cochlea, for example in the case of our own voice or when the head is under water. The inner ear also contains an organ that records the posture of our body, allowing us to keep our balance. This part of the inner ear is referred to as the labyrinth (see figure on p. 242).

Békésy studied almost all aspects of hearing. He started by examining the basilar membrane. This had been done before in particular by the mid-19th century polymath Hermann von Helmholz. He had published a book of considerable impact *On the Sensation of Tone as a Physiological Basis for the Theory of Music*. By the introduction of clever techniques Békésy was capable of preparing the separate and intact hearing organ in conditions which had never been available before. Dissections were made using a high-speed drill with the organ submerged in water, which was continuously exchanged. Once he had finished his dissection Békésy stated "I found the inner ear so beautiful under the stereoscopic microscope that I decided I would just stay with that problem. It was beauty and the pleasure of beauty that made me stick to the ear."

In the beginning of his work Békésy experienced some difficulties because he did not have an M.D. degree. He had difficulties of getting access to heads of cadavers for his studies, but as his studies progressed, effective collaborations were established. Rumors about his general insight into basic problems of communication engineering and especially his studies of the function of the ear started to spread. He received invitations for employments outside Hungary. For a year Békésy worked in Berlin, but he rapidly returned to Budapest, because he was worried about his health. It seems that he had a tendency to depression and to hypochondria and what made things worse was that he completely lacked confidence in doctors.

Békésy's studies of the patterns of vibration in the membranes of the cochlea led to major advances and in 1928 he was able to publish his first article and possibly the one with the greatest impact[5]. During his whole scientific career Békésy published almost 150 articles. It is striking that he was the sole author of almost all of them. Only in five publications did he have a co-author. It is also of interest that out of the 21 references in his Nobel lecture[4] only one is to a publication by himself. All his early publications were in German — he was bilingual because his mother spoke German — but after 1947 Békésy published almost exclusively in English. The publications deal exclusively with studies of various aspects of hearing, except for a few articles written between 1964 and 1966 which present data from studies of another sense, that of taste. His first paper from 1928 had already made him known to the scientific community and he received several invitations for future collaborative work. One of them came from Professor Robert Barany in Uppsala, the 1914 Nobel laureate in physiology or medicine, briefly mentioned in my previous book[6]. Like Békésy, Barany was of Hungarian origin and he also was engaged in studies of the inner ear, but in his case they concerned the labyrinth part and its functions. Békésy was flattered by the offer to become Barany's assistant, but could not picture himself surviving in "this extremely dark and cold" place in Sweden and declined.

His work was recognized by a number of prizes during the 1930s. In 1939 he became professor of experimental physics in Budapest. This led to responsibility for several laboratories and access to talented assistants and students. It was a very productive period and a true harvest time for Békésy. But then came the Second World War and under the foreign occupation, discussed in the previous chapter, the situation went from bad to worse and most of the laboratories where he worked were destroyed. There was no improvement of his situation in his occupied home country after the war. He became very depressed and could not see a way forward. He knew from his deep insights into history that Budapest over the centuries, after having been destroyed, had always managed to rebuild itself. This, however, did not help him at the time. He decided to take the ultimate step and leave his beloved home country. Possibly, the fact that he remained a life-long bachelor and did not have a family or other relatives to take responsibility for facilitated his decision.

The Swedish Connection

Békésy decided to leave for Sweden. He had already worked in Sweden for a year in 1939 and since then he had developed two particular contacts in this country. These were Yngve Zotterman and Gunnar Holmgren. In 1946 Zotterman had become professor of physiology and pharmacology at the Veterinary School in Stockholm but until then he had developed his science at the Karolinska Institute, during later years as an associate professor. Zotterman was a neurophysiologist who already as a young scientist had developed pioneering studies of nerve conduction. For a while he collaborated with Edgar D. Adrian in Cambridge, who had shared the 1932 Nobel Prize in physiology or medicine with Charles S. Sherrington "for their discoveries regarding the function of neurons". Zotterman was particularly interested in the sensory function of skin, especially in relation to pain and heat, but he also studied the neurochemistry of taste buds. He had met Békésy already in 1937 in Budapest and became fascinated by his research. Zotterman reported about his interesting scientific contact to Holmgren, who was a professor of ear nose and throat diseases and also since 1931 the vice-chancellor of the Institute. In addition he was chairman of the Nobel Committee 1938–1940. Holmgren had a stern personality but was a researcher deeply involved in science. It was he who in collaboration with the Red Cross had managed to get Barany, mentioned above, released from a prisoner of war camp in Russia during the First World War and arranged for him to come to Sweden in order to receive his Nobel Prize. When Holmgren heard from Zotterman about Békésy's exciting research he

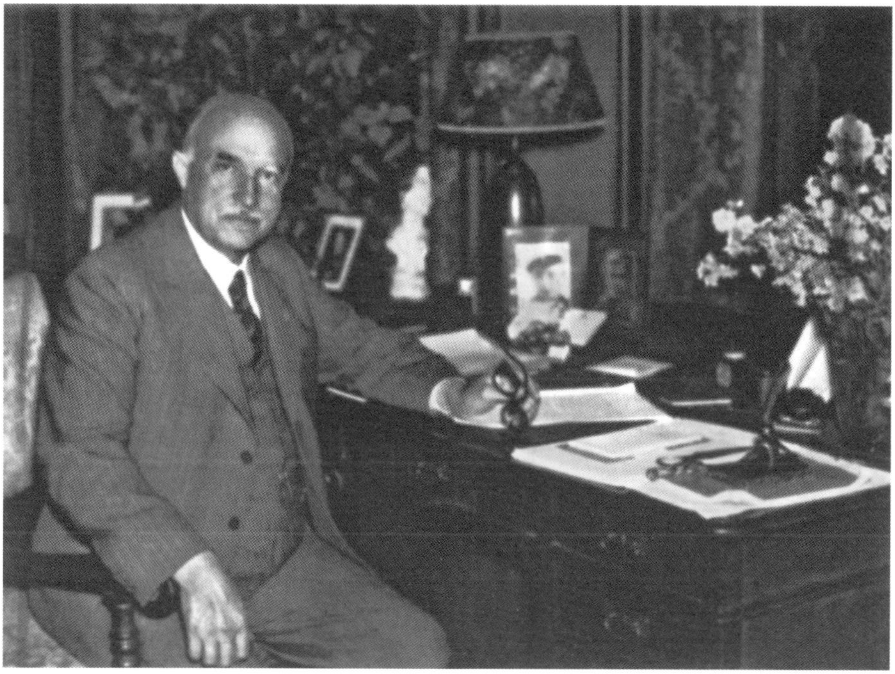

Gunnar Holmgren (1875–1954), Vice-Chancellor of the Karolinska Institute, 1931–1940. [Courtesy of the Karolinska Institute.]

became enthusiastic and invited him to Stockholm. Békésy came to Stockholm for a short time in 1939 and initiated collaborative work at the Institute and the Royal School of Technology, but then returned to Hungary in spite of the rapidly escalating international turmoil in central Europe.

After the war Holmgren took new initiatives to get Békésy to Stockholm. He had good contacts with members of the Swedish government and managed to secure from the minister of social affairs, Gustav Möller, a salary for one year for Békésy. Depressed and scared by the tragic developments in Hungary he arrived in Stockholm in 1946. Upon arrival Békésy was greeted by a number of colleagues who wanted to help him. He established collaboration with research groups at the Royal School of Technology and he became a Visiting Professor at the Karolinska Institute. However, the shortage of resources for Békésy's research made him leave Sweden already after only a year. Still, he managed to make some important contributions during this year by developing a new type of audiometer which was operated by the patient. This instrument allowed the distinction between hearing defects that are due to damage to the cochlea or are due to other factors. This technique turned out to have applications also outside the field of hearing. In 1947 Békésy accepted a position at the

Psycho-Acoustic laboratory at Harvard in the US. He was given a particular responsibility as Senior Research Fellow, which allowed him to concentrate exclusively on his research, without carrying any teaching duties. His patron professor S. S. Stevens, who like his Swedish hosts had already visited Békésy in Budapest in 1937, also tried to minimize the administrative burden that he had to carry. A very productive period ensued, but occasionally Bekesy looked back on his days in Budapest, reflecting that the discoveries he had made at that time were more fundamental than those he made later.

Békésy was very critical in evaluating his own work and he was also sensitive to the criticism of others. His fellow Hungarian the chemist George Olah, who received the Nobel Prize in chemistry in 1994 "for his contribution to carbocation chemistry", has quoted Békésy in an interview with István Hargittai[7] as follows:

> He (Békésy) wrote that what all scientists need is to have a few good enemies. When you do your work and write it up and you send it to your friends, asking for their comments, they are generally busy people and can afford only a limited time and effort to do this. But if you have a dedicated enemy, he will spend unlimited time, effort and resources to try to prove that you are wrong. Békésy ended up saying that his problem in life was that he lost many good enemies who became his friends.

Holmgren did not give up hope of tempting Békésy to come back to Sweden. He persuaded the Swedish government to establish a personal professorship for him at the Karolinska Institute, but eventually Békésy decided to stay at Harvard. Besides the fact that the conditions for research was superior at Harvard Békésy was worried about the political situation in Europe and did not like to live too close to the Soviet Union. He stayed at Harvard for 19 years, after which he unpredictably settled in Hawaii for the remainder of his days. During his time at Harvard, Bekesy was elected to membership in the U.S. National Academy of Sciences. On this occasion he was sent a questionnaire in order to provide biographical information about himself. One question was "Major interest?" His answer was short, "Art." Another question was a little longer "Major influences which determined the selection of your particular field of science?" Again he gave a short answer, "Pure accident." Békésy also received a large number of honors of which his Nobel Prize in 1961 was the most spectacular. It offered a renewed connection with Sweden.

A Discovery that Caught the Ear of the Nobel Committee

Békésy's development of his science was unique in his technical-mechanical approach measuring different physical parameters. Not surprisingly he was nominated for a Nobel Prize both in physics and in physiology or medicine in 1950. Without making any specific evaluation the Nobel committee of physics upon the occasion of Békésy's initial nomination for a prize noted the following:

> Professor von Békésy whose name for the first time this year is included among those nominated to a Nobel Prize in physics, is known for his pioneering contributions in the field of physiological acoustics. By the development of anatomical methods of preparation and by the use of modern physical methods of analysis it has been possible for him to make significant contributions to the theory of hearing. Although von Békésy in an extraordinarily skilful way has employed physical methods of measurement, it has not been possible for the committee, however, to identify that his publications present any discovery or invention within the field of physics that would justify a Nobel Prize in physics.

Later nominations for a prize in physics therefore were also disregarded with reference to the original conclusion of the committee. The importance of his discoveries was obviously in the field of hearing physiology and hence also for the understanding of various kinds of defects in hearing functions. Over the years Békésy was proposed 20 times for a prize in physiology or medicine before he finally received his prize.

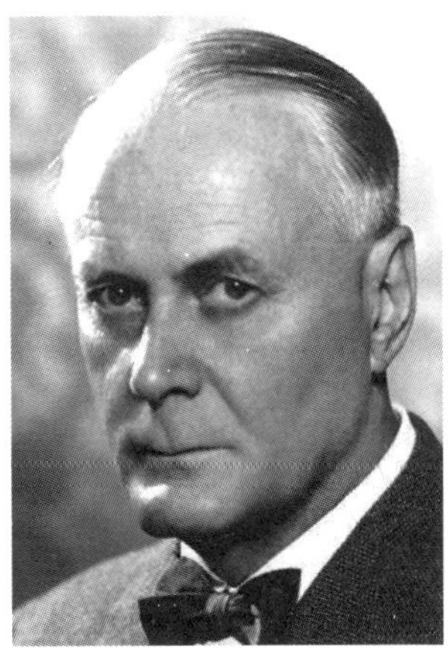

Ragnar Granit (1900–1991), recipient of a shared 1967 Nobel Prize in physiology or medicine. [From *Les Prix Nobel en 1967.*]

The first nomination, submitted in 1950, was from Dr H. Frenzel in Göttingen, Germany. The brief proposal highlighted Bekesy's contribution to physiological acoustics and compared it to that of Helmholtz. The committee considered the nomination important and let Professor Ragnar Granit, who had held a personal research chair in neurophysiology at the Institute since 1946, make a full investigation. Granit, born in 1900, originally came from Finland where he also started his powerful career. He gained experience of working in the US and the progress of his research allowed him in 1940 to choose between a position at Harvard and at the Karolinska Institute. He decided to stay in Scandinavia. When he arrived at the Institute he was already a world authority on the neurophysiology of the visual system. His discoveries in the studies of this system of sense were eventually recognized by a Nobel Prize in physiology or medicine in 1967. He shared the prize with Haldan K. Hartline and George Wald as will be further mentioned below. Thus Granit was a well-qualified judge of Békésy′s findings.

He reviewed the field of acoustic physiology over his 13-page report and noted that the impressive advances in the field were based on contributions by physicists, like Békésy, and physiologists. The longstanding, high-class research by Békésy was highlighted, but it was noted that the nature of his long series of important findings might make it difficult to discern individual specific steps of discovery. The review therefore focused in particular on specifying such major advances in knowledge and to evaluate them in a historical perspective. The so called resonance theory, originally formulated by Helmholtz and after him studied by many researchers, was approached by Békésy in a very concrete way. He built models, at first relatively simple and then more complex. Step by step Békésy was able to make a series of fundamental observations concerning for example which part of the basilar membrane in the cochlea responded to sounds of different frequencies. Already by using his first model he was able to demonstrate that exposure to high-frequency tones activated regions close to the oval window whereas the lower the tone was, the further along the basilar membrane the resonance impacted the membrane (see figure on p. 242). Granit then proceeded to describe how Békésy, after having published his first revolutionary data in 1928, continued to apply his findings to material dissected from human cadavers. In time alternatives to the dominant theory of a resonance model already formulated by Helmholtz were proposed. As illustrated in Békésy's Nobel lecture[4] he concluded that out of the four different theories proposed, the most valid one was the theory referred to as *travelling waves*. Granit cited a number of publications from the 1940s that illustrated how knowledge in this field was advancing. He emphasized that a particular strength of Békésy's work was his deep insight into the physical aspect of acoustics combined with his advanced technical skill allowing him to develop ever more relevant models. The review concluded in the following way:

> Békésy's contribution appears to me without question to belong to the category of discoveries which one grants straightforward admiration.

> Intellectually it is of the highest class and it is by way of background supported by publications in the field of acoustics, all of high quality. For my part I found his contribution worthy of a prize.

The committee agreed with Granit and declared that Békésy's work merited a prize, but the 1950 prize went to the discoverers of the hormones of the adrenal cortex (Ref. 6, Chapter 6).

In 1954 there were two nominations of Békésy, one extensive (6 pages) from R. Mittermaier, Marburg and one from N. Henning, Erlangen. In the beginning of the nomination by Mittermaier it was mentioned that the functions of the inner ear had not been considered since 1914, when a prize was given to Barany. However, the prize awarded to him was for the second major function of the inner ear, the balance apparatus, and the motivation was "for his work on the physiology and pathology of the vestibular apparatus". The committee concluded that a considerable amount of new information had accumulated since Granit's evaluation four years earlier. He was therefore requested to make a supplementary review of Békésy's research.

Granit noted that whereas Békésy in his previous studies had mostly concerned himself with the physical aspects of hearing, in his more recent publications he had focused on the conversion of the mechanical energy into electrical signals and on how the so-called microphonic potential, the output, was generated. In technically elegantly designed experiments it was possible for Békésy to measure energy potentials using microelectrodes. He demonstrated that the microphonic action did not represent a direct translation of mechanical energy. The tissue must also contribute some energy. The critical part in generating the microphonic action was demonstrated to be the tectorial membrane. The general conclusion was that the cochlea did not by itself transform mechanical energy into electric energy but that the organ of Corti was its own electrical generator of the microphony potential. It had been demonstrated by other scientists that the nerve impulses emerge in a phase relationship to the microphonic potential. In summary there can be said to be two phenomena, one qualitative and one quantitative, that needed to be measured. One was the pitch, the frequency, of the sound which led to the activation of a set of neurons originating at a certain region of the cochlea, and the other was the intensity of the stimulation. The identification of the former, the so-called tonotypic axis of the cochlea, represented an important discovery with consequences for the future development of cochlear implants. The latter phenomenon, the intensity of stimulation, was found to be expressed as different temporal nerve firing patterns. The observation that evolution had led to the existence of independent potential generators to facilitate the conversion of mechanical energy to electrical energy was found in parallel studies also to apply to other mechano receptors in the body, like for example in muscles.

Granit concluded lyrically that Békésy was a master of techniques in designing his experiments, including even an element of *l'art pour l'art*. Still he was not convinced that the new discoveries that had been added on their own would merit a prize, but this was not required since Békésy was clearly already worthy of a prize because of his earlier fundamental contributions to the field of the physiology of hearing.

In 1955 there were two more, relatively detailed nominations by L. Ruedi from Zurich and A. Hilding from Minneapolis. The committee asked Granit to analyse these nominations, but he concluded that the additional information provided did not motivate another review. In 1956 there were four nominations of Békésy from Germany and two years later there were as many as seven nominations from different parts of the world, Heidelberg, Munich, Pecs, and Boston and Medford, Massachusetts. Two nominations also included a second name. Some nominations were quite elaborate and included references, in one case exceeding more than 70 items. The position of Békésy as the world authority on hearing at the time was obvious from his publications in *Science*[8] — "Current status of theories of hearing" — and in *Scientific American*[9] — "The ear".

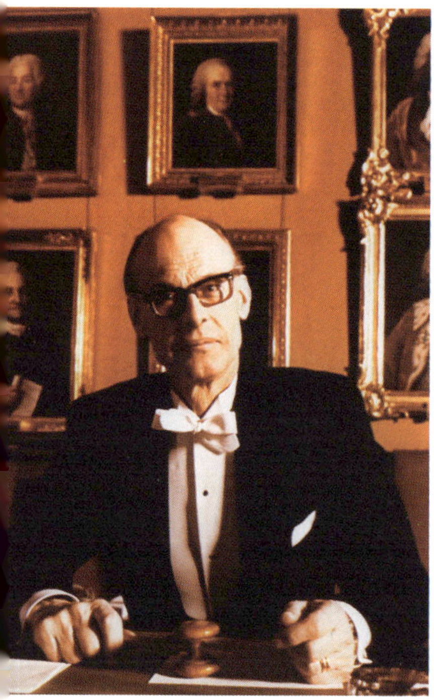

Carl Gustaf Bernhard (1910–2001). Picture taken in 1973 when Bernhard was president of the Royal Swedish Academy of Sciences. He is dressed in tails and sits below the portrait of Linnaeus, one of the founders of the Academy. [From the collections of the Academy.]

The committee chose to use a new reviewer in 1958. It was the professor of physiology Carl Gustaf Bernhard born in 1910. He had done his PhD thesis at the Karolinska Institute in 1940 on the neurophysiology of vision. In 1948 he was appointed professor and chairman of physiology, a responsibility he carried until 1971 when he transferred to the Royal Swedish Academy of Sciences to become its Permanent Secretary. He therefore became one of my predecessors in this function and also an important mentor for me in the management of Academy affairs. At the time when he was to leave the Karolinska Institute I heard him justify this step at a meeting of the

College of Teachers in the following way: "I have been tempted by an older lady than the Karolinska Institute." The Institute had been established in 1810, whereas the Academy started its activities as early as 1739.

Bernhard's review was very comprehensive and detailed. It covered 18 pages. He first noted that Békésy's work had already repeatedly been declared worthy of a prize by the committee. He also remarked that the central motivation for a prize to Békésy was his demonstrations of the pattern of movement of the basilar membrane when the ear is exposed to pure tones and, as a new component, the conclusive demonstration of a durable state of electrical polarization in the organ of Corti. As previously mentioned, these seminal findings represented only a few among the many observations made by Békésy over the years. Bernhard then followed the timeline of Békésy's scientific contributions, expressing admiration for his technical proficiency and also for his systematic and imaginative analysis of each and every step in the mechanisms of hearing, including also bone transmission. Comparisons were made with the contributions by others to mark out the priority of much of what Békésy had done. Among other matters he discussed the alternative theories for activation of the basilar membrane, already alluded to above. The experimental evidence for highlighting the theory of "travelling waves" as the preferred alternative to the other three dominating theories, including the resonance theory introduced by Helmholtz already in 1863, was presented. Bernhard also discussed the forces that activated the hair cells and emphasized that it is not a pulling of or a compression of the cells by the tectorial membrane, but the shearing that occurs in their position as a consequence of their association with two membranes, both influenced by the spatiotemporal waves in the fluid. This was what activated the release of nerve impulses.

Towards the end of his evaluation Bernhard expressed his admiration for Békésy's research. He stated:

> Without doubt there are explicit reasons for the pronouncement that Békésy's analysis of the functions of the middle and inner ear are of decisive importance for our present knowledge about the physiology of hearing. His elegantly performed experiments have led to irrefutable discoveries, which have been verified by other techniques. The validity and reliability that characterizes data that Békésy has generated is certified in all of the literature and the way he approaches his problems is often characterized by his colleagues in the field — and for good reasons — as that of a genius. I can easily understand why several of the

nominators position his name *au par* with Helmholtz when it comes to contributions in the field of hearing physiology. In the nominations many have referred to his consequential analysis of all the steps in the transmission mechanism.

Afterwards Bernhard repeated the major discoveries made by Békésy and stated that his candidature to a Nobel Prize had been markedly strengthened. He also cited from a recent review at the time by H. Davis which had stated "Our knowledge of just how the basilar membrane, the organ of Corti and the tectorial membrane vibrate under the influence of sound is due almost entirely to the studies of one man, Georg von Békésy." Finally he reiterated that Békésy's findings represented a remarkable singlehanded contribution by one man and that it had practical consequences in clinical medicine in the development of new methods for differential diagnosis. His conclusion was that it was highly desirable to award a Nobel Prize to Békésy. However, it would be three more years before he received his prize.

The Decisive Year of 1961

Times were changing at the Karolinska Institute. New disciplines became established and new professors were recruited. The traditional disciplines like physiology or chemistry had to fight harder to become successful in getting their Nobel Prize candidates selected. This was a time of frequently divided opinions in the committee and hence problems in formulating a unanimous proposal. In 1958–1960 proposals in the fields of microbial genetics, nucleic acid biology (Ref. 6, Chapter 7) and immunology (Chapters 1 and 2) were given priority.

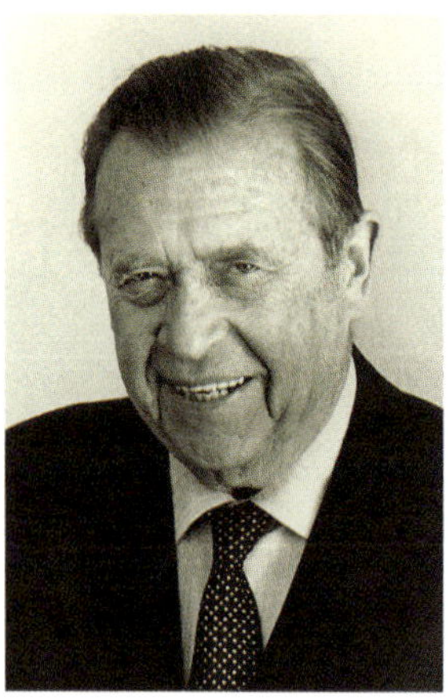

Carl-Axel Hamberger (1908–1988), professor of audiology at the Karolinska Hospital. [Photo by Lennart Nilsson, courtesy of Hamberger's son Bertil Hamberger.]

There was one nomination for Békésy in 1959 and three more in 1961. Among the latter Mittermeier repeated and expanded his 1954 nomination and yet another nomination came from a professor of audiology at the Karolinska Hospital, Carl-Axel Hamberger. Hamberger was a powerful representative not only for his specialty of ear, nose and throat diseases, but also for clinical medicine in general. He had been trained at the Karolinska Institute and after a period at the University of Gothenburg, he was called back in 1960 to Stockholm to become professor and chairman at the Institute and at the Karolinska Hospital. He became a member of the Nobel committee the following year and hence could personally follow up his comprehensive nomination of Békésy. He remained on this committee for many years exerting considerable influence and he was still a member when I joined the committee in 1973. Together with the previously mentioned secretary Gustafsson (Chapter 3) he formed what literally was a pair of "heavyweights" in the committee.

The discussions about the 1961 Nobel Prize seem to have been exceptionally intense and polarized. When the committee finished its meeting on September 28 no conclusion had been reached. Another meeting had to be held. On October 19 the committee reported to the college of teachers that it had not been possible to come to a unanimous agreement. Out of the 12 members, a narrow majority of seven voted for John Eccles, Alan Hodgkin and Andrew Huxley, whereas the remaining five, professors Gard, Hamberger, Klein, Luft and Malmgren preferred Békésy. The members of the faculty agreed with the minority and Békésy received the prize. One might say that this was a "sound" decision. 1961 was the second time that Eccles had been passed over (Chapter 2). He had to wait for two more years, since in 1962 the discovery of the double helix structure of DNA was recognized (Chapter 8).

Following its usual practices at the time, the Karolinska Institute sent a telegram to Békésy's laboratory to inform him of its decision to award him the 1961 Nobel Prize. However, this telegram did not immediately reach Békésy since he was on his way to New York to receive another scientific prize at the Waldorf Astoria. When he arrived in New York, he followed his normal habit of always visiting the New York Public Library. Eventually he walked to the Waldorf Astoria to receive his local prize but was surprised to find the lobby filled with reporters, TV cameras, microphones and spotlights. A single person, Dr Hooper, recognized him and brought him to the attention of the assembled mass media. Békésy turned away and was confused about all this attention for such a minor scientific prize. Then Hooper said "But, Dr Békésy, do you not know that you have received the Nobel Prize?" Once his ignorance had been erased he could attempt to handle the situation. His first question was "Who else?" When he learnt that he was the single recipient he noted with satisfaction: "That's better." He then received his local prize, ate the official lunch and returned to the public library.

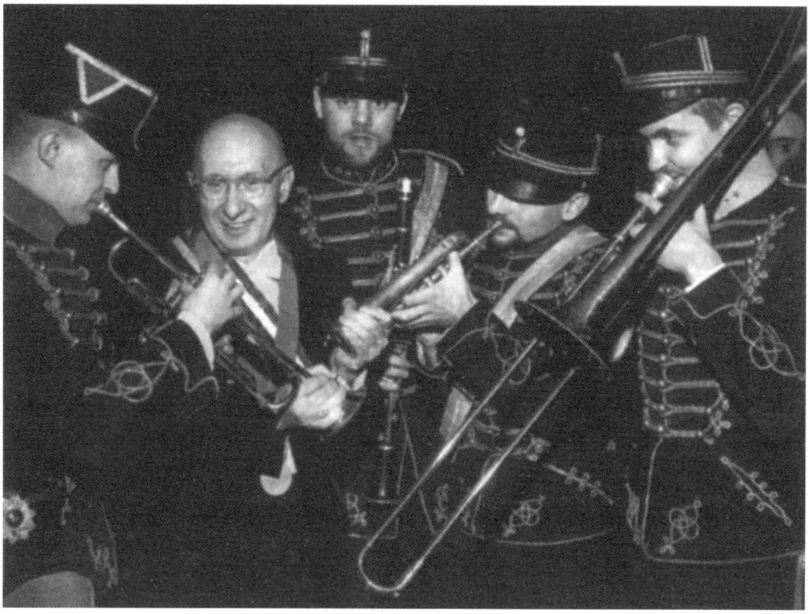

Students at the Karolinska Institute paying tribute to Békésy. [From Ref. 10.]

During the week in Stockholm, Békésy was taken care of by Bernard. He has written about this charming and, because of Békésy's shyness, sometimes complicated responsibility in his autobiography[10]. It all worked out well and Békésy managed the frequent contacts with the press well, although he was never fully at ease in interview situations. He preferred face-to-face contacts with people who shared his interests. However, being a gentleman, he put up with the various expectations of him during the unique conditions of the Nobel week. Some tails were hired for him and he used these at the Nobel Prize ceremony, the banquet and the ensuing party — the "nachspiel" — arranged by the students association as well as during the Royal dinner, the following day.

The Prize Ceremony

The laudation for Békésy at the Nobel Prize ceremony was given by Bernhard[11]. He followed a tradition maintained at the Karolinska Institute for many years, namely to speak without notes. My own experience from giving the introductory speeches in 1976 and 1989 is that accepting this challenge can be rewarding. Bernard gave an animated presentation, which contained a fine characterization of Békésy's series of impressive contributions. Firstly, he mentioned aspects of how we hear our own voice. A comparison was made of how we experience a fog-horn on a boat depending upon whether we are out on the deck or inside the boat. This example had been used by Békésy as an illustration of this kind of situation, reflecting an individual experience gained by many. When I was 9–14 years old I went to a special music school, the Adolf Fredrik's music classes. We did a lot of choral singing and as a part of that we did studio recordings for Swedish Radio at its original address, Kungsgatan (King's street) 8 in central Stockholm. I was very surprised on one occasion when I listened to one of our recordings, which also included a solo sung by me. I did not recognize my own voice! The impressions of listening to your own voice transmitted directly via the bones of the head to the cochlea or via air waves are completely different. This is a phenomenon that Békésy examined more directly in some of his studies.

The continuation of Bernhard's presentation is so well formulated that it deserves to be cited verbatim.

> According to the saga, Heimdal was able to hear the grass sprout. Our ability is perhaps not of that kind, but our ear is anyhow sensitive enough to record the bounce of an air molecule against the ear drum, while, on the other hand, it can withstand the pounding of sound waves strong enough to set the body vibrating. Moreover, the ear is capable of a selectivity which permits a close analysis of sounds the various qualities of which determine the characteristics of the spoken word and of instrumental and vocal expressions in the universe of music.

It should be added that Heimdal, mentioned in the first sentence, was one of the Asa (Æsir) Gods in Nordic mythology and that the original full statement was "His hearing was so good that he could hear the grass sprouting and the wool grow on sheep." The same figure of speech occurs in different forms in other texts. The Swedish author Jascha Golowanjuk, of Russian-Jewish background born in Uzbekistan, has written in his book *Silverpopplarna* (The Silver Poplars): "… could hear how the grass was growing and how the clouds were sailing in the sky."

Bernhard went on to describe the fundamental steps in hearing and the role of earlier discoveries and contributions of others. He then continued:

> von Békésy's distinction is, however, to have recorded the events in this fragile biological miniature system. Authorities in this field evaluate the elaborate technique which he developed to this purpose as being worthy

> of a genius. By microdissection he reaches anatomical structures difficult to access, uses advanced teletechnique for stimulation and recording, and employs high magnification stroboscopic microscopy for making apparent complex membrane movements, the amplitudes of which are measured in thousands of a millimeter.

He then continued by describing how Békésy had managed to explain the quality of the localized impression that sound waves make on the basilar membrane, with the highest crest of the waves impacting the region near the apex of the cochlea at low frequency tones and near its base at high frequencies. In conclusion, the beautiful studies of the shearing effects of the activated hair cells and the conversion of mechanical into electrical energy amplified by the endonuclear potential discovered by Békésy were finally mentioned. Altogether it was a very appropriate tribute to the work of a single man, impressive in its total involvement and in its remarkable series of achievements.

Despite his reserved personality Békésy was a good lecturer. He demonstrated this by his banquet speech at the festivities in the Golden Hall of the City Hall after the Prize ceremony[12] (Chapter 2). In this presentation he made the following statement:

> But aside from these concrete accomplishments, Sweden has attained something much more difficult, namely, the ability to make judgments of the value of scientific achievements over many decades, judgments that are internationally accepted in spite of the different customs, opinions, and interests of the different nations. In the Olympic Games, we can measure time differences and distances, but in science an objective judgment is much more difficult to make. How can they do it? I know only one way, the method used by art lovers to differentiate between originals and counterfeits, and that is to compare and compare and compare. Comparing has helped me to distinguish between the outstanding and less important scientific works. I think the Nobel Prize committee probably *does more reading and comparing than any other scientific body in the world* (my italics). I think we are all grateful for this tremendously unselfish work which is hardly visible in the splendor of this festive occasion. Since the Swedish people make their judgements so slowly and carefully, I used to be afraid of their criticism. Later I learned to respect their criticism, though, because they showed me where my work could be improved.

A Different Kind of Nobel Lecture

Békésy's talent as a speaker also became apparent the following day when he gave his Nobel lecture[4]. As was apparent he had a keen sense of humor and could interpolate into his lectures an anecdote or aphorism when appropriate. The lecture was called "Concerning the pleasures of observing, and the mechanics of the inner ear". The first paragraph had a discrete subtitle "Trying to do science in an unscientific way" and to a major extent dealt with his interest in the arts. The audience became somewhat confused when, in the early part of his presentation, he showed a statue of a baboon from 1,400 years BCE and a stone monkey from China that was 1,600 years older still. They might have been wondering where the lecture would take them. However, in all fairness it should be mentioned that Békésy also gave a brief introduction about the basis for hearing. This factual part of the presentation was gently transformed into a discussion about how to do science, which provided him with an opportunity to show even many more of his favorite art objects. He discussed the quality of fantasy in relationship to the question, "Why is it so difficult to imagine something new?" which led him to the remark that he

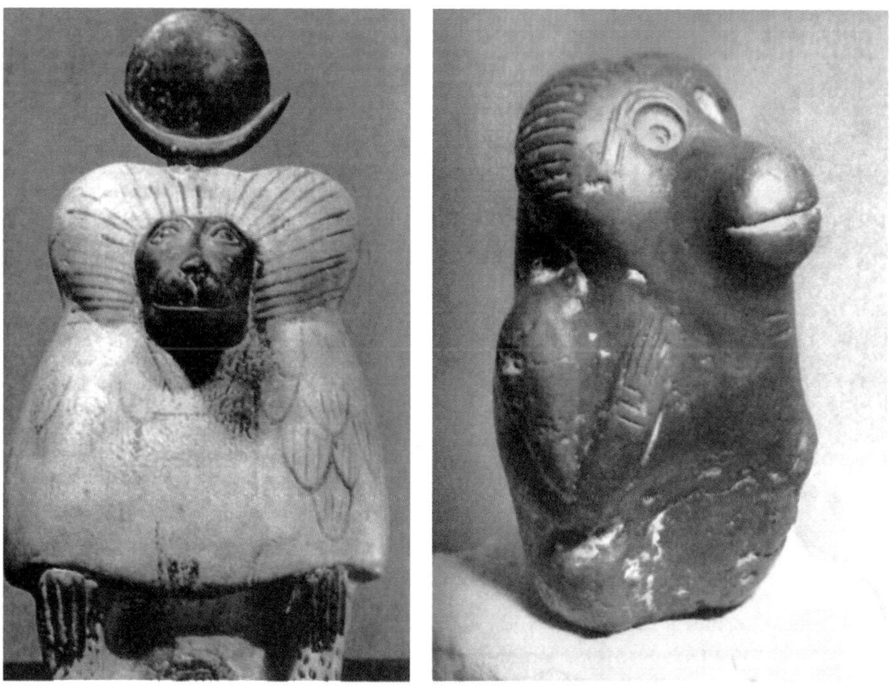

Unusual objects depicted at a Nobel lecture[4]; a baboon of limestone and silver from Egypt, ca. 1,400 BCE and a black stone monkey from Bogas-Koi, ca. 3,000 BCE.

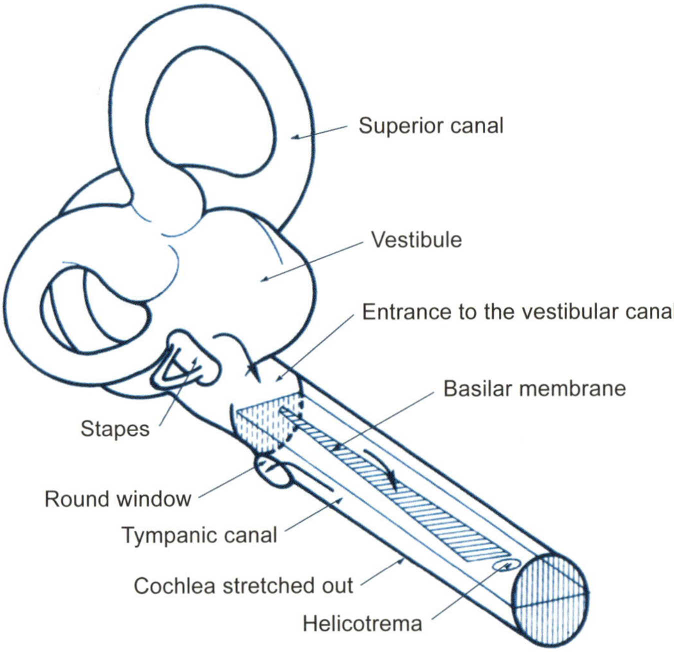

Schematic diagram of the inner ear showing the basilar membrane on which the sensitive nerve cells are located. The vibrations of the eardrum are transmitted through the stapes to the inner ear. [From Ref. 4.]

had gathered inspiration from Leonardo da Vinci. This icon of his did not try to outdo Nature by his art but to let his fantasy become stimulated in a process of learning from Nature. After having shown and discussed some 10 pictures of his favorite art he returned to his advanced model building and the impressive results that the use of this had allowed him to gather. A reference was given to one of his later mechanical models of the cochlea. It was constructed simply from a rubber membrane mounted on a metal frame. This simple model allowed him to demonstrate that among the different theoretical models for types of deformation of the basilar membrane, the travelling wave appeared to be the correct one as already mentioned. But he developed his model further. He also wanted to mimic the nerve supply. To do this he first tried frog skin, but soon gave up on this. Eventually he simply used the lower part of his own arm to register the maximum of the travelling wave! He used two cycles of tone in order to determine the effect of the pitch of the tone. The outcome of this ingenious arrangement was spectacular. In his own words: "Thus the century-old problem of how the ear performs a frequency analysis — whether mechanically or neurally — could be solved; from these experiments it was evident that the ear contains a neuromechanical frequency analyzer, which combines a preliminary mechanical frequency analysis with a subsequent sharpening of the sensation area." The last paragraph of his printed presentation included one more spectacular observation. The place where the local stimulation was recorded was found to be surrounded by an area of strong inhibition. This phenomenon has become consolidated to be a general mechanism in sense physiology and applies not only to the skin, but also to the ear and to the eye. It is referred to as *lateral inhibition*. The specific signal is amplified by suppressing the signaling from its surrounding.

A Meeting of Minds

It must have been a special occasion and challenge for a very solitary person like Békésy to come to Stockholm for the Nobel festivities and to be the central person in such a spectacular event. He was used to a lonely life, but this was of his own choice. His closest "friends" were his art objects. Throughout his life he collected such objects and also books, as we have already mentioned. They were his dearest companions. He could spend hours trying to understand the inner meaning of his art objects and assimilating their inherent beauty. As mentioned above, they gave him inspiration and also guided him in his science. He wanted his experiments to be beautiful and his conclusions to be emotionally appealing and very often they were. The ingenious solutions to various problems selected by evolution often have such a character — simplicity and function generally go together — and we interpret the revelation of them as beautiful. This subjective reaction follows from the fact that we admire optimized function at the same time as beauty is in the eyes of the beholder — us. This has been formulated by Lawrence Durrell in the working material included in the volume *Balthazar* of *The Alexandria Quartet* in the following way: *Science is the poetry of the intellect.*

To be a King — or of course a Queen — surprisingly, also can be a lonely occupation. Your responsibilities are decided by your role as head of state and the choices to be made in the execution of different representative functions, which very often are not of your own choosing. Thus a King needs some demanding occupation besides the daily routine responsibilities to refresh his mind and to develop his talents, whatever they may be. King Gustaf VI Adolf, the grandfather of the present Swedish King, was a scholar. He was referred to as a "professorial amateur professor". When he had finished

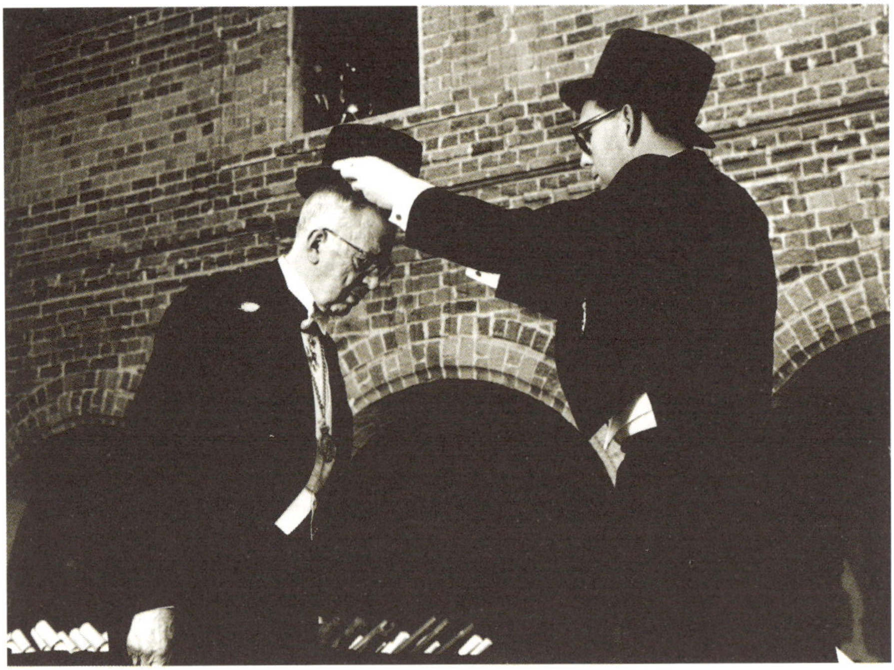

The Swedish King Gustaf VI Adolf (1882–1973) receiving an honorary doctorate from the Karolinska Institute in 1966. The promoter is Arne Engström, further presented in Chapter 8. [Courtesy of Wilhelm Engström.]

his academic studies he became an honorary member of the Royal Swedish Academy of Letters, History and Antiquities and some decades later he served as its president. He also became a member of the British Academy and a member of the Papal Archeological Academy. During his long life he was awarded honorary doctorates at eight universities in Sweden and abroad. The last honorary doctorate was awarded in 1966 at the Karolinska Institute. The reasons for this wide academic appreciation was the fact that the King was a highly respected amateur archaeologist actively involved in excavations in different parts of the world. On these occasions he referred to himself as the Count of Gripsholm, to retain anonymity. Many of these excavations took place in Italy, in particular in places of old Etruscan settlements. Other places where he participated in excavations were in Greece and even in the Far East, like in South Korea. He was also interested in Chinese art and his collection of East Indian porcelain can be seen at the East Asian Museum in Stockholm. In their love for art the King and Békésy had a shared preoccupation. Their common interest in art from the Orient, immediately and naturally fostered contacts. They did not only meet at the prize ceremony but according to the traditions at the dinner in the Royal Castle on the day following the Nobel Prize

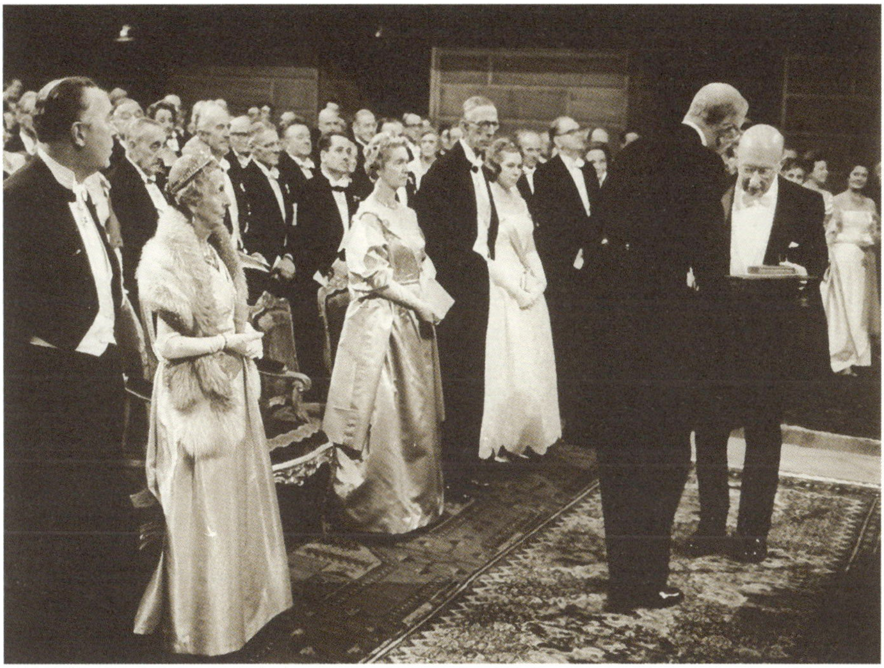

Békésy receiving his Nobel insignia from the hands of His Majesty King Gustaf VI Adolf. [© Scanpix Sweden AB.]

ceremony. This dinner is a fairy-tale event and deserves some extra comments.

The Royal Palace in Stockholm is the largest in northern Europe and includes 660 rooms with windows. Many of the rooms used for festive representative events have a unique quality. My involvement as one of four Lord Chamberlains-in-Waiting since 2000 has provided privileged insights into these exquisite environments. The Nobel dinner has its particular charm with flaming logs in the big fireplaces of the reception room where the royal family passes by all the guests and greets them individually welcome as they stand in a large circle in the room (p. 381). The meal is served in an accompanying room with a beautifully-laid table with exquisite porcelain and cutlery arranged precisely to within a millimeter. The meal consists of high-quality dishes, generally including game shot by the King himself, and excellent wines from the well stocked royal wine cellar which combines to provide an unforgettable feast. The menus of both the exquisite banquets in the City Hall and the dinners in the Royal Palace have been published[13].

At the dinner Bernhard mentioned Békésy's interest in art to the King, who immediately invited Békésy to pay another visit to the castle the following day. At this private audience they discussed the various objects that Békésy

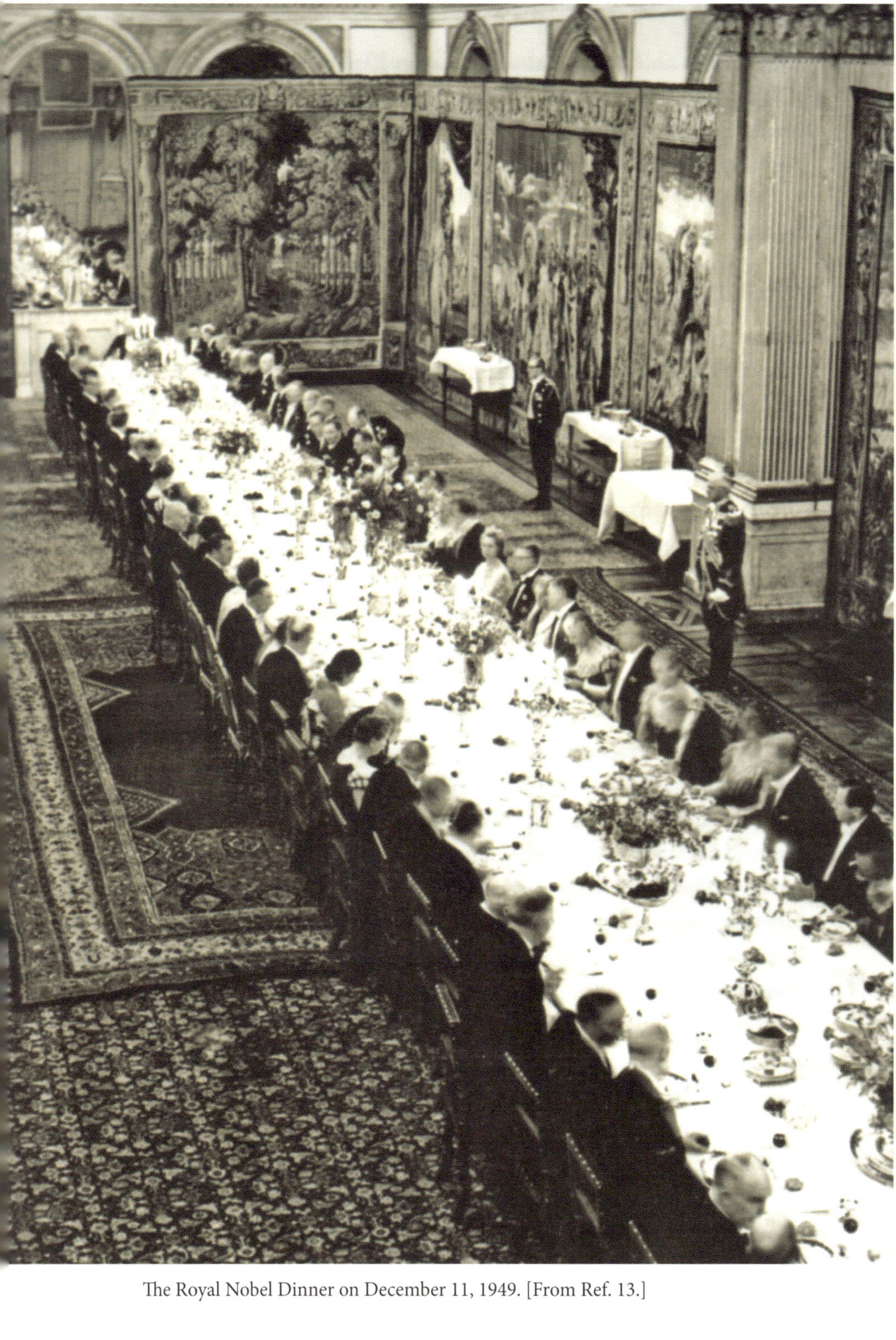

The Royal Nobel Dinner on December 11, 1949. [From Ref. 13.]

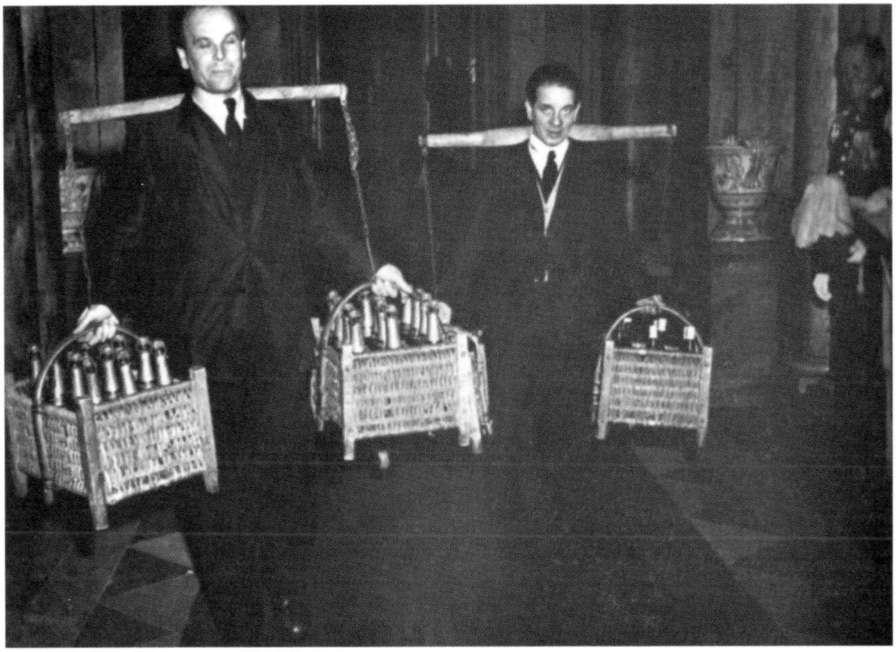

In the absence of elevators the precious wines for the Royal Dinner are carried by use of yokes to the upstairs dining room. [From Ref. 16.]

had accumulated over decennia and also both admired the objects collected by the King.

A number of years later, on August 16, 1970, Békésy wrote a letter to Ståhle, the above-mentioned Executive Director of the Nobel Foundation. It read in part: "A few days ago while browsing through my books, I found the catalogue of Chinese art of His Majesty King Gustaf VI Adolf. It brought back to me the interesting hour I was permitted to spend with His Majesty when I received the Nobel prize…. All this brought back to me discussions of nine years ago. I never forgot the question of what the Nobel Prize winners do with their prizes. I did not really spend it, I systematically bought art objects with it and the value of these objects became in the last years a multiple of the Nobel Prize." Later on he continued: "Two weeks ago I was in Philadelphia and there they put all items of one collector in a separate room. It is the most fascinating experience, since the way items were selected and fit together showed one thing that big museums could not show "love for the objects". It is the same sensation that His Majesty's selection gave me." This was written in 1970 but since 1966 Békésy, supported by Zotterman, had contemplated bequeathing his art collection to the Nobel Foundation.

Our Senses and Nobel Prizes

Our senses are critical for our communication with the external world. Aristotle provided the traditional classification into five senses — seeing, smelling, tasting, touching and hearing — but our body also has other physiological capacities serving as senses. These are capacities to register balance, movements of different kinds, temperature, pain, hunger, thirst etc. There is a broadly integrated somato-sensory "feel" system of high complexity in our body.

Our senses can be evaluated from two different perspectives. One is the physiological capacity to register various physical and chemical parameters and the other is the processing of the information collected, the integrated interpretation by the brain, the *perception*. Békésy's research mainly provided information about the first part, although he did analyze the generation of signals to be transmitted to the brain in the cortical organ. It is difficult and perhaps not even meaningful to compare the impact of loss of different senses. However, hearing, the sense selected by Békésy for his studies, has a particular quality. The deaf-blind American author and political activist Helen Keller has said "Blindness cuts us off from things but deafness cuts us off from people." Thus not to hear is a serious handicap with a compounded impact on life.

Because of the critical importance of our senses in our daily life and, when malfunctioning, in disease, discoveries of their ways of operating have been recognized by Nobel Prizes in physiology or medicine. As already described the inner ear contains two anatomically connected but physiologically separate senses, the organs for hearing and for balance, and advances in knowledge on both of these have been recognized by the prizes awarded.

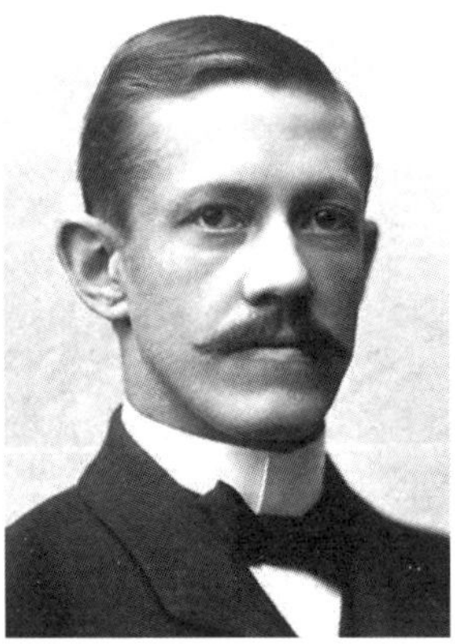

Allvar Gullstrand (1862–1930), recipient of the 1911 Nobel Prize in physiology or medicine. [From *Les Prix Nobel en 1911.*]

The understanding of the fundamental sense of seeing has increased markedly during the previous century and three Nobel Prizes in physiology or medicine have highlighted the advances. The first one was to the Swede Allvar Gullstrand who was recognized "for his work on the dioptrics of the eye". By his science he had elucidated the formation of optical images on the retina by light passing through the lens. He was a highly respected professor of ophthalmology at Uppsala University and with his broad knowledge he was also very active as a member of the Nobel Committee for physics at the Royal Swedish Academy of Sciences; a full member 1911–1929 and its chairman for the last eight years. Together with Svante Arrhenius he managed to delay the recognition of advances in theoretical physics[14]. It was first in 1923 that they were overruled by the other members of the committee, supported by the members at large at the Academy, and Albert Einstein was able to receive the 1922 prize and Niels Bohr the 1923 prize.

The next prize for studies of eye physiology was awarded in 1967 to Granit, already encountered above, Haldan K.Hartline and George Wald "for their discoveries concerning the primary physiological and chemical visual processes in the eye". They had performed beautiful studies using electrophysiological methods examining single nerve fibers, techniques pioneered by Edgar D. Adrian, who had received his own shared Nobel Prize in 1932, and the already mentioned Zotterman. The possibility of registering electrical responses in the retina stimulated by light had already been discovered in 1865 by Frithiof Holmgren, incidentally the father of Gunnar Holmgren, who tried to recruit Békésy to work in Sweden. The father was the originator of the electroretinogram (ERG). The retina contains two kinds of light receptors, the rods and the cones, which are the source of electrical impulses conveyed to the brain. The cones are the source of our capacity to distinguish colors. The polymath Thomas Young, living at the turn of the 19th century, had already postulated that the there should be three main types of color-receiving structures. As techniques for critical studies developed, this was further substantiated more than 100 years later by Selig Hecht, who was the mentor of Wald at Columbia University in New York. When the techniques to register electrical impulses from individual neurons in the brain were developed later, a still deeper insight into functions of perception in the brain became possible. This led to one half of a Nobel Prize in physiology or medicine in 1981 to David H. Hubel and Torsten N. Wiesel in 1981 "for their discoveries concerning information processing in the visual system".

The olfactory sense has also been recognized by a Nobel Prize, albeit relatively recently. It was in 2004 that a Nobel Prize in physiology or medicine recognized the work by Richard Axel and Linda B. Buck "for their discoveries of odorant receptors and the organization of the olfactory system". Using advanced molecular techniques it was possible to identify the number of receptors for smell in the upper nose in different species and how this chemosensory world was represented in the brain. Smell is the most original of all the senses. It is a matter of distinguishing different chemical compounds, something even the original cells in the formation of cellular life needed to learn to do. A critical factor in managing such a function is to have receptor molecules at the surface of the cell. The importance of the existence of receptors was already repeatedly discussed in Chapters 1 and 3. Studying the complete genomic nucleotide sequence in mice and man it was possible to identify 1300 odorant receptors in mice and 500 in humans. These numbers should be put into the perspective of a total number of genes of about 20–25,000 in these mammals. Thus about 5% of all genes in mice are involved in separating olfactory signals! This emphasizes the unique importance of this sense. However, there are many hundreds of thousands of different kinds of smells. In order to separate all of these, again the mechanism of combinatorial diversification discussed in Chapter 3 for generation of an essentially endless number of antibody specificities, needed to be used. Still, as far as smell is concerned, it is not a matter of generating an endless number of variants of homologous genes. Instead it is the pattern of reactivity of a certain odorant with receptors with various specificities and location in the olfactory mucosa that orchestrates signals to the brain. In the brain these signals are integrated into a pattern of combinatorial differentiation identifying a specific smell. In elegant studies Axel and Buck demonstrated the topographical imprints in the brain of different olfactory stimuli. The imprints do not reflect the chemical relationships and systematization of the molecules that elicit the specific smell signal. Instead it is the importance that a particular signal has to the host that counts. Is it a smell that signals a risk of poisoning or is it an important signal connected with mating, etc.?

The olfactory epithelium represents the only site in the body where extensions of neurons leading directly to the brain tissue are exposed to the surrounding environment. As discussed in chapter 5 in my previous book on Nobel Prizes (Ref. 6, Chapter 5) and as briefly mentioned in Chapter 1, it was believed that poliovirus could only replicate in nerve cells and that therefore the virus must have entered the body via the olfactory epithelium. Belief in this dogma was so strong and the disease considered such a threat that trials in children were launched to explore the effect of destroying the epithelium by an etching treatment as a means of protecting against polio. Of course this did not prevent the attack by the virus, but the capacity for olfaction was sadly lost.

No futher Nobel Prizes have been awarded to recognize discoveries of the mechanisms of other senses. The area of taste might have been considered. The four basic tastes — salty, sweet, bitter and sour — have been well recognized for a long time, but the existence of a fifth category of taste buds detecting a sensation called *umami* has also been found more recently. The name derives from two Japanese words for delicious and taste. The term was already introduced in 1908 by the Japanese Professor Kikunae Ikeda, who was studying the taste of L-glutamate. However, it was not until 1985 that it was officially recognized that it represented a separate fifth basic quality of taste. It is now accepted as important to consider this quality of taste in excellent cooking. Activation of umami receptors stimulate salivation and generally improve the taste of food. Hence the English word "savor" to describe the particular sensation of an attractive taste. Apparently the discovery of a fifth kind of taste was not considered to be of the magnitude required for recognition by a Nobel Prize, besides the fact that its discoverer has been dead for a long time. It is now time to return to Békésy.

A Final Home in Hawaii; East Meets West

At the mature age of 67, Békésy made one more move — which was to be his final one — with regard to his work and home environment. Surprisingly he decided to go to the other side of the world from his home country Hungary. He went to Honolulu, Hawaii. The university in that city arranged an endowed chair in sensory sciences for him, sponsored by the Hawaiian Telephone Company. His reasons for moving are unclear. A contributing factor was a fire in Memorial Hall at Harvard. His laboratory was in the basement of this building and the incident led to loss or damage by water of a large part of his research documentation. He was not attracted by the prospect of moving into a new ultra-modern building to substitute for the one destroyed by the fire. Maybe he was just in search of a new academic environment.

His two obsessions, his science and his art remained the essence of his life for the six more years he was granted. Life on the remote Pacific islands was rejuvenating. He became more closely acquainted with the oriental way of living and he developed new and enriching contacts. In particular he treasured his contacts with the physiologist Yasuji Katsuki and the author Yasunari Kawabata. Kawabata received the Nobel Prize in literature in 1968. The motivation was "for his narrative mastery, which with great sensibility expresses the essence of the Japanese mind". He was the right person to describe to Békésy the refined Japanese culture reflecting carefully nursed long-lasting traditions. Some of Kawabata's writing was done at the famous hotel Hiiragiya Ryokan in Kyoto. A few years ago I had the enriching experience of staying together with my wife in the room in this Japanese hotel, an environment of refined esthetics, where Kawabata did his sublime writing. His exit from life was tragic. Four years after he received his Nobel Prize he gassed himself to death, probably a suicide.

In 1970 Békésy reflected on his experience of living in Honolulu. He wrote:

> I spent three years here and I think it is the most interesting place I have ever been. It is international to a degree which is almost hard to understand. There are groups from Asia, Australia, America, and Europe and they still are able to survive and respect each other. At the same time it forces me to realize that the whole way of thinking, working, taste, and so on, is completely different in the East and in the West. It cannot be erased by organizers or even by big wars. It is there, it is thousands and thousands of years old. I maybe know it better and realize it better than many other people because I collect old art objects and it took me years to understand the difference between Japanese ways of thinking and Chinese ways of thinking, that there is a real difference. There are so many cultures with their own histories and own ways to evaluate life .... It is in Hawaii where I realized first how complicated the world really is and how difficult it is to understand the other man's opinion, even if somebody does everything to understand it.

Throughout life Békésy retained a deep feeling for his original home country. However after 1946 he was never to return to Hungary, not even in 1969, when he was awarded an honorary doctorate from the University of Budapest. He was very proud of this recognition but chose to receive his diploma at the Hungarian Embassy in Washington. This was referred to in a speech given at the memorial service three years later by the president of the University of Hawaii, Harlan Cleveland.

> Those of us in Hawaii who knew him are saddened by the loss of a friend, but the whole world has lost one of its first citizens, an authentic creative genius in the medical sciences. The word "genius" is used rather frequently these days, but to meet Dr von Békésy was to realize again that there are intellectual giants who tower over the merely brilliant as great mountains tower over high buildings. His work on the delicate machinery of the human ear formed the firm scientific basis for most recent advances in the treatment of deafness, and also showed the unity of design in sensory systems in nature.

And his closing words were:

> His honors in otology, psychology, acoustics and medicine are too many to be listed here, but one of them meant more to him, perhaps than the Nobel Prize. This was the award from Budapest, which could be regarded as something of an apology from that proud and troubled country to one of its most distinguished sons.

A Gracious Will

Four months after the letter Békésy wrote to Ståhle in 1970 he signed a will in which he bequeathed his whole collection of art to the Nobel Foundation. However, his books were to remain in Honolulu. Stig Ramel (p. 101), Ståhle's successor in 1972, became responsible for retrieving the collection of art that had come into the possession of the Foundation, when Békésy died the same year. He has described this vividly in his memoirs[15]. Together with Mr Joseph H. Guttentag, an American lawyer at the law firm Surrey, Karasik and Morse, Washington D.C., he visited Honolulu in January 1973. The way Ramel described his experience of entering Békésy's apartment deserves to be cited verbatim:

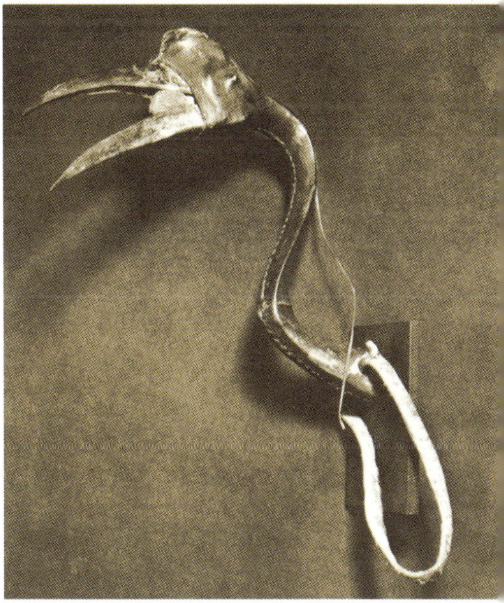

Hunter's decoy in the form of a ground hornbill head. Hausa and other northern tribes, Nigeria. [From Ref. 13.]

> We were the first to enter after (Békésy's) death and when we turned on the light we found the rooms filled from floor to ceiling with pieces of art. It was the feeling of entering an Egyptian sepulchral chamber, gold glittered through the dust, fantastic African face masks were staring at us and everywhere there were Indian sculptures, Chinese vases and Japanese paintings. On my retina remains forever etched an African bird's mask with its long beak stretching in a threatening way towards us and high up on a bookshelf an elegant Japanese tea pot in coral colored lacquer (p. 256). For a week we supervised the packing of the many hundreds of items — not only supervised, we did in fact

ourselves participate in the packing and carrying together with the local porters, whose pace of work we tried to increase a few degrees by providing a good example. I asked Joe what fee he, as a lawyer of one of the leading bureaux in Washington, used to apply when he worked as a porter. He assured me that he was the most well-paid porter in the USA.

After this experience Ramel felt as if he knew Békésy in person although he never met him in real life. His impressions were strengthened by the contacts he had with Békésy's scientific colleagues and other acquaintances in Honolulu. He was in particular intrigued by Walter Karpus, who prior to Hitler's take-over in Austria had been a chicken farmer. Karpus was engaged as Békésy's instrument builder and accompanied him through life to Boston and Honolulu. Ramel summarized his impressions in the following way: "I had never met him (Békésy) in life, but now I met him in death, and he became immensely alive to me."

Ramel personally supervised the transport by air of the 43 boxes and noted that he had never before or ever after paid as much for excess weight as on this occasion. When arriving at Arlanda airport he even described how he entered the airport by the baggage conveyor belt, but that may be a tall story.

Once the collection had arrived in Stockholm a very comprehensive work of valuation and cataloging started. This was led by assistant professor Jan Wirgin at the East Asian Museum in Stockholm working together with experts from British Museum. A full display of Békésy's whole collection was given during the Nobel Week of 1974 and the catalogue of that exhibition[2] demonstrated the very high quality of the large number of items included. As mentioned in the introduction of this chapter a beautiful piece of Békésy's collection of art has been selected to be retained at the office of the Nobel committee at the Karolinska Institute. This is just one among a few selected pieces for that office and some additional pieces can also be found in the anteroom to the board meeting room at the house of the Nobel Foundation at Sturegatan 12 in Stockholm. It was the Swedish Nobel laureate Sune Bergström, Chairman of the Board of the Nobel Foundation 1975–1987, who made this selection. Because of these unique assets, the atmosphere at both these offices provides excellent examples of a successful mixing of intellectual pursuits and esthetics. Besides the beautiful piece shown on p. 221, other pieces collected by Békésy and displayed at the office of the Nobel committee are a bronze relief, also from Benin, and a Bodhisattva head from Cambodia. There are also other interesting pieces of art in this office. In 1998 Bergström and his wife

Maj donated two Indian ink paintings by a Chinese artist called Gao Xingjian. Two years later Gao received the Nobel Prize in literature! In a corner of a large office there is a small picture by the famous Swedish artist Peter Dahl. It is a great piece of art depicting an act of intercourse and one may wonder how it has found its place in this collection. During Lindsten's time as secretary of the committee (p. 116) he started a very pleasant tradition. The first encounter between the Nobel Prize recipients of the year and the committee responsible for selecting them took place in a charming smaller art museum, the Thielska Gallery. There we were treated to an excellent dinner. The front of the menu was an original piece of art (two new motifs each year, limited edition of 25 copies). I have framed all these pieces of art and attached the menu on the back of the picture. The evening was also enriched by presentations by the curator Ulf Linde of selected paintings, including some of the most famous ones from Edvard Munch's oeuvre, and live music performed *en chambre* by outstanding Swedish artists. The only remuneration the artists received was two tickets to the Nobel Prize ceremony and to the banquet. One year Lindsten had invited Dahl to contribute a picture. When we saw the motif he had selected we became somewhat concerned. Could we expose this to our — frequently American — scientists? A small group of us decided to reject it, a very particular case of allocation to a Nobel *Salon de Refusés*. This event was picked up by the Swedish press and a monthly journal called *Ottar* focusing on sexual education could not understand that we with our medical background found it offensive to show an act of intercourse. After this digression it is time to return to the Békésy collection.

The different parts of the Békésy collection, except for the few items mentioned above, can now be found, separated into the different geographical origins of the objects at three museums in Stockholm; the East Asiatic Museum — about 200 objects; the Mediterranean museum — also about 200 objects (some especially allocated to the Gold room); and finally also at the Ethnographic Museum — slightly more than 50 objects. So in the end Békésy's whole collection did not end up in the one room, in accordance with his wishes expressed in his will — "It is my desire that my art object collection be represented intact if at all possible," but it is well maintained for the future and its quality can be enjoyed by the public. In fact anyone can browse the various items on the web at http://www.varldskulturmuseerna.se/sv/forskning-samlingarna/sok-i-samlingarna. Objects at the East Asian Museum can be found under "Nobelstiftelsen", at the Mediterranean Museum under "bek" and at the Ethnographic Museum under "Békésy". In his book, Ramel referred[15] to how he occasionally went to the East Asian Museum to see the coral-red tea pot and reminiscence about his contacts with Békésy, his virtual friend.

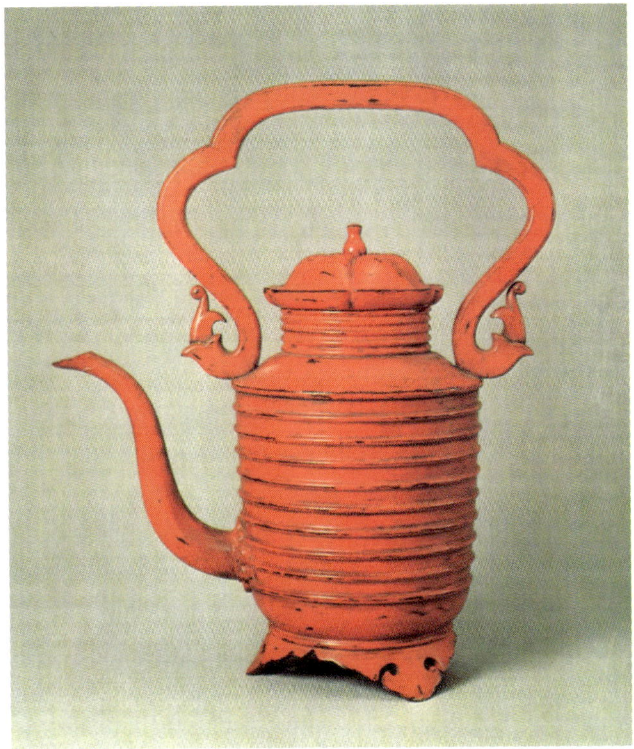

Ewer of negoro lacquer, Momoyama period. Late 16th century, Japan. [From Ref. 16.]

Chapter 7

Unraveling the Complexity of Protein Folding

To Fold or Not Fold
A Question of Function
New Tools of Nature

In 1962 Nobel Prizes in both chemistry and physiology or medicine were awarded to scientists using X-ray crystallographic data. The pioneers in three-dimensional studies of complex proteins — Max F. Perutz and John C. Kendrew — and the decipherers of the DNA double helix — Francis H. C. Crick, James D. Watson and Maurice H. F. Wilkins — were recognized for their groundbreaking observations. Technological developments allowed the visualization of large macromolecular structures central to the functions of life. Major improvements in understanding complex protein structures and the biggest discovery in biology of the 20th century, the recognition that DNA carries the genetic information, were rewarded.

The light microscope was the first technical device developed for studies of the invisible world of nature. However, because of the wavelength of light there was a limit to the smallest size of structures that could be identified by use of this instrument. An important further development was the use of electrons, qualitatively different from electromagnetic irradiation like visible and ultraviolet light. An electron beam has a much shorter wavelength and hence allowed the characterization of very small structures too, like virus particles. Electron microscopy was developed in the 1930s, but it was not recognized by a Nobel Prize in physics until 1986. In that year, half the prize was awarded to the 80-year-old Ernst Ruska "for his fundamental work in electron optics, and for the design of the first electron microscope". However, to "see" even finer structures, like individual atoms and molecules, a form of electromagnetic radiation with a much smaller wavelength than visible light needed to be used. A previously unknown form of such radiation was discovered serendipitously in 1895 by W. Conrad Röntgen, who was to receive the first Nobel Prize in physics in 1901. This was X-rays. They provided an opportunity to increase the resolution. It became possible to examine atomic elements and complexes of them in three dimensions. One could "see" molecular structures, even in their details.

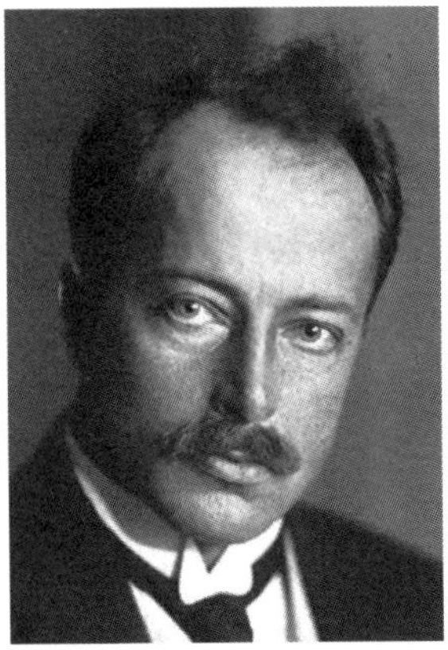

Max von Laue (1879–1960), recipient of the 1914 Nobel Prize in physics. [From *Les Prix Nobel en 1914*.]

The usefulness of the rays found by Röntgen for characterization of crystalline structures was already recognized by two Nobel Prizes in physics in 1914 and 1915. In 1914 Max von Laue was awarded the prize "for his discovery of the diffraction of X-rays by crystals". A year later, a father and son called Bragg, William Henry and William Lawrence respectively, received the same prize "for their services in the analysis of crystal structure by means of X-rays". The background to their shared prize was recently discussed[1]. In these early studies the objects examined were crystals of inorganic substances. The son Bragg was only 25 years old at the time of this extraordinary recognition, the youngest recipient ever of a Nobel Prize. The important Bragg's Law employed in forthcoming crystallographic studies was named after him and not after his father. Lawrence Bragg came to play a major role for the development of crystallography over many decades to come, including the advance into studies of ever larger molecules of organic nature. He was a central actor, also as a nominator for candidates to Nobel Prizes, in the developments presented in this and the following chapter. His life has been described in a biography appropriately called *Light Is a Messenger*[2].

The symmetry of crystals had been noted for centuries, but they were not scientifically investigated until the 17th century. Johannes Kepler noted the hexagonal symmetry of snow flakes and the Danish Catholic bishop and scientist Nicolas Steno demonstrated in 1669 that the angles between the faces of quartz crystals remained constant. The symmetrically arranged atoms in a crystal can scatter X-rays primarily by their interaction with electrons. This scattering can be registered as an electron density pattern recorded on a photographic film. In practice the crystal is mounted on a rotating device

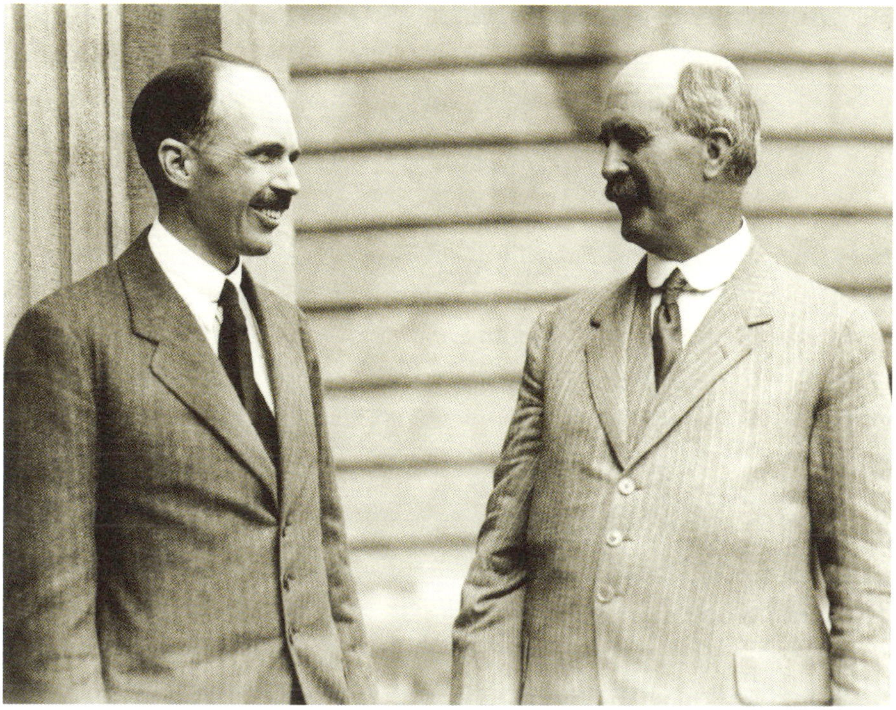

William Lawrence Bragg with his father, William Henry Bragg, 1930s.
[Credit: Smithsonian Institution Archives. Image SIA2007-0340.]

and the reflections generated are photographically recorded. It is possible for scientists examining these diffraction patterns to deduce the three-dimensional nature of the entities forming the crystal. Different crystals have different symmetry and the characteristics of this can be derived by identification of their so-called unit cell, which allows a definition of the particular space group of the structure. In the *International X-ray Tables* prepared in 1924 by William T. Astbury and Kathleen Lonsdale, whom we will meet later, a total of 230 different kinds of space groups had been defined. A number of supplementary techniques and mathematical algorithms were developed over time to interpret and resolve increasingly more complex structures. X-ray crystallography has become central in the development of different fields of science since crystals can be formed by many kinds of inorganic chemical materials — salts, metals, minerals — as well as a wide array of organic molecules of varying degrees of complexity. The technique was a tool originally developed by physicists and later adopted by chemists.

Crystallographic analyses of complex biological molecules started to develop in the 1930s but the discoveries made of the structure of an increasingly higher level of complexity took a long time to develop. Technical improvements and the introduction of new kinds of mathematical processing required the management of large volumes of data. Ways to manage this mass of data needed to be introduced. The development of computers in the aftermath of the Second World War was of decisive importance for the advance of the field. Because of the need for many steps of development, Nobel Prizes in chemistry recognizing the characterization by use of X-ray crystallography of structures of important biochemical substances were not awarded until 1962 and 1964. The development of increasingly more advanced techniques has made it possible to progressively unravel the structure of more and more complex molecules and even functional aggregates of such molecules. A number of Nobel Prizes in chemistry awarded in the present century have recognized these important further developments.

The Great Sage

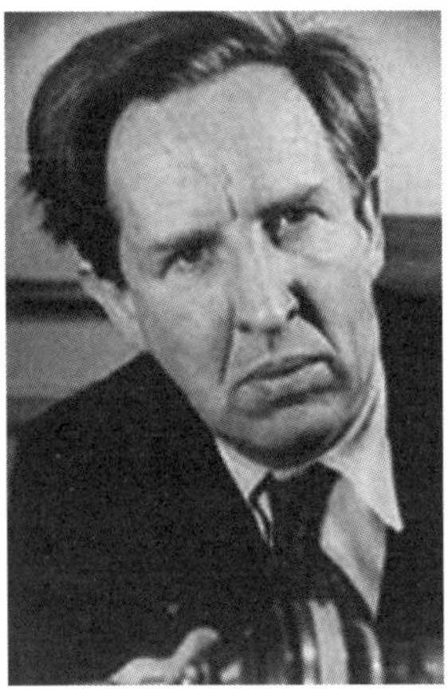

John D. Bernal (1901–1971).

John D. Bernal has been referred to as one of the most charismatic and controversial figures of 20th-century Britain. He became known for his energy and exuberance. Not only was he a qualified scientist and mathematician, but he was also extremely well versed in the arts, literature, politics and history — hence his nickname *the great sage*. He has been fictionalized by the author C. P. Snow as the character Constantine in his novel *The Search*.

Bernal was born in 1901 in Ireland to a father of mixed Italian and Spanish/Portuguese Sephardic Jewish origins and a well-educated mother from Antrim in Northern Ireland. His upbringing in a Catholic and patriotic environment also fostered a passion for science. Together with his mother he planned his own education from the age of 12 onwards. When he was an undergraduate some 10 years later in Cambridge he rejected his religion and became engaged in ultra-left-wing politics. He developed a faith in the societal experiments of the Soviet Union and its leader Stalin, but this faith was shaken when the Soviets invaded Hungary in 1956. Still, he retained his belief in the political ideology of communism throughout his life and was also heavily involved in various peace efforts. In 1953 he received the Stalin Peace Prize and between 1959 and 1965 he was the president of the World Peace Council.

His private life was highly convoluted and unconventional involving many women, three of whom he acknowledged to have fathered children with. His approach to science also seemed to have had a manic streak. He spurned an endless number of ideas but often it became necessary for his collaborators to follow up the spontaneous initiatives. In spite of these limitations he became the father of the branch of molecular biology devoted to the three-dimensional structure of complex organic molecules. He and his collaborators demonstrated the potential of the developing tool of X-ray crystallography. They wanted to understand the structure and function of the molecules of life.

Besides his important contributions to science he is at least equally known for his philosophical studies of the social aspects of science (p. 412). He published books expressing his basic tenet that the fruits of science are to be shared by everyone and that properly used they will greatly improve the fate of mankind. Bernal's multicolored life, which ended in 1971 has been biographically presented[3].

The Birth of a New Branch of Science

In 1923, when Bernal had graduated from Cambridge he started to work with Bragg senior, now Sir William, at the Davy Faraday laboratory at the Royal Institution in London. Bernal did conventional crystallographic studies of graphite and metals, but in the same laboratory Astbury had initiated some pioneering studies of organic material. It was at this time that it was first suggested that possibly some organic materials might also have an organized structure like the elements of a salt crystal. Studies of the central structure of natural fiber-like hair showed repeated reflection patterns indicating an orderly molecular structure. Bernal brought along the impressions of Astbury's findings when in 1927 he moved back to Cambridge to become its first lecturer in structural crystallography. He approached a number of different organic materials and his first breakthrough came in studies of sterols, complex molecules that include vitamin D and cholesterol. In further studies he was able to show the structure of different enzymes, like pepsin, and even some very early impressions of the complex structure of a plant virus, tobacco mosaic virus (p. 361).

Bernal started to train students, who later went on to receive the Nobel Prize in chemistry. The first one was Dorothy Crowfoot (Hodgkin) who joined him in 1934 both in scientific and private adventures. In science together they developed a new approach studying hydrated crystals, viz. organic materials in an environment closer to their natural state. They initiated the first studies of a complex protein, the hormone insulin. Max Perutz from Austria joined Bernal in 1936. The story goes that on his arrival in Cambridge, Perutz asked Bernal: "How can I solve the secret of life?" The answer was, "The secret of life lies in the structure of proteins, and X-ray crystallography is the only way to solve it." Much later, in his Nobel lecture[4], Perutz stated: "I started my X-ray work on crystalline proteins in the Cavendish laboratory under J. D. Bernal in 1937, just after he and Dorothy Hodgkin had demonstrated (a *Nature* publication on insulin in 1934; *my remark*) that protein crystals can be made to yield sharp X-ray diffraction patterns which extend to spacings of the order of interatomic distances."

In 1937 Bernal moved to become Professor of Physics at Birkbeck College, University of London, because of opinions held by Ernest Rutherford, the discoverer of the atomic nucleus and the 1908 Nobel Prize recipient in chemistry (p. 165). Rutherford disliked Bernal intensely and therefore blocked his possibility of obtaining tenure at Cambridge. In the same year Bernal became a Fellow of the Royal Society, only 36 years old. Developments at the London College were delayed because of the intervention of the Second World War. Bernal was involved in the exotic project Habbakuk initiated by Geoffrey Pyke aiming at building aircraft carriers using pykrete, a mixture of wood pulp and ice, but in particular he made decisive contributions to the preparation and success of the invasion in Normandy. He was trusted enough to become a close assistant to Lord Mountbatten, in spite of the fact that he openly declared his solidarity with Communist regimes. Perutz, as we shall see, politically did not fare that well.

Bernal continued to inspire young students looking for routes into science. He put Kendrew on the track to become a crystallographer as a result of contacts they had established during the war. Much later Aaron Klug came to work with Bernal on the enzyme ribonuclease and finally in the mid-1950s Rosalind Franklin, whom we will meet again in the next chapter, joined him to study TMV. Klug, mentioned briefly in my previous book[5], received the Nobel Prize in chemistry in 1982 for his crystallographic work in part concerning TMV, whereas Franklin was never nominated for her critical work on the crystals of DNA because of her untimely early death in 1958. Bernal who gave many forthcoming Nobel laureates critical inspiration was never himself discussed as a candidate for a Nobel Prize. He was in fact nominated by a French colleague for a prize in physics in 1959, but the proposal did not include any justification and it was not further reviewed by the committee. Bernal also appears in the Nobel archives in 1948 when he was one among many nominators of Patrick M. S. Blackett for a prize in physics, which he also received this year. In 1957 and 1959 he nominated Hodgkin for a prize in physics, to be further discussed below.

Probably Bernal's strength was to provide inspiration, but he may have lacked the tenacity that was needed, not least in X-ray protein crystallography, to bring a complex research project to fruition. In a review in the *London Review of Books* in 2000 Perutz wrote, "He (Bernal) was a prolific source of ideas and gave them away generously. During the long, lean years when most of my colleagues thought I was wasting my time on an insoluble problem, Bernal would drop in like the advent of spring, imbuing me with enthusiasm and fresh hope." What Bernal lacked in tenacity Hodgkin as well as Perutz displayed all the more. They were, to use Medawar's terminology, obsessionalists.

The Lady of Crystals

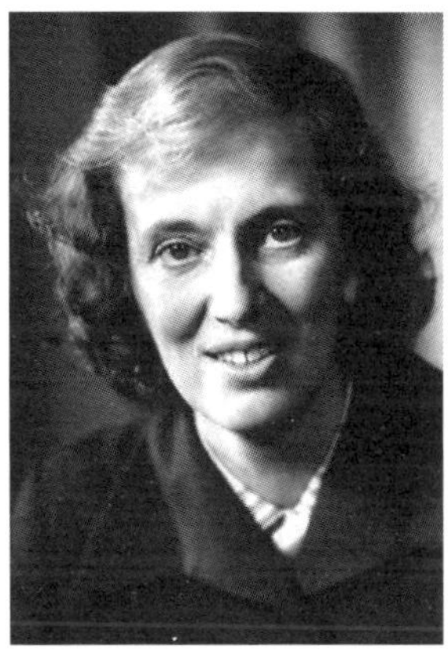

Dorothy Crowfoot Hodgkin (1919–1994), recipient of the 1964 Nobel Prize in chemistry. [From *Les Prix Nobel en 1964*.]

Dorothy Crowfoot Hodgkin, was born in 1910 in Cairo, where her father was engaged in educational projects. He was an archaeologist and classical scholar and his work also deeply involved her mother, who among other things was a qualified botanist. Thus Dorothy was brought up in a rich academic environment and she wavered between different potential intellectual pursuits, being close to becoming an archaeologist prior to eventually selecting chemistry. She studied chemistry at the all-female Somerville College, Oxford. Her interest in chemistry and crystals started early in life and in her Nobel lecture[6] she referred to her reading of a book for children popularizing science. In this book Bragg senior made a statement that "X-rays increased the keenness of our vision over 10,000 times." When she joined Bernal in Cambridge in 1932 she accelerated her academic career in earnest. She spent two happy and productive years there before returning to Oxford where she remained the rest of her academic life. In 1936 she became a research fellow at Somerville College and in 1960 she was appointed Wolfson Research Professor at the Royal Society. She changed her family name when she in 1937 married Thomas Hodgkin. They had three children together but like Bernal's marriage the relationship was far from conventional. The family had major political ideological involvements. Her husband Thomas, like Bernal, was a member of the communist party. Dorothy Hodgkin was also attracted to leftish politics, primarily on humanitarian grounds and not as a card-carrying Communist.

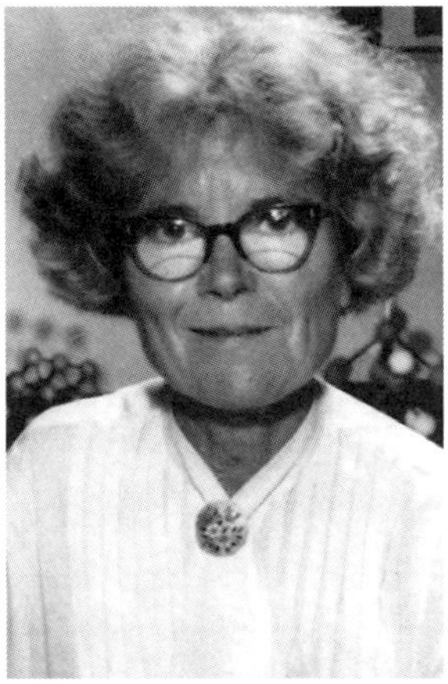

Kathleen Lonsdale (1903–1971).

In 1947 she was elected a fellow of the Royal Society. She was not the first woman to be given this honor. Two years earlier, following a statutory amendment, two female fellows had been admitted. These were Marjory Stephenson, a biochemist studying bacterial metabolism, and Kathleen Lonsdale, mentioned above. Lonsdale was a good friend of Hodgkin, a fellow crystallographer and authority in the field who had determined the structure of benzene. She had also been of great assistance to Hodgkin in her early work on penicillin. Under Lonsdale's watchful eye crystals were grown in her London laboratory and brought to Oxford. She was also a Quaker and a pacifist.

One of Hodgkin's own students in 1940 was Margaret Roberts, the future Prime Minister Margaret Thatcher. In the 1980s Thatcher installed a portrait of Hodgkin at 10 Downing Street, the British Prime Minister's residence. An excellent description of Hodgkin's life and her achievements can be found in a biography by Georgina Ferry[7].

Hodgkin's pioneering contributions to our understanding of molecules of moderate size for natural reasons in time preceded the eventual deciphering of the structure of large protein. However, her work was first recognized by a Nobel Prize in 1964, two years *after* the prize in chemistry to Perutz and Kendrew, the researchers unraveling the three-dimensional features of large proteins. The circumstantial reasons for this delay will be further discussed below. Because the Nobel Prize chemistry committee might have chosen to award her a prize prior to the recognition of the structure of more complex protein molecules, Hodgkin's Nobel Prize will be fully discussed in this chapter. However, this will be done without access to the Nobel archive materials of 1963 and 1964, due to the 50 years' secrecy rule.

Hodgkin's crystallization work, initiated by the contacts with Bernal, in parallel with Astbury's work, opened up the field of studies of the three-dimensional structure of organic molecules. Her encounter with Bernal was an example of a lucky accident — meeting on a train, some friends advising her to contact him — as emphasized in her Nobel Lecture[6]. The field of crystallography was then taken up by many other scientists, including a fair representation of women, as the development of techniques allowed the examination of increasingly more complex organic molecules. This was expressed by Bragg in one of his nominations of Hodgkin for a Nobel Prize in the following way:

> She has always led in the application of what might be called the classical approval of X-ray analysis as distinct from the new methods of Perutz and Kendrew which they applied to protein. The sterols, penicillin, vitamin B12 are landmarks in X-ray analysis, and all were due to Mrs Hodgkin.

A Scientist Obsessed by Hemoglobin

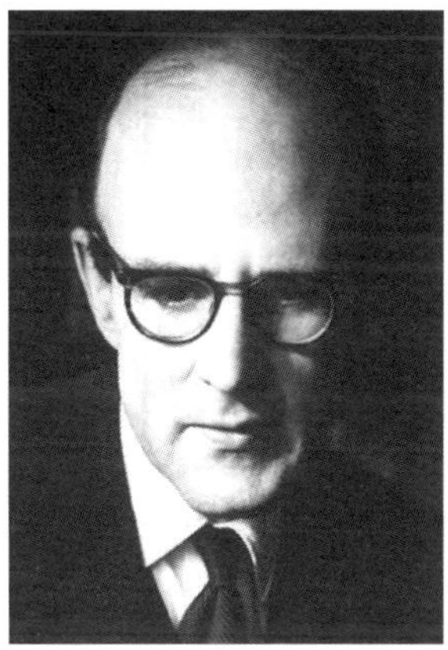

Max F. Perutz (1914–2002), recipient of the shared Nobel Prize in chemistry in 1962. [From *Les Prix Nobel en 1962*.]

Max Perutz was a scientist with a very focused and intense career. He was recognized as a researcher with strong motivation and a unique capacity to stay with the problem he had decided to solve. In addition he was an impressive manager of front line science, besides also having deep humanistic societal commitments. His life has been excellently described in another biography by Ferry, a book called *Max Perutz and the Secret of Life*[8].

Perutz was born in Vienna in 1914. His parents were highly assimilated Jews, faithful Catholics, who had never set foot in a synagogue. For generations the family had been textile manufacturers, which provided a good financial background to a solid bourgeois life. In the absence of academic scientific traditions it was suggested that Perutz should study law to prepare him for the family business. This never came to be because an alert schoolmaster took notice of the talented boy and stirred his interest in chemistry. In 1932 he entered the University of Vienna where, in his own words, he "wasted five semesters in an exacting course of inorganic analysis". Organic chemistry seemed all the more interesting to him and in particular he was excited to hear about the work in Cambridge by Sir Frederick G. Hopkins, the recipient of the 1929 Nobel Prize in physiology or medicine "for his discovery of the growth-stimulating vitamins". Perutz therefore decided to do work for a PhD in that particular university setting.

Having his expenses paid by his father he started work with the larger-than-life figure of modern science, Bernal. However, Perutz's first contacts with Cambridge were not what he had hoped for. Bernal was not present on his arrival and it took time for him to get an introduction to the laboratory and to learn the techniques of crystallography. In addition he found that he had landed in a politically very charged environment with a definite leftish orientation. But politics was not for Perutz. His experiences from Vienna had left him distrustful of any form of politics, be it oriented to the left or to the right. Still Perutz soon came to like the Cambridge atmosphere and it became the place where he was to stay for the rest of his life.

The first task that Bernal gave him was to analyze salt crystals of iron rhodonite. This task may not have stirred his imagination but possibly he was attracted by it because as a mountaineer he had an interest in mineralogy. He soon managed to generate some data and was even encouraged to present his provisional results at a meeting arranged by the Royal Society. This he took on with gusto but his enthusiasm quickly cooled when he saw Friedrich Paneth in the audience. Paneth, as has become apparent from Chapter 5, was a world authority on research into minerals and radioactivity.

After a while Perutz was able to start his work on organic molecules, but Bernal's support of his early work did not last long because of his move to London in 1937. The Cavendish Laboratory was in a holding mode since its illustrious head Rutherford had just died. Fortunately this led to Sir Lawrence Bragg being appointed Cavendish Professor of Experimental Physics in 1938, a position he kept until 1953. He became a staunch supporter of Perutz and his efforts to characterize the complex hemoglobin molecule. But why hemoglobin?

Perutz's choice of hemoglobin as the subject of his crystallographic studies was partly fortuitous. He wanted to tackle an important biological problem. Then he remembered that his cousin Gina was married to a professor of chemistry in Prague. His name was Felix Haurowitz and Perutz took the train to visit him in his home town. Since 1925 Haurowitz had been working on the physiology of blood with a particular interest in the specific protein hemoglobin that gives blood its red color. Perutz learned that there were different forms of hemoglobin and that several kinds of these molecules had been crystallized. At the time Haurowitz was developing very important experiments that were to demonstrate that hemoglobin changed its structure every time it took up and released oxygen. The molecule with and without oxygen gave different crystal structures. Perutz first suggested that he might start by solving the molecular structure of hemin, which can be obtained from broken-down hemoglobin. Haurowitz then pointed out to him that the complete formula of hemin was already known and in fact it was this finding that was the basis for the 1930 Nobel Prize in chemistry to Hans Fischer from Munich "for his researches into the constitution of haemin and chlorophyll and especially for his synthesis of haemin". Thus Perutz's goal should be to study the whole molecule.

Haurowitz did not have any crystals available but recommended Perutz to contact the biochemist Gilbert Adair in Cambridge. When he got back to Cambridge contact was established and eventually Perutz received material for his first studies. It was small crystals of horse methemoglobin, a form of the protein that develops when blood is left exposed to the air. In time Perutz managed to set up his own chemical laboratory and to grow his own crystals. At this time Perutz had already learned from discussions with his fellow students that he would be almost crazy to approach a molecule of this size. At the time the largest molecule, the structure of which had been solved contained 58 atoms. The complete hemoglobin is a combination of four iron-containing molecules composed of a total of about 10,000 atoms! Helped by Bernal's enthusiastic backing, Perutz, undeterred, took on the quixotic project. Using the crystals he had managed to produce he got his first results. They were encouraging in that the rotating crystals gave distinct reflections and a regular array of sharp spots could be observed on the photographic film. This showed that the atoms in the crystal were arranged in a repeating regular pattern and that the molecule had a two-fold axis of symmetry. It only remained to interpret the meaning of this pattern, something that turned out to require a very long scientific odyssey, a life-long journey. Thus it came to last far beyond the time of recognition of the important advances made in the project by the Nobel Prize in 1962.

When Hitler annexed Austria in March 1938 the situation for the Perutz family changed dramatically. They all became refugees with Max in Cambridge and his parents in Prague to where they had fled. Eventually it was possible for Max to bring his parents to England, but the situation this created was not uncomplicated. Professionally Max was very well supported, not least by Bragg's involvement with him as a person and with his research, and still clouds lingered on the horizon. Towards the end of 1939 Winston Churchill initiated discussions in the British government about how to filter out the foreign aliens that might be a threat to the country.

Perutz carried on with his early research, and at Christmas he was presented with a book that changed his professional outlook. It was *The Nature of the Chemical Bond and the Structure of Molecules and Crystals* written by Linus Pauling[9]. He referred to this book as the most exhilarating he had ever read. In his own words:

> His book transformed the chemical flatland of my earlier textbooks into a world of three-dimensional structures.... Pauling's imaginative approach, his synthesis of structural, theoretical and practical chemistry, his capacity of drawing on a wide variety of observations to prove his generalizations and his vivid writing drew the dry facts of chemistry together into a coherent intellectual fabric for me and thousands of other students for the first time.

In 1940 Perutz successfully submitted his thesis on the early results of crystallographic studies of the structure of hemoglobin. Two months later a policeman knocked at Dr Perutz's door carrying an arrest warrant.

He was interned together with a large number of other refugees, many of whom had an academic background, first near Liverpool and later in a more sealed-off setting surrounded by barbed wire on the Isle of Man. Perutz tried to indirectly mobilize his scientific peers Bragg and Bernal to see if they could help to secure his release. In June the internees were transferred to a camp in Canada. This camp eventually hosted more than six thousand men, a fraction of whom were refugee academics. Perutz was very disheartened by his internment and expressed his situation in the following way:

> To have been arrested, interned and deported as an enemy alien by the English, whom I regarded as my friends, made me more bitter than to have lost freedom itself. Having first been rejected as a Jew by my native Austria, which I loved, I now found myself rejected as a German by my adopted country.

There was a complete detachment from the outside world in the encampment, but one way of using their time meaningfully was the establishment of a "camp university". Of course Perutz taught the principles of X-ray analysis of crystals.

There were many influential supporters of Perutz engaged in finding ways of arranging for his release with reference to his stature as a first-class scientist of importance to both Great Britain and potentially also to the United States.

Bragg's involvement was the most critical for the developments. He wanted Perutz back and in November the "foreign alien" finally got a cable from his father that the Home Office had ordered his release. After a cumbersome trans-Atlantic journey Perutz arrived in Liverpool on a bleak January morning. The completeness of his freedom was almost overwhelming. He was filled with emotion on the train ride back to Cambridge. Without further ado he was back at the bench in the laboratory. His salary was now paid by a grant from the Rockefeller Foundation. He was happy to pick up on his uphill battle to unravel the structure of hemoglobin. Its secrets were slowly revealed, but there remained a need for improvement of techniques to resolve the large structure. In the private sphere life was altogether brighter. Perutz found his life partner in Gisela Peiser. She was a German refugee, one year younger than him, and they met when she started to work in the office of the laboratory.

Via Bernal Perutz became involved in warfare research, in particular the Habbakuk project already mentioned above. In fact the name of the project was misspelled. It had been taken from the Old Testament prophet Habakkuk, who according to Voltaire was a man "capable of everything". As a mountaineer Perutz was interested in properties of glaciers and the interaction of ice and other materials. His contributions to the project were limited but his involvement led to his first trip to the United States. He became very excited about his contact with New York and his interactions with crystallographers in that city. At the time he also became a British citizen. After having spent almost a year on the Habbakuk project Perutz was back in the Cavendish laboratory at the beginning of 1944. As the Second World War finally came to a cataclysmic end he started to expand his research group and in late 1945 there was an important addition.

Enter Kendrew

In an interview with Istvan Hargittai[10] Perutz described his first encounter with Kendrew:

> In 1945, he walked into my office, a young man in his smart wing commander's uniform. He asked if he could come and work with me as a research student. I was flattered because I never had a research student, let alone one who had distinguished himself already in the War.

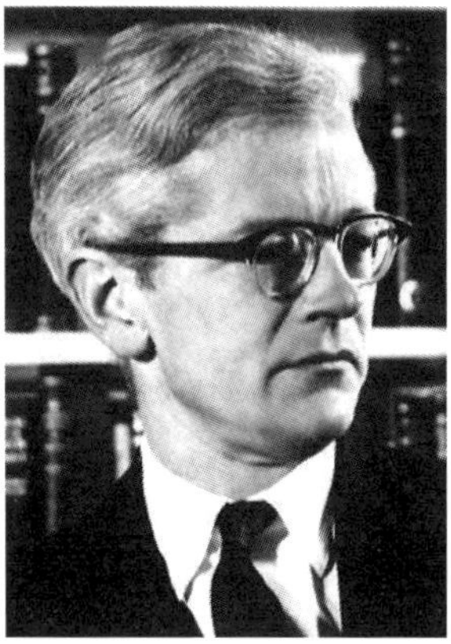

John C. Kendrew (1917–1997), recipient of the shared Nobel Prize in chemistry in 1962. [From *Les Prix Nobel en 1962*.]

But there was also a problem. How would it be possible to carve out a partial problem from the broad approach to the structure of hemoglobin so that the data obtained after some three years work could be used in a PhD thesis?

Kendrew was born in 1917, and was thus only three years younger than Perutz. He came from an intellectual family and got his schooling in Oxford and Bristol before he went to Trinity College, Cambridge as a Major Scholar in 1936. It was Bernal who towards the end of the war encouraged him to get involved in biological problems. He was also stimulated in his approach to science by contacts with Pauling in the US at about the same time. Pauling's involvements in studies of the peptide bonds in proteins were crucial for the advances eventually made by Perutz and Kendrew as we shall see.

Kendrew entered the laboratory with a certain natural authority and has been described as upright, confident, well-organized and efficient. He and Perutz were to collaborate for twenty years but soon after his Nobel Prize in 1962 Kendrew phased out his experimental science and became a highly successful science administrator. By way of contrast, Perutz, who was very successful in his own right in organizing the science efforts at the world famous Laboratory of Molecular Biology at the Cavendish laboratory, always stayed in close contact with the laboratory work. The two scientists were very different personalities, and possibly therefore might have complemented each other well.

In mid-1946 it was decided that Kendrew should attempt to work out the structure of myoglobin. This is a protein which can store and release oxygen and it serves the same function in muscles as hemoglobin does in blood. One advantage of myoglobin when it came to studying its three-dimensional structure was that it is only one-fourth of the size of hemoglobin — in total about 1,200 atoms versus 4,800 atoms. Sperm whale myoglobin was selected for Kendrew's studies, because of its propensity to produce useful crystals.

The group plugged on with their work and Kendrew was able to present his PhD thesis in 1949, but the group was still waiting for a major breakthrough. In the autumn of the same year Crick, whom we will get to know in more detail in the next chapter, joined the group at the laboratory. Using his incisive intelligence he came to have a major importance not only in solving the structure of DNA, but also in mapping the complex three-dimensional structure of large proteins. The problem was to advance from two to three dimensions in mapping out all reflections. Patterns had been found but there was a need for new approaches to model building to interpret the thousands of reflections in terms of phases. One important change occurred when Pauling and his colleagues, in particular Robert Corey revealed the fundamental features of the peptide bond and the alpha helix, which turned out to be a critical modular structure occurring as a part of many proteins.

The Genius of Chemistry

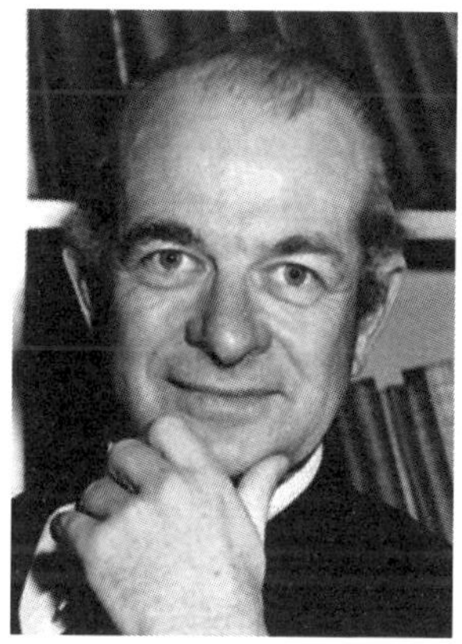

Linus C. Pauling (1901–1994), recipient of the 1954 Nobel Prize in chemistry. [From *Les Prix Nobel en 1954*.]

Pauling was a scientist and peace advocate well known to the public even today, perhaps mostly for advocating high doses of vitamin C to prevent respiratory infections. However that represented only a very minor part of his many wide-ranging projects. The unique attribute he should be remembered for is that he, as a single recipient, was awarded both a Nobel Prize in chemistry in 1954 and another prize in peace in 1962 for his humanitarian achievements. He gained an impressive authority in the field of biochemistry, as already referred to. His eventful existence has been documented in a book called *Force of Nature: The Life of Linus Pauling*[11].

Pauling was born in Oswedo, Oregon in 1901 but the family soon moved to Condon, where his father was a pharmacist. He had a close relationship with his father, who encouraged the intellectual development of his precocious son. Sadly his father died when Linus was only eight years old and regrettably his relationship with his mother did not have the same fiber. It lacked emotional warmth. To get away Pauling lived for periods with his grandfather, a German-speaking laborer, in Condon. Pauling referred to this environment, allowing contacts with Indian children and cowboys, as his spiritual birthplace. In this milieu he felt full of energy and confidence in himself, but according to his own formulation he was "... bookish and shy; that he was tongue-tied around girls". During his student years he developed his entrepreneurial talents delivering newspapers, working in a butcher shop, operating a movie projector on weekends, etc. Because of his background

Pauling felt both an insider and an outsider. He was always ready to challenge orthodoxy.

He studied at the Oregon State College and received a B.Sc. in chemical engineering in 1922. He was then appointed a Teaching Fellow at the California Institute of Technology (Caltech) and after being a graduate student there 1922–1925 he received his PhD Early on he became interested in the fundamental question of the nature of the chemical bond. His approach had an impressive scientific breadth. It involved many disciplines and methodological approaches including the relatively new field of X-ray crystallography. He was both an experimentalist and a theoretical scientist and rapidly developed into become the leading chemist of his time. His major book, already referred to above, was read as a bible by students and young researchers, including Perutz. Pauling applied his wide knowledge to both inorganic and organic chemistry. In the latter he became interested in the structure of proteins. Using crystallography he was able to demonstrate during the late 1940s a canonical structure of proteins, their alpha-helix twisting. He had already in 1931 become professor and Chairman at Caltech, the same year as he became the first recipient of the Langmuir Prize — the highest American Chemical Society Award in Pure Chemistry.

In the archives of the chemistry Nobel Prize, Pauling is a very prominent candidate. This giant of chemistry was nominated for a Nobel Prize in chemistry almost every year from 1940 onwards. In 1954 there were as many as 13 nominations, six of which came from previous Nobel Laureates, including Svedberg (p. 180) and Tiselius (p. 280) who were members of the committee. Pauling had been evaluated many times and the reviews had had different foci covering his wide-ranging research. Thus the reviews in 1940 focused on his studies of the chemical binding, in 1944 on his examination of biologically active compounds, in 1950 on molecular structure and chemical binding, and in 1952 on proteins and their building stones. In 1954 an overview was carried out of his whole production. The reviews in 1952 and 1954 were made by Gunnar Hägg, a

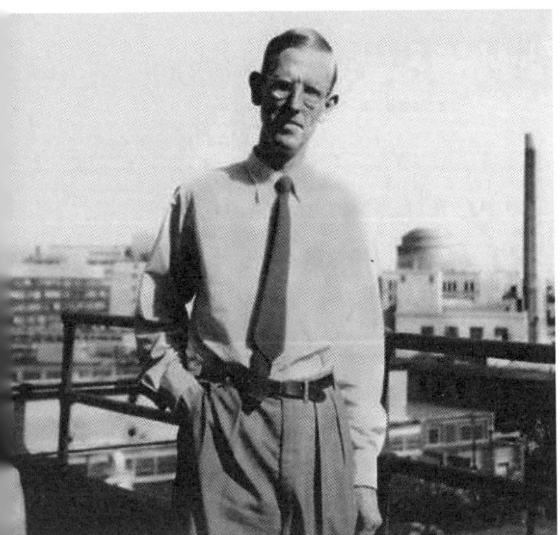

Gunnar Hägg (1903–1986). [Photo by Ivar Olovsson.]

professor of general and inorganic chemistry at Uppsala University. He was a well-respected scientist with a particular focus on crystallography. Among students of chemistry in Sweden at the time he was particularly well-known for his textbooks, one of which also was published in English in 1969, with the title *General and Inorganic Chemistry*. Hägg was an adjunct member of the committee in the years 1952, 1954 and also in 1962. Between 1965 and 1976 he was a full member of the committee and thus came to have central functions in the Nobel work for many years (p. 279).

Pauling had been declared worthy of a prize since 1950, but the question was which one of his different discoveries should be recognized by the prize. The committee decided in 1954 to focus on his original fundamental work on the chemical bond and less on the application of this knowledge to complex molecules. It used the prize motivation "for his research into the nature of the chemical bond and its application to the elucidation of the structure of complex substances".

Since the prize was not for his more recent discoveries, Robert Corey as a possible joint recipient of the prize did not need to be evaluated by the committee in 1954. However, the committee could not refrain from taking notice that "Pauling's theories on structure therefore, perhaps more than any other contribution, have played an important role in the development of protein chemistry in later years." This attitude was also reflected in the presentation speech at the Prize ceremony by Hägg[12]. Towards the end of this speech he emphasized the role that Pauling's fundamental discoveries had had for the interpretation of the complex structures of the large protein molecules. He specifically cited the expected complexity of hemoglobin with its 8,000 atoms and also mentioned the identification of the important alpha helix module of proteins. Also Pauling mentioned protein structures at the end of his Nobel lecture[13].

Critical Turning Points in the Understanding of the Structure of Hemoglobin

One day in 1950, Bragg challenged Perutz and Kendrew to consider more seriously helical structures. The main sources of information they had drawn from were Astbury's early pictures of hair, as an example of a helical structure, and emerging studies by Pauling and collaborators, as just mentioned. One limitation of Astbury's studies was that the light beam had always been at a right angle to the fiber axis. Only later was it appreciated that changing the angle by tilting the sample could provide important supplementary information. In addition the preconceived belief at the time that there should be an equal number of whole amino acid residues per turn of a helix held back the conceptualization of new principle forms of structures. The Cavendish group believed it might be four, but eventually it turned out not to be a whole number. There are 3.7 residues in a turn of the Pauling-Corey alpha helix.

One Saturday morning in June of 1951 when Perutz was in the library to do his reading up on recent literature he found in two issues of the Proceedings of the National Academy of Sciences, no fewer than eight articles by Pauling and collaborators, especially Corey, which led to the definition of the alpha-helix structure. Immediately Perutz understood that Pauling was right and that sadly he had misjudged his own data. He had been misled by the incorrect interpretations of the repeat structures of Astbury's studies of hair and a preconceived idea that the so-called amide groups in the amino acids were not planar but oblique. It soon dawned on Perutz that it would be possible to prove the correctness of Pauling's model using material that was available in the laboratory. His examination of a *tilted* horse hair showed that predictable but previously unrecognized reflection spots could be identified. Acknowledging the existence of the alpha-helix structures in the hemoglobin molecule allowed further advances in the understanding of the complex molecule. Perutz could now open his mind to new possibilities, no longer being corralled by inherited knowledge.

On Monday morning Perutz took his newly taken picture of the horse hair into Bragg's office and jubilantly shared with him the new results. Bragg asked him what had stimulated him to undertake the experiment. He was told that it was because he was so angry and disappointed with himself for not having seen what Pauling had discovered. Bragg's terse reply was "I wish I'd made you angry earlier!" This sentence was later used by Perutz as a title of a volume of essays on science and scientists[14].

When Crick joined the group at the Cavendish laboratory he originally had plans to use X-ray crystallography to study protein structure, but he did not find a suitable object. However, he developed opinions on the interpretations of the hemoglobin molecule by Perutz and his colleagues. Using his analytical intelligence he argued that for theoretical reasons the "hatbox" model preferred at the time was wrong. In fact the critique, provided under the rubric *What Mad Pursuit* — a title taken from John Keat's *Ode on a Grecian Urn* — was rather devastating. In parentheses it can be mentioned that Crick liked this title and used it again later in a biographical book, as we shall see. The patterns examined by Perutz and Kendrew for some time needed to be extensively reinterpreted. A new approach to solving the so-called "phase problem" was needed. One way of doing that, as suggested by Crick was to use a method called isomorphous — Greek for unaltered form — replacement, a technique previously used for smaller molecules. This had been considered earlier, but most large protein structure crystallographers had dismissed the idea. The general belief was that the heavy atoms intended for use would not have a measurable effect in a larger molecule. Bragg himself had formulated it bluntly in a *Nature* article: "No heavy atom could stand out in such a crowd." This belief turned out not to be right.

In 1952 Perutz, in collaboration with Vernon Ingram, made a major breakthrough. Ingram later made critical findings contributing to the opening of the field of molecular medicine, which will be further discussed in the next chapter. The two scientists examined the diffraction patterns of hemoglobin in both an unlabelled form and in a form labeled by two mercury atoms and saw critical and informative differences. According to Perutz's own words:

> I found the exact intensity which knowledge of the absolute intensities had led me to expect. I raced up three floors to Bragg's office and asked him to come down to the darkroom. As we looked at the two pictures, we realized that the phase problem which had baffled us for the last 16 years was at last solved, and Bragg went around generously telling everybody that I had discovered a goldmine.

Eureka moments were rare in the development of crystallographic work, but this was one of them. Perutz referred to it as his life's most important discovery. A general picture of the three-dimensional structure of hemoglobin could now be deduced, but the challenge for the coming work was to increase the resolution. In fact at the time of recognition of Kendrew's and Perutz's work in 1962 the resolution obtained in the studies of myoglobin was much better than in the studies of the much larger hemoglobin molecule. In his Nobel lecture[15] Kendrew emphasized his limited insight into the scope of the problem he had embarked on and referred to it as "a case of ignorance being bliss". It took until the breakthrough in 1953, when Perutz discovered the possibility of applying the isomorphous replacement method that both his and Kendrew's projects could move on.

In a historical perspective it became possible step by step to comprehend the different phases in the maturation of a complex protein. The first insight was the appreciation of the existence of a *primary structure*, the necklace of amino acids in varying numbers, as beautifully illustrated by Frederick Sanger's studies of the two protein chains of insulin. He was awarded his first Nobel Prize in chemistry in 1958 "for his work on the structure of proteins, especially that of insulin". Later it was understood that there were certain kinds of preferred modular *secondary structures* such as the alpha helix demonstrated by Pauling and, as discovered still later, also so-called anti-parallel beta structures, in some cases referred to as beta barrels. In its final folding a protein takes on a *tertiary structure*, which allows it to express its specific function. The final folding of a protein, be it spontaneous or assisted by so called chaperone proteins, is still today only partly known and the protein folding problem remains a major challenge to scientists. There is room for many perturbations with smaller or larger parts of a protein remaining in an unfolded state and potentially only taking on a certain shape at time of interaction with its target.

Understanding the Structure of Myoglobin

As already mentioned Kendrew, like a number of other scientists, was lured into crystallographic studies of large organic molecules by Bernal. The early studies of myoglobin emphasized that it was a fortunate choice because of its fundamental structural similarity to one-quarter of the hemoglobin molecule studied by Perutz. The myoglobin molecule has 153 amino acid residues associated with a single heme group containing iron. However the attempt to apply the isomorphous replacement method to myoglobin required some empirical experimentation since it lacked the sulphydryl groups present in hemoglobin, which were the structures used for attachment of mercury. Eventually it was possible to generate a number of heavy atom substitutes by different chemical modifications of various parts of the molecule. A large number of reflections were collected and different phases of the patterns observed were derived.

The first computers that started to become available after the Second World War were an important asset and with time crystallography became ever more — in practice indispensably — dependent on advanced computers managing volumes of data vastly in excess of what single individuals might handle. A good use was made by the Cambridge team of the best computers at the time, EDSAC II and IBM 7090. The pocket calculators of today are much more powerful than these early pre-transistor machines. I remember once as a student seeing the local representation of these early computers at the Stockholm University. It was called BESK — binary electronic sequence c(k)alculator and it occupied two floors in the building at Drottninggatan 95 in the middle of the city. One was occupied by the complex set-up of radio tubes and the other floor housed the fans that were needed to remove all the heat generated by the tubes. The engineers operating the machine were proud to demonstrate that it could sing the most famous Swedish snaps drinking song *Helan går*, sometimes jokingly referred to as the Swedish "national anthem".

As Kendrew described in his Nobel lecture[15] it was decided to approach the structural analysis of myoglobin in three stages. The first stage was finished in 1957 and involved 400 reflections allowing a total resolution of 6Å. Parenthetically it can be mentioned that 1 Å = 1×10^{-10} meter; a unit introduced by the Swedish physicist Anders Ångström, whose life in the mid-19th century overlapped with that of Alfred Nobel. Two years later Kendrew and his collaborators had increased the resolution to 2 Å by collecting and analyzing 10,000 reflections. In a third step the number of reflections was increased to about 25,000 with the aim of reaching a resolution of 1.4 Å. This final step would also allow the identification of the small hydrogen atoms. At the time of the prize the last phase of the study had not as yet been completed. The characterization of the myoglobin molecule was facilitated by the fact that it was represented by alpha helix modules in 75 percent of its structure, a good deal higher than the percentage in most other proteins. It was also of great help for the interpretation of structure when in the later phase of the studies the amino acid sequence of the protein became known. It was determined by a research group at the Rockefeller Institute using the technique developed by Sanger in his characterization of the insulin protein. The complex structure of the molecule was demonstrated by an arrangement of glass plates layered equidistantly to each other. Each plate depicted the density map of one cross-section of the molecule. Today computer-aided technologies have made it much simpler to illustrate the three-dimensional structure of large and complex molecules. They can easily be viewed from different angles on a computer screen.

The Delayed Nobel Prize to Hodgkin

It would seem more logical to have given a Nobel Prize in chemistry to Hodgkin prior to the one to Kendrew and Perutz. She was Bernal's first successful student and she pioneered crystallographic studies of different important biological molecules — sterols, penicillin and vitamin B12 — of lesser complexity than the protein polypeptides. The most likely explanation for the fact that she received her prize two years after the protein crystallographers was the special situation that developed in 1962. As will be discussed below and in the next chapter both the Nobel Committees in chemistry and in physiology or medicine confronted realities that prompted them to jointly recognize the paradigmatic shift in emphasis on the central biological roles of proteins and nucleic acids. On this occasion it was considered urgent to recognize the momentous discovery of the structure of DNA and in that context it was very appealing to award in parallel the crystallographic revelations of the complexity of large proteins. The deliberations by the committees on these matters will be further discussed below and in the next chapter.

Hodgkin was nominated for a Nobel Prize in chemistry for the first time in 1950 by Joseph D. H. Donnay, a well-known crystallographer at John Hopkins University, Baltimore. He referred to her determination of the crystallographic structure of penicillin. Her contributions in this area were reviewed by the chairman of the committee, Arne Westgren. He was an important scientist in the Nobel work, who was born in 1889 and developed his academic career at Uppsala University under the supervision of Svedberg, introduced in Chapter 5. Westgren obtained his PhD in 1915 and after this he went on to become a pioneer in the application of X-ray diffraction methods in physical metallurgy. In 1927 Westgren was appointed professor of general and inorganic chemistry at the University of Stockholm. He became a member of the Royal Swedish Academy of Sciences in 1933 and ten years later he left his position at the university to become permanent secretary at this Academy, a full time employment. He retired to become former permanent secretary —

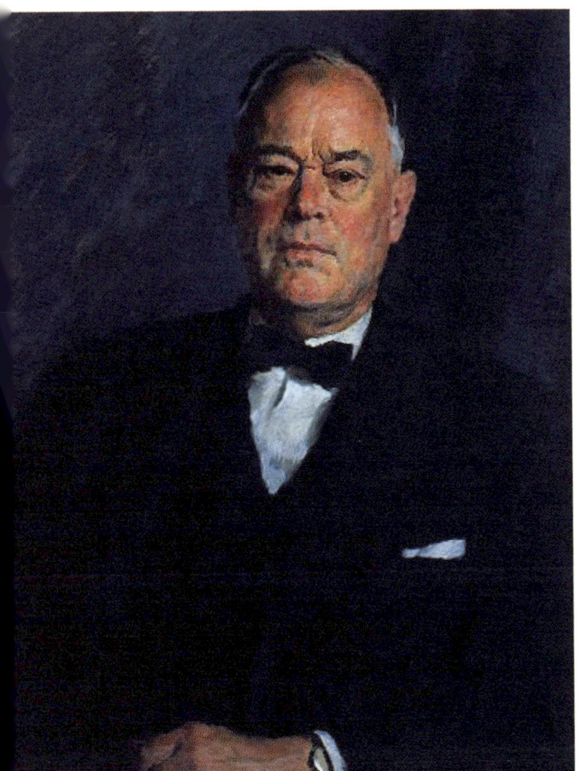

Arne Westgren (1889–1975). Portrait at the Royal Swedish Academy of Sciences.

a title I myself enjoyed using — in 1959, but he remained deeply involved in the work of the Nobel Committee for chemistry even after this.

Westgren's association with the work of the Nobel Committee for chemistry started already in 1926 when he became its secretary. It should be noted that one need not be a member of the academy to serve as a secretary of a Nobel Committee. Of course one does not have any voting rights, neither in the committee nor, unless one is a member, in the final selection of the prize recipients by the academy *in pleno*. In 1943 he became a member of the committee and left the secretary's position. A year later he took over the chairmanship of the committee from Svedberg. He retained this highly influential position for as long as 22 years, six years beyond his retirement from his leadership position at the academy. His overview of the dynamically changing field of chemistry must have been unique.

As mentioned earlier[5], the committee for the Nobel Prize in chemistry was remarkably stable over two decennia from the mid-1940s. Its most long-lasting member was Svedberg. He became a member in 1926, the same year in which Westberg became secretary. That Svedberg became a member in

Longtime members of the Nobel Committee for chemistry between 1926 and 1976.

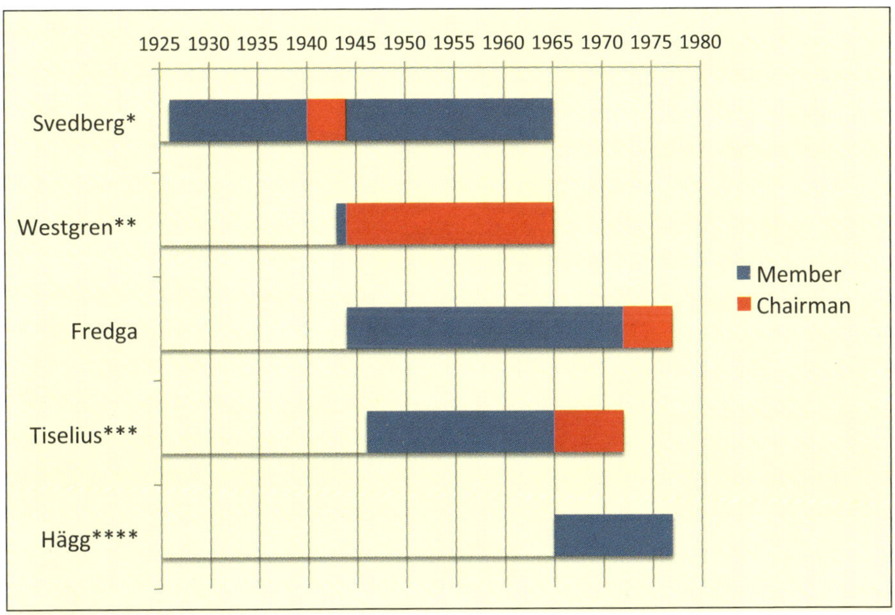

* Nobel Prize in chemistry in 1926.
** Secretary of the committee since 1926.
*** Nobel Prize in chemistry in 1948.
**** Adjunct member of the committee in 1952, 1954 and 1962.

this particular year might appear puzzling since he received his Nobel Prize the same year. An explanation for this conundrum has been given in Chapter 5. Svedberg remained on the committee until 1964 when he turned 80 years old, a total of 38 years!

Two other longtimers were Arne Fredga (1944–1976) and Arne Tiselius (1946–1971) (he died in the latter year), to be further introduced in Chapter 8. One can discuss the strength and weaknesses of such long-term memberships. Today the maximum mandate is twice three years, which may be preceded and possibly also followed by an annual appointment to an adjunct membership. Because the committee for physiology or medicine nowadays perpetually works with ten adjunct members, longer-term involvements by individual scientists

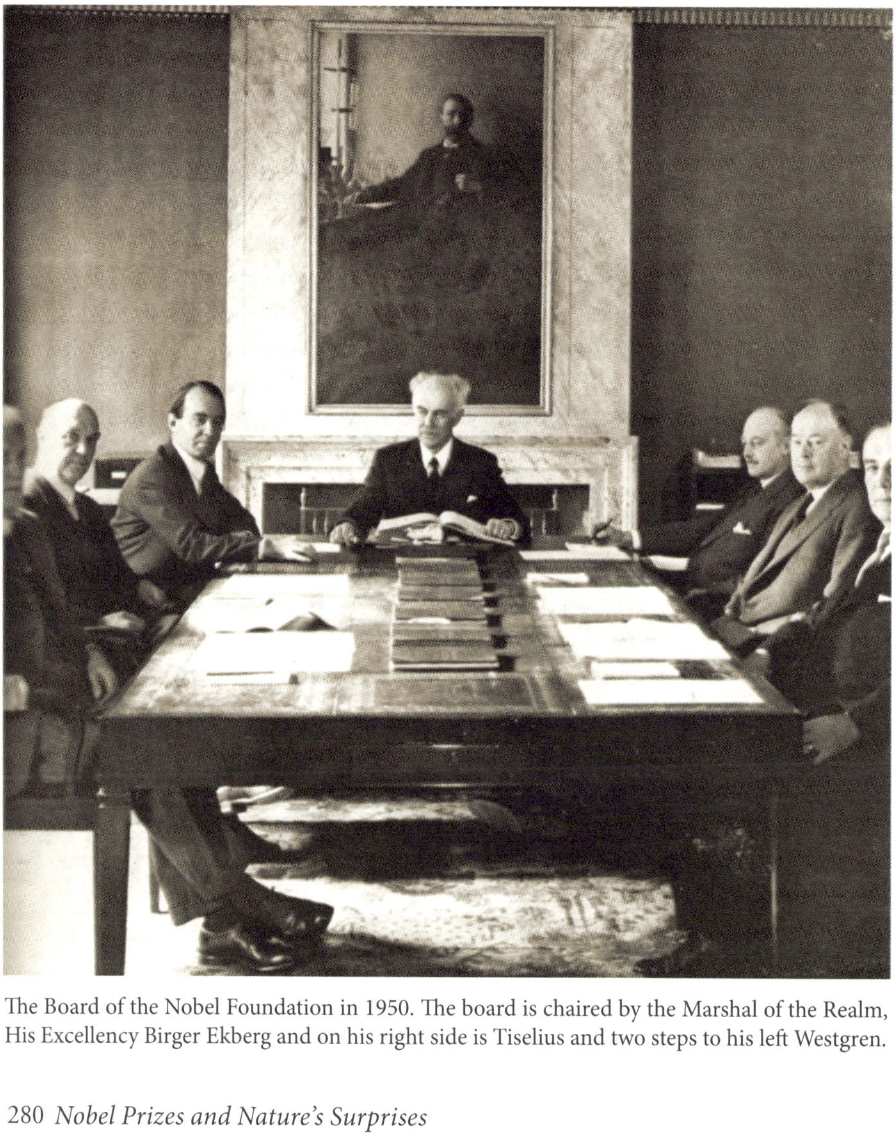

The Board of the Nobel Foundation in 1950. The board is chaired by the Marshal of the Realm, His Excellency Birger Ekberg and on his right side is Tiselius and two steps to his left Westgren.

on the committee today are much more common at the Karolinska Institute than at the Academy.

Besides membership of committees there are also other functions in the Nobel system where members of the academy and professors of the Karolinska Institute can serve. The picture above shows a meeting with the board of the Nobel Foundation in the jubilee year of 1950. Tiselius, the vice-chairman (1947–1959), is sitting on the far left and Westgren in the middle on the right-hand side. Ten years later Tiselius became the chairman of the board a responsibility that he carried for five years (1960–1964). He will be discussed more extensively in the next chapter.

Bragg, the critical nominator of candidates in the field of crystallography (see tables on pp. 289 and 333), had frequent contacts with Swedish scientists over many years, also, surprisingly, during the Second World War. These contacts were in part arranged by an organization called the British Council founded in 1934. The Council was created to promote a wider appreciation of British culture abroad. One way of doing this was lecture tours by scientists and culture workers. During the war there were only four European countries (besides Sweden, Iceland, Portugal and Spain) which could receive lecturers. In 1943 Bragg flew to Stockholm and visited Uppsala for a lecture. In the picture below he can be seen in company with a number of the central actors in the chemistry committee, Svedberg, Fredga, Tiselius and Hägg.

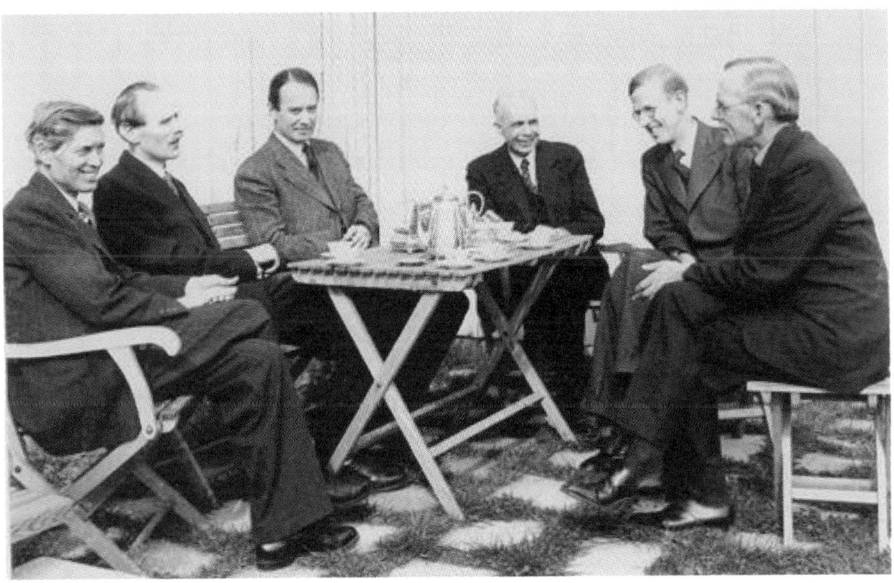

A unique gathering in Uppsala in 1943. From left: Svedberg, Fredga, Tiselius, Bragg, Hägg and a local physicist Axel E. Lindh. [Photo by Ivar Olovsson.]

Let us now return to the review in 1950 of Hodgkin's studies of the structure of penicillin by the veteran committee member Westgren. Being himself a crystallographer he was able to fully appreciate her work. He complimented her perseverance and great skill in the investigations, but he questioned whether the results obtained justified all the effort invested. The understanding of the structure of penicillin at the time apparently had not facilitated the development of methods to chemically synthesize the substance. Thus the conclusion was that the work proposed for recognition did not have sufficient importance to justify a Nobel Prize.

In 1956 Hodgkin was nominated again. In fact she was nominated for a prize in physics or in chemistry, but because she had not made any independent significant methodological contributions it was decided to exclude her from being discussed for a prize in physics. This time the nomination concerned her pioneering work on the structure of vitamin B12 and the nominator was the respected British crystallographer Sir Robert Robinson. Westgren made another evaluation. Again he was very impressed by Hodgkin's scientific efforts and stated:

> Mrs Hodgkin's determination of the (three-dimensional) structure of the B12 molecule is undeniably an impressive achievement, which bears witness to a rare tenacity and much ingenuity. The challenge (taken on) is more difficult than any other of a similar kind resolved by the same X-ray crystallographic approach.

The reviewer wondered to what extent her successful studies had spurred other researchers to tackle similar problems. His conclusion was that it remained to be seen if this would be the case or not. The final recommendation was to wait and see before a decision about a prize was taken, in particular since the structural studies of vitamin B12 had not as yet been concluded. Parenthetically it can be mentioned that I, during my second year of medical studies in 1957, was so impressed by the beauty of the chemical structure of vitamin B12 that I had a drawing of its formula with the central cobalt on the door of my study. In this context it could be reiterated that vitamin B12, composed of 181 atoms, is a much smaller structure than Kendrew's myoglobin molecule, 2,600 atoms representing 153 amino acids.

In 1957 Bernal made a comprehensive nomination over four and a half pages with reference to several articles by Hodgkin for a prize in physics emphasizing that the structural analysis of vitamin B12 had been completed the previous year. Following earlier recommendations the committee of physics transferred this material to the committee of chemistry. The latter committee in addition received renewed proposals to award a prize for the results of the studies of the structure of vitamin B12 by three separate nominators. In one of these nominations it was recommended that she should share the prize with Alexander R. Todd, who eventually became the single Nobel Prize recipient in chemistry for that year. However he did not receive his prize for his contribution to the structure of vitamin B12, but "for his work on nucleotides and nucleotide coenzymes" discussed earlier[5]. No further evaluation was made of Hodgkin in this year.

The next time she was proposed was in 1959. Bernal again nominated her for a prize in physics and in addition there were two nominations of Hodgkin alone addressed directly to the chemistry committee and another one, which proposed that she should be combined with Kendrew and Perutz (Table 7.1, p. 289).

Westgren did an additional review of Hodgkin's more recent work and he also made remarks on the proposal to combine her with Perutz and Kendrew. He stated that the situation regarding Hodgkin's candidacy had not changed much since his previous evaluation three years earlier. The structural analysis of vitamin B12 had essentially been brought to conclusion and Hodgkin was the single dominating figure in this field of research. It was believed that this important advance would incite fellow crystallographers to examine other biologically relevant substances, but there had not been any rapid expansion of this field of research during the three years that had passed. Westgren sought for an explanation of this in the fact that crystallography is an exceptionally cumbersome form of research requiring years of strenuous work. Scientists who are willing to make such a sacrifice are rare, with Hodgkin as a shining exception. In a later historical context[16] Westgren returned to his admiration of Hodgkin. In a description of her scientific efforts he referred to her "... unbounding perserverance, extraordinary imaginative and brilliant intuition".

As will be further discussed below, Westgren believed in this year that the protein crystallographic studies by Kendrew and Perutz had not as yet been developed extensively enough and that therefore it would be best to delay the decision-taking on a prize. By way of contrast he considered Hodgkin's work mature enough to be recognized by a prize. But still he wanted to wait. As to the possibility of combining the three scientists in one prize he stated:

> As a matter of fact the X-ray analyses of complex organic molecules by the Oxford and Cambridge schools might not have so much in common

> that a joint recognition would be considered advisable. A division of a prize between more than two scientists should if possible be avoided.

The last sentence emphasized that still at this time the Nobel committees were trying to keep the number of prize recipients to one or possibly two.

In 1960 Bragg, the father figure in the field of crystallography took a tactical initiative. He nominated Hodgkin, Perutz and Kendrew for a prize in physics, a nomination supported by Cyril N. Hinselwood from Oxford (Table 7.1, p. 289) and Watson, Crick and Wilkins for a prize in chemistry. The nomination for a prize in physics included a very extensive review of the history of the developments of the subfields of crystallography and also referred back to the 1914 and 1915 prizes in physics to von Laue and to himself and his father, respectively. Although it was a joint nomination, the protein crystallographers, Perutz and Kendrew were discussed separately from Hodgkin. In his cover letter Bragg wrote:

> Dr M. F. Perutz and Dr J. C. Kendrew, the leaders of the Molecular Research Unit in the Cavendish Laboratory at Cambridge, which is supported by the British Medical Research Council, have succeeded in solving the problem of determining the structure of the vastly complex protein molecules, haemoglobin and myoglobin, by X-ray analysis. It seemed almost impossible only a few years ago that such structures, containing thousands of atoms, could be determined directly, but this has now been achieved as the culmination of many years of patient investigations. I enclose a summary of the work and supporting papers.
>
> The other outstanding contribution is that made by Mrs Dorothy Hodgkin, in solving the structures of complex organic molecules such as Vitamin B12, $C_{63}H_{88}N_{14}O_{14}PCo$, and her previous contribution to the analysis of the penicillin molecule. The work on B12 was a real *tour de force*. It is generally recognized that, as a feat of analysis by the established trial-and-error methods of X-ray analysis it stands alone, and Mrs. Hodgkin is widely acclaimed as the foremost exponent of this art. The solution of the protein structures, on the other hand, was made possible by elaborating new methods of attack.

Bragg's nomination contained a lot of additional supporting material. It can be noted that he always referred to Perutz and Kendrew in that order and it is clear from his text that he considered Perutz as the leading figure and hence that alphabetical order should not be used. This attitude was adopted by the Nobel committee and when a prize was awarded Perutz's name preceded Kendrew's. Bragg's admiration of Hodgkin was emphasized by the formulation "...come from Mrs Hodgkin's laboratory at Oxford but these papers on penicillin and B12 will, I hope, suffice as illustrations of her genius." An illustration of Bragg's admiration for Hodgkin can be seen on p. 301. On the blackboard he has written "B12 Intelligence = Dorothy Hodgkin".

Besides Bragg's and Hinselwood's nominations there was also one more nomination each of Hodgkin and of Perutz, the latter as a part of a nomination also including two other candidates. After a discussion between the committees in physics and in chemistry it was decided that the latter committee should take charge of the crystallographers. No further evaluation was made this year and the candidates were put on hold.

In 1960 Hodgkin was also nominated for a prize in physiology or medicine by the professor of internal medicine at the Karolinska Institute, Henrik Lagerlöf. She was nominated together with Lester Smith and Karl Folkers, who had made critical contributions to the isolation and chemical characterization of vitamin B12. A review of Hodgkin's central contribution was made by Arne Engström (p. 347), a professor of medical physics and adjunct member of the committee. Since he had a dominating role in the evaluation of the discoverers of the structure of DNA, he will be introduced more extensively in the next chapter. Engström was impressed by the successful three-dimensional characterization of the structure of vitamin B12, but remarked that this molecule is much smaller than the proteins structures examined by Perutz and Kendrew. He noted that the progress in solving the structural problem of vitamin B12 was aided by the identification of the chemical composition of the vitamin including the identification of cobalt in the molecule, something that facilitated the structural analysis using the heavy atom approach. The conclusion of the review was that "there is no question about the fact that solving the crystalline structure of vitamin B12 is highly worthy of a prize. However, the question remains if the chemists who have made a critical contribution by determining the chemical composition of the molecule should not be included."

In 1961 Bragg repeated his nomination of Perutz, Kendrew and Hodgkin, but this time he addressed it directly to the chemistry committee (Table 7.1, p. 289). There were also proposals of the first two nominees by a number of other nominators, as further discussed below. In the case of Hodgkin the committee did not take any further action. It referred to its previous evaluation and decision. Hodgkin was also nominated for a prize in physiology or medicine together with Perutz and Kendrew by a Swedish professor of biochemistry from Göteborg, Einar Stenhagen. The archive materials from the committee give some contradictory information. It specifies that another special investigation of Hodgkin should be made, but apparently this was not done. Presumably Engström argued that there was not much to be added to the review he had made the previous year. Most likely the committee therefore relied on this previous evaluation when it stated in its summary that Hodgkin's determination of the structures of penicillin and vitamin B12 was worthy of a Nobel Prize.

Finally in 1962, when crystallographic studies of proteins and DNA came to dominate the prizes, the chemistry committee again passed by Hodgkin with reference to its prior considerations. There was no external nomination of Hodgkin this year, but she was nominated by the chairman of the committee, Westgren. This procedure, most often in the form a of a nomination by the secretary representing the committee (Ref. 5, Chapter 6), is used even at the present time to ensure that an important candidate will be available for discussion in a particular year even in the absence of a nomination from an external invited nominator.

Hodgkin had to wait another two years before she eventually received her Nobel Prize in chemistry. Whether during this time she might also have been seriously considered for a prize in physiology or medicine remains to be seen. In the absence of access to archival material one can only speculate about the nominations and the potential ensuing deliberations and initiatives taken by the committees. It seems likely that Bragg repeated his nomination of Hodgkin, since the chemistry committee had not agreed to combining her with Perutz and Kendrew as he had suggested. Furthermore it is not unlikely that the latter two scientists themselves nominated their fellow shining star crystallographer, most likely for a prize in chemistry. It has been stated[17] that Perutz himself felt uncomfortable that his prize preceded Hodgkin's. She had been longer in the field and in addition he might have — rightly (?) — considered her achievements superior to his own.

Although in essence all the fundamental information about the three-dimensional structure of vitamin B12 had been determined in 1959 it is possible that some of the additional information that Hodgkin and collaborators published in 1961–62 may have given a boost to her candidature. Probably there was therefore another review of the progress of her work. The fact that it took two years and not just one year to finally award her the delayed and well-deserved Nobel Prize may have a simple explanation in that the chemistry committee for obvious reasons might have been reluctant to give a prize in the same sub-discipline two years in a row. The 1963 Nobel Prize in chemistry recognized Karl Ziegler and Giulio Natta "for their discoveries in the field of the chemistry and technology of high polymers".

When the 54-year-old Dorothy Hodgkin came to Stockholm to receive her Nobel Prize it was an exceptional event. The appearance of a single female recipient of a prize in natural sciences has only occurred on two other occasions in the long history of the Nobel Prizes; in 1911 when Marie Curie came to receive her second Nobel Prize, this time in chemistry and as a single recipient; and in 1983 when Barbara McClintock received her prize in physiology or medicine "for her discovery of mobile genetic elements". Hodgkin was an inspiring role model for female scientists at a time when the general field of science was dominated by men. However it should be added that the subfield of crystallography for some reason attracted a relatively large number of highly competent female scientists, as will also become apparent from the next chapter.

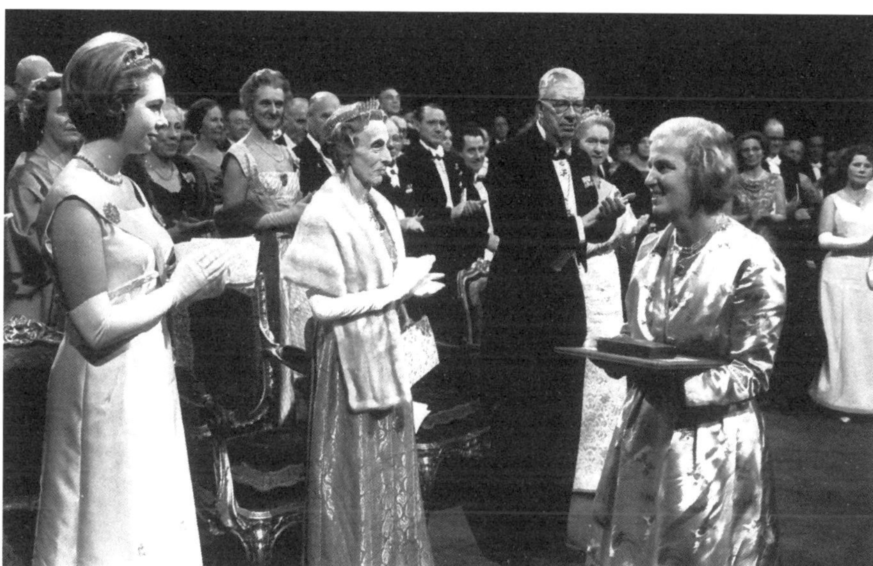

Hodgkin receiving her Nobel Prize. [© Scanpix Sweden AB.]

Hägg, who had given the laudation addresses to Pauling in 1954 and, as we shall see, to Perutz and Kendrew in 1962, also gave the introductory speech at the 1964 Nobel Prize ceremony[18]. He presented some historical background to the developments in crystallographic studies of organic molecules, but he did not refer to the prize two years earlier to Perutz and Kendrew. Instead he stated close to the end:

> In 1956, after eight years' work, Mrs Hodgkin and her collaborators had clarified the B12 structure. Never before had it been possible to determine the exact structure of so large a molecule, and the result has been seen as a triumph for X-ray crystallographic techniques. It was also, however, a triumph for Mrs Hodgkin. It is certain that the goal would never have been reached at this stage without her skill and exceptional intuition.

Although Hodgkin had to wait two years for her prize, since she was not recognized on the same occasion as Perutz and Kendrew, there was a reward. Instead of receiving only one-third of the prize money she was able to collect the whole sum! Of course money does not count in scientific recognitions, but still.

Protein Crystallography Comes of Age

There were special circumstances which led to that the structural analyses of the two dominant forms of molecules of life — DNA and proteins — were recognized by Nobel Prizes in 1962. As we shall see it was tempting to reward simultaneously the dramatic new insights into the structure of the digital information molecules and the tools whose synthesis they directed. Discussions of a prize recognizing protein crystallography started in 1951 when Perutz was nominated by a Japanese colleague for his studies of horse hemoglobin (see Table 7.1, p. 289). The committee noted that, at the International Congress of Crystallography which had been held recently in Stockholm, X-ray crystallographic studies of proteins had been the focus of interest. The discussion had been led by Bernal, referred to as the father of the field, and his interactions with the crystallographers at the Cavendish laboratory had been mentioned. Among these Perutz was cited as having made observations that had attracted much attention in his studies of horse hemoglobin. However, it was noted by the committee that it was too early to consider a possible recognition of his still rather incomplete results.

It would take until 1959 before Perutz, now together with Kendrew as well as Hodgkin, was again was nominated for a prize. As already mentioned the chairman of the committee, Westgren, made an evaluation. Concerning the protein studies it was noted that they had turned out to be much more cumbersome than originally expected but that, as a result of the enduring

Table 7.1. Nominations for Nobel Prizes in chemistry and in physiology or medicine for the characterization of the structure of large proteins. (Names of candidates within parentheses indicate the use of somewhat different motivation.)

Year	Chemistry Nominated	Chemistry Nominator	Physiology or Medicine Nominated	Physiology or Medicine Nominator
1951	Perutz	Y. Morino, Tokyo		
1959	Perutz, Kendrew (Hodgkin)	C. Martius, Zürich		
1960	Perutz, Kendrew (Hodgkin)	W. L. Bragg, Cambridge (x) C. N Hinselwood, Oxford (x)	Perutz, Kendrew (Ingram) Perutz (Crick)	J. McMichael, London E. J. King, London
1961	Perutz, Kendrew (Hodgkin) Perutz, Kendrew (Corey) Perutz, Kendrew Perutz, Kendrew Perutz, Kendrew	W. L. Bragg, Cambridge L. Pauling, Pasadena F. Sanger, Cambridge H. Zahn, Aachen I. Nitta, Osaka	Perutz, Kendrew (Hodgkin)	E.Stenhagen, Göteborg
1962	Perutz Perutz, Kendrew (Corey) Perutz, Kendrew Perutz, Kendrew Perutz, Kendrew	A. Butenandt, Münich L. Pauling, Pasadena J. Roche, Paris G. R. Pomerat, New York H. A. Scheraga, Ithaca	Perutz, Kendrew	H. Theorell, Stockholm

(x) Nomination originally submitted for a prize in physics, but transferred to the chemistry committee.

and imaginative studies, important progress had been made. Since the work was ongoing and additional results were expected to be presented in the near future it was considered premature to seriously discuss recognition by a Nobel Prize. This situation remained unchanged the following year when Bragg, supported by Hinshelwood, made his first nomination of Perutz, Kendrew and Hodgkin to receive a prize in physics, as already referred to above. It is stated in the biography of Bragg[7] that he waited to nominate the protein crystallographers until they had obtained results of sufficient magnitude to make them strong candidates for the prize. This had consequences also for the simultaneous nomination of the discoverers of DNA as we shall see. The chemistry committee, which had taken over the nomination for a prize in physics, concluded that major advances had been made but wanted to suspend judgment regarding priority for a prize.

The committee reflected on the proposal it had received the same year directly from Bragg to consider Watson, Crick and Wilkins, as will be discussed further in the next chapter. After extensive deliberations it proceeded to make the following summary:

> One other circumstance needs also to be considered. In his proposals Bragg gives preference (in recognition by a prize) for work by Perutz and Kendrew on the structure of proteins and for the structural studies by Dorothy Hodgkin of penicillin and vitamin B12. These are according to his opinion the foremost among the achievements in X-ray crystallography in recent times. He has proposed the three researchers for a joint prize in physics because they have made their analyses mainly by use of physical methods. However the importance of the results they have obtained decidedly belongs within chemistry and their possible recognition by a prize should be in chemistry. Viewed from a chemical perspective Perutz' and Kendrew's investigations of globular proteins are as important in general as the nucleic acid research by Watson, Crick and Wilkins. However, the former as well as Dorothy Hodgkin's contributions rank higher (sic, my remark) than those made in the field of nucleic acids and viruses since it has been possible to build on (derive the data from) an experimental material, which is much more plentiful and thus more complete than for example the one that Wilkins and Franklin and Gosling (note that only crystallographers are mentioned — Watson and Crick were considered to be neither crystallographers nor chemists; my remark) has been possible to produce. Their (Perutz, Kendrew, Hodgkin) analyses thus provide more solid evidence and are more penetrating.

The conclusion by the chemistry committee in 1960 therefore was that before considering the candidature of the nucleic acid researchers a final decision had to be taken on a prize for Perutz, Kendrew and Hodgkin. Apparently the chemists preferred to award a prize to these crystallographers. But they retained a wait-and-see policy.

In 1960 Perutz and Kendrew together with Vernon Ingram were also nominated for a prize in physiology or medicine. There was also one additional separate nomination for a prize in this field for Ingram and another for Perutz, in the latter case together with Crick. The historically important crystallographer Astbury had also been nominated in an extensive proposal for a prize. Engström made a *preliminary* evaluation of Astbury together with Kendrew.

The year before he already had made the same kind of evaluation of Astbury's work and concluded that there was no need for a complete investigation. This time his conclusion was different. Since there had been major advances in the work he recommended a follow-up by a more comprehensive review. He undertook this review himself. It summarized the powerful advances in understanding of protein structures, making the important distinctions between the different levels of protein folding from primary to tertiary structures. He then discussed the pioneering contributions by Astbury in his studies of thread-like structures like keratin, myosin, collagen etc. His conclusion was that Astbury had had a central role in developing the field of *biomolecular structure*, a term he himself had coined. Engström therefore proposed that Astbury's contributions could be worthy of a prize and that possibly he should be combined with Kendrew and Perutz. However although Engström in his preliminary evaluation, which also included Kendrew, recommended that he should also be subjected to a complete investigation, this was not done. The final decisions by the committee of physiology or medicine this year was that Astbury, in contrast to Engström's recommendation should not be considered for a prize and it did not make any comments on Perutz and Kendrew.

In 1961 the temperature had risen further and there was an increased number of nominations for a prize to the protein crystallographers. Bragg repeated his nomination, which still also included Hodgkin, but this time it was sent directly to the chemistry and not to the physics committee. Pauling who had seen a copy of Bragg's nomination the previous year endorsed the candidacy of Perutz and Kendrew but substituted Hodgkin for his own collaborator Corey. He also nominated him as a potential recipient of an undivided prize. There were three nominations for Perutz and Kendrew alone, one of which came from their prestigious laboratory colleague Sanger. Finally there was one more nomination of Perutz alone in a proposal that also included two separate other names. In spite of this wide support for a prize the committee stayed with its wait-and see policy. It wrote:

> The committee thus still retains a position of expectancy as concerns the question of a possible recognition of Perutz and Kendrew, who with such success have tackled the problem of the structure of proteins. When the (three-dimensional) structure of myoglobin and hemoglobin has become more completely determined and the question of a prize in this field again has been brought to the fore, which can be expected to be in the near future, it seems to the committee that a review should

be instigated concerning the early work in this field by Corey, who this year has been nominated for the first time.

The Nobel Prize in chemistry in 1961 went to Melvin Calvin "for his research on the carbon dioxide assimilation in plants" an important applied form of chemistry. One of the nominations of Calvin had been by Hevesy (Chapter 5).

There was also a discussion about the crystallographers in the committee for physiology or medicine. It had received a nomination from the Swede Einar Stenhagen, professor in medical biochemistry, originally at Uppsala University, but since 1959 at the University of Göteborg. He proposed Hodgkin, Perutz and Kendrew because the molecules they studied had major medical importance. As already mentioned this resulted in Hodgkin being declared worthy of a prize, but no further analyses of Perutz and Kendrew were made and they are not mentioned in the summary report by the committee.

In 1962 the Nobel laureate and member of the committee Theorell submitted a nomination with two alternative proposals. The first was for Konrad Bloch and Feodor Lynen who, two years later, received the prize in physiology or medicine and the other nomination was for Kendrew and Perutz. One may ask why there were no outside nominations for these candidates for a prize in physiology or medicine. After all the molecules they examined had a considerable physiological and medical importance. It appears to have taken time to let physiology develop into a biochemical specialty.

Engström was selected to make a complete review of the latter two candidates. He gave a very readable presentation of the developments of crystallography of biological molecules. He emphasized the increasing degrees of complexity in the analyses depending on the size of the selected molecular target; Hodgkin's Vitamin B12 90 atoms; Kendrew's myoglobin 2,600 atoms and Perutz's hemoglobin about 10,000 atoms. Engström reviewed the importance of progressively more complex mathematics and the role of increasingly efficient computers in deriving the phase pattern and identifying the unit cell from the diffraction pattern. Substitution techniques were discussed and the importance of identifying particular modular structures like alpha-helixes was described. Finally Engström also noted the critical importance of identification of the amino acid sequence of the target protein in solving the complex structure at high resolution. One example was the importance of identification of positions of the amino acid proline, which uniquely allowed the formation of turns of the string of amino acids. Engström finally noted the state of the art and concluded that Kendrew had reached further than Perutz because of the relatively simpler structure of myoglobin compared with hemoglobin. On the other hand, knowledge about the structure of myoglobin markedly facilitated the advances in understanding of the structure of hemoglobin because of the principal similarities between the two complex molecules. The conclusion of this 1962 review was "John Cowdery Kendrew's and Max Ferdinand Perutz' contributions are of the highest class and they are extraordinarily worthy of receiving a Nobel Prize". The committee agreed with Engström that Kendrew and Perutz were deserving of a prize, but it was eventually recommended that the prize in physiology or medicine this year should focus on the discovery of the structure of DNA, the subject of the next chapter.

It should be emphasized that there is one major difference between the archive materials available at the Karolinska Institute and at the Royal Swedish Academy of Sciences briefly alluded to earlier. The archive materials at both institutions include all nominations as well as all the reviews made during a particular year. At the Karolinska Institute the minutes of the final September meeting of the committee used to be attached. They included names of the candidates that had been reviewed and the conclusions as to whether they were considered to be worthy of a prize or not. There was also a final proposal by the committee for the preferred prize recipient(s). When opinion was divided the number of committee members, and their names, preferring one candidate or another were recorded as exemplified in Chapters 2 and 6. At the present time, presumably for reasons of secrecy there is no information in the archives of the deliberations of the committee. The outcome of the discussions by the committee in September is presented verbally to the Nobel Assembly.

At the Academy the archive materials, following long traditions, is much richer and of much greater value to historians of science. The yearly paper-bound book at first presents the list of nominators and nominees. Hereafter comes what in Swedish is referred to as "kapprock", a Swedish term that is not easily translated. The closest translation would be "cloak" or "overcoat". Originally it was the term for a coat with several cape-like collars for males. The English actor and author David Garrick used such a coat when acting as a wagoner and hence the name Garrick occasionally has been used to name it. With time the Swedish word has become of use in a number of metaphorical contexts, for example, a certain covering document accompanying a larger documentation, summarizing a certain request or proposal. The "kapprock" of the annual summary volumes of the work of committees for Nobel Prizes in physics or chemistry contain an extensive summary of the deliberations about a large number of candidates or groups of candidates active in a certain sub-discipline. At the end it gives a specific recommendation for prize recipients for the year. In 2012 the summary of the chemistry committee covered some 50 pages and that of the physics committee was about twice that long.

As described earlier the respective proposals are scrutinized by the class of physics and the class of chemistry of the Academy before they are subjected to a final vote by all members of the Academy present at the meeting at which the prize recipient(s) of the year is selected. Regrettably the documentation by the committee at the Karolinska Institute does not include a "kapprock". During my time in the Nobel committee at the Institute, starting in 1973, the secretary of the committee Gustafsson (p. 114) took personal notes and I believe his successor Lindsten also did this. Hopefully there might have developed a tradition to make such unofficial notes and they will be archived for future use by historians.

Towards the Finish Line

In the critical year of 1962 the spectrum of nominations for a prize in chemistry was similar to the previous year with three proposals for Perutz and Kendrew (Table 7.1, p. 289), but in this year given by different nominators. In addition Pauling repeated his nomination of the two candidates for half the prize with the remaining half to be used for recognizing Corey. There was also a nomination of Perutz alone. Bragg did not repeat his proposal and as mentioned above Hodgkin did not receive any outside nomination. The committee selected its adjunct member Hägg to do a new review, including not only Perutz and Kendrew, but also Corey. Corey's contributions had already been reviewed extensively by Hägg ten years earlier, in connection with a proposal for recognizing Pauling's impressive contributions by a prize in chemistry, and again in 1954 the year of Pauling's prize. Hägg extended his analysis and gave a presentation over five pages of historical advances in chemical insights that led to the postulation of the existence of the alpha-helix structure. Over another five pages he presented the history of the developments of protein structure analysis at the Cavendish laboratory.

In his review of Kendrew and Perutz he noted that major developments had taken place since the previous review by Westgren in 1959. In particular understanding of the structure of the myoglobin molecule had advanced because of the progressively increased resolution and also the access to knowledge about the amino acid sequence of the molecule as presented in 1961. The presence of alpha helix structures was demonstrated and the existence of stretches between them allowing a bending of the molecule and the formation of a compact structure. The location of the heme group with its central iron atom could also be located in the convoluted molecule. For the first time the tertiary structure of a larger protein had been defined.

Hägg discussed to what extent the crystallographic form of the molecule would be expected to be similar to that of the physiologically active molecule. He gave arguments for the belief that valuable information on function could be deduced from knowledge about the structure of the "frozen" crystallized molecule. He then noted that also Perutz and his collaborators had made considerable progress in their work on hemoglobin since 1959. Because they were working with a four times larger molecule than the one examined by Kendrew it had not been possible for them to move as fast. However, fortunately understanding of the myoglobin molecule had provided considerable help in interpreting the structure of the hemoglobin molecule. Furthermore, as in the case of myoglobin, separate chemical studies in 1961 had revealed the amino acid sequence of the two kinds of polypeptides that build up the hemoglobin molecule.

Hägg's conclusion was that awarding a Nobel Prize to Perutz and Kendrew was highly motivated and he concluded his review in the following way:

> It is possible that these circumstances (that the hemoglobin structure is four times larger than the myoglobin structure) will restrict the possibilities to fully explore the hemoglobin molecule to the same extent as the myoglobin structure. However, Perutz's contributions in this field are so great and his importance also for Kendrew's work is so apparent that it obviously is not possible to exclude him when the question of a prize for Kendrew is discussed. If Kendrew's myoglobin work had not been carried out, recognition of Perutz on his own for his hemoglobin work would soon have become appropriate. It is possible that in such a situation one could have waited one or more years until the results had become more secure and rich in details. Since it is now possible to appreciate Perutz's results in relation to (insights into the structure of) the myoglobin (molecule) and in addition (one) knows his importance for Kendrew's research, such a delay is completely uncessessary.

He finally added that Kendrew and Perutz had *not introduced any principally new approaches* (my italics) in their work. However, they had worked in a very skilful way and the introduction of heavy atoms into the molecules they had been studying had been crucial for the advance of their work. As mentioned in Chapter 3 Medawar had made a distinction between analytical and synthetic discoveries. He used the crystallographic determination of the three-dimensional structure of a complex molecule as an example of the former category. A Nobel Prize in chemistry can be given for a discovery or for an improvement. Apparently Perutz's and Kendrew's impressive findings were judged to belong in the latter rather than in the former category. As will be discussed in depth in the next chapter the committee had a major dilemma in 1962, because it also had an opportunity to give an award for the *discovery* of the double-helix structure of DNA. The fact that the chemistry committee decided to prioritize the work on protein structures must be considered to reflect a certain degree of conservatism because it wrote in its summary:

> To this should be added the exceptionally apparent direct and indirect importance of Crick's, Watson's and Wilkins's publications for a large number of presently relevant research problems, which hardly have any counterpart in the consequences of Kendrew's and Perutz's in fact admirable work.

The committee cited extensively from Hägg's review in its summary. As concerned Corey's contribution it wrote:

> When Pauling himself now recommends Corey for recognition by a prize, it shows his great appreciation of his (Corey's) involvement as a collaborator. However it is difficult to avoid the suspicion that Pauling to some extent overrates Corey's importance in a noble-minded eagerness to also get him rewarded. He exaggerates when he says "It is clear that the conclusion reached by Kendrew about the alpha helix in myoglobin could probably not have been reached if Corey had not carried out his fundamental investigations of the precise dimensions of the polypeptide chain.

The unanimous conservative conclusion by the committee in their selection of Perutz and Kendrew as the prime candidates, apparently reached by harmonious discussions in this, for many years well-coordinated group, was:

> ...(in this selection) it has been considered that their (Perutz' and Kendrew's) contribution represents one of the most important results which has been obtained by use of the X-ray diffraction methods since these were introduced 50 years ago by von Laue and W. H. and W. L. Bragg. During the time that has elapsed since then, this fundamentally important field within the discipline of chemistry has not been given attention by the conferment of a Nobel Prize. To this should be added that the presently rapidly increasing efficacy of X-ray analysis makes it possible to analyze ever more complex structures, not the least of biologically important substances. It can be expected that in this field, new and important results (will be presented), which also may be considered to be recognized by the award.

This visionary statement has turned out to be correct and after the follow-up prize to Hodgkin in 1964 there have been many Nobel prizes for crystallographic clarification of the structure of amazingly complex macromolecular aggregates. At the time of writing a decision was taken to award the 2012 Nobel Prize in chemistry to Robert J. Lefkowitz and Brian K. Kobilka for their studies of G protein coupled receptors. As late as 2011 Kobilka managed to reveal the three-dimensional structure of both the transmembraneous receptor, a polypeptide chain passing seven times through the lipid bilayer and the G proteins on the inside of the membrane that conveys the outside signal to the interior of the cell. Crystallographic studies have revolutionized the field of molecular biology and the progress brings to mind a statement by the illustrious Nobel Prize (shared) recipient in physics in 1965, Richard Feynman. He wrote: "What I cannot see (construct) I cannot understand."

In 1962 there was an illustrious group of Nobel Prize recipients, three of whom will be presented in the next chapter. Perutz and Kendrew were addressed by Hägg in a laudatory speech at the prize ceremony[19]. He gave a background to their painstaking work emphasizing the importance of the 1953 advance when Perutz succeeded in marking hemoglobin by heavy atoms. He finished his speech somewhat hyperbolically:

> ...It is fairly certain that the knowledge which will thus be gained of these substances which are so essential to living organisms will mean a big step forward in the understanding of life-processes. It is thus abundantly clear that this year's prizewinners in Chemistry have fulfilled the condition which Alfred Nobel laid down in his will; they have conferred the greatest benefit on mankind.

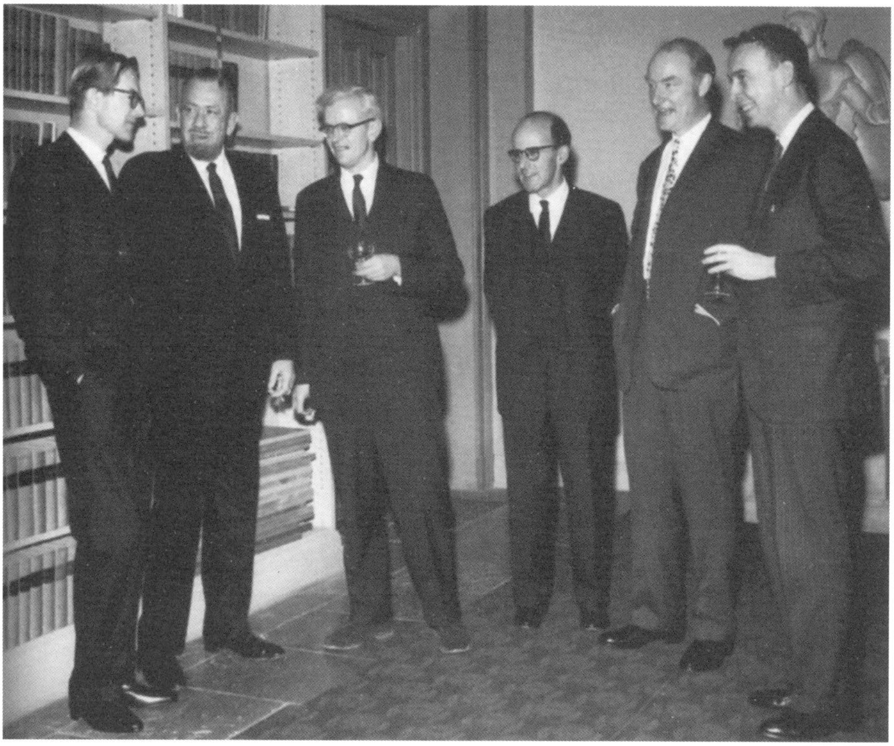

All the Nobel laureates present in Stockholm in 1962. From left: Wilkins, Steinbeck, Kendrew, Perutz, Crick, Watson. [© Scanpix Sweden AB.]

In his Nobel lecture[4] Perutz acknowledged that they had not yet reached the final goal. He said:

> Please forgive me for presenting, on such a great occasion, results which are still in the making, but the glaring sunlight of certain knowledge is dull and one feels most exhilarated by the twilight and expectancy of the dawn.

Perhaps he was thinking of Isaac Newton who once, when he was asked about how he made discoveries, gave the following answer "By always thinking about them. I keep the subject constantly before me and wait until the first dawnings open little by little into the full light."

Science endeavors represent a never-ending journey. Opening one door to a previously closed room of knowledge usually shows that there are two or more additional doors to open. Of course some doors lead to rooms that are more important and larger than others and provide possibilities for the opening of a huge number of new doors. A major discovery is recognized by its impact. Opening up a new field of research can usually be identified by the rapid increase in publications in the research area that has unexpectedly become available.

Life after the Nobel Prize

The future lives of the three crystallographers after they had received their Nobel Prizes in 1962 and 1964 took different courses. They left major imprints by their various involvements in science, in science administration, in writing and in humanistic engagements.

A Female Scientist and Humanist

Hodgkin retained her devotion to science even after she had received the Nobel Prize. She remained a dedicated "bench chemist". Sadly, already during her Cambridge days Hodgkin had started to develop problems with her joints, first mainly her hands and later her feet. She was diagnosed with rheumatoid arthritis and needed to use a wheelchair during the later phase of her life. In spite of this she continued to persevere in her work. Her most important project was the characterization of the structure of insulin, which she had initiated together with Bernal already in 1934. Thirty-five years later she and her collaborators were able to publish the complete three-dimensional structure of the hormone.

Besides the Nobel Prize her pioneering crystallographic work was recognized by the Copley Medal from the Royal Society in 1976, its most prestigious award, for the first time given to a woman, and the Lomonosov Gold Medal in 1982. In 1965 she received a unique honor, the highest royal order in the United Kingdom, the Order of Merit. She was only the second woman ever to receive this order, the first one being Florence Nightingale in 1907. After Hodgkin's death in 1994 she was recognized on two occasions by commemorative stamps. In 1996 she was selected as one of five "Women of Achievement" in Great Britain and in 2010 she was one of the ten most illustrious scientists depicted on stamps to commemorate the 350th anniversary of the Royal Society.

From her parents Hodgkin had learned the ethics of selflessness and service to humanity. She was what her biographer Ferry[7] aptly referred to as "a quintessentially English woman whose humanity recognized no national borders". Her main contribution in these realms was her involvement in the Pugwash movement. She was chairman of this organization between 1976 and 1988 and took many important initiatives. One example was when she challenged all living Nobel scientists to sign a Pugwash Declaration against nuclear weapons. Eventually she managed to persuade 111 of her fellow laureates to put their names to the proposed declaration. She received the Lenin Peace Prize in 1987. Because of her leftish humanitarian involvements she was not allowed to enter the US without a CIA visa waiver. She died at the age of 84.

A Great Science Administrator

Very soon after their joint Nobel Prize, Kendrew and Perutz started to take different career paths. Already during the 1950s Kendrew had demonstrated a considerable talent for the building of science organizations. He formed a great team with Perutz in the early phase of development of the Medical Research Council Laboratory of Molecular Biology at the Cavendish Laboratory. He had been elected a Fellow of the Royal Society in 1960, but after receiving the prize he prioritized developing his talents for organization and diplomacy, abandoning his experimental science. Already in 1959 he had founded the *Journal of Molecular Biology*, and he remained for many years its editor-in-chief. It still remains one of the leading journals in its field today. He became one of the founders of the European Molecular Biology Organization in 1963 and in 1974 he was successful in persuading European governments to establish the European Molecular Biology Laboratory (EMBL) in Heidelberg. He became its first director and his fellow laureate Perutz became the first chairman of its council, by way of contrast one of the few committee works he himself was involved in. Today EMBL is still a great laboratory. It remains a monument of Kendrew's devotions. Kendrew also had a number of different involvements in the International Council of Scientific Unions over some 15 years, including being its President. At the age of 80 he died of prostate cancer.

A Scientist with Wide-Ranging Involvements

In contrast to Kendrew, Perutz could never leave his science. He continued to work on the structure of oxy- and deoxy-hemoglobin to understand how it functions as a transporter of oxygen. In 1970 it became understood what the mechanisms were. Later on he was engaged in studies of protein aggregates in neurodegenerative diseases. In fact during the last week of his life, before dying of skin-derived Merkel cell carcinoma in 2002, he submitted a manuscript on such aggregates in Huntington's disease. But he also managed to achieve so many other different things.

In 1947 he was made head of the newly established Medical Research Council Unit for Molecular Biology, a laboratory originally located at the Cavendish laboratory and supported by its leader since 1938, W. L. Bragg. His importance for the development of Perutz's hemoglobin project, frequently referred to above cannot be overrated. Perutz devoted the first paragraphs in his Nobel lecture to praising him. Possibly he had learnt at that time that it was Bragg's nominations which eventually led to the crystallography prizes in 1962. Regrettably Bragg could not attend the Nobel Prize ceremony in 1962, because he was being operated on for prostate cancer at the time. However, he was to have many additional good years. In 1965 he returned to Sweden

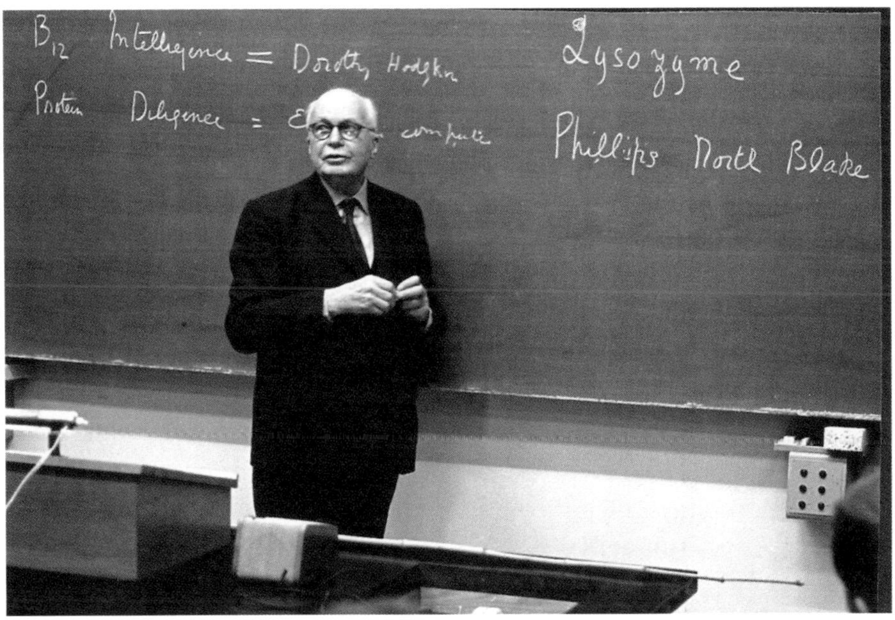

Bragg lecturing on the occasion of his visit to Stockholm in 1965 celebrating the 50th anniversary of his Nobel Prize. [Photo from Ref. 1.]

to celebrate the fact that 50 years had passed since he and his father together had received the Nobel Prize in physics. He gave lectures and had impressive stories to tell from his rich life[2]. There are very few laureates who have an opportunity to come back to Stockholm to celebrate the 50 years jubilee of their prize, but we will meet one more in the next chapter. Bragg died in 1971 and Perutz's epitaph on the occasion deserves to be cited. He wrote:

> When reviewing scientific work I sometimes paraphrase people's papers, but when I tried to paraphrase Bragg's I always found that he had said it much better. Bragg's superb powers of combining simplicity with rigor, his enthusiasm, liveliness and charm, and his beautiful demonstrations conspired to make him one of the best lecturers on science that ever lived… (His) approach to science was an artistic, imaginative one… Nowadays cynics want us to believe that scientists work only for fame and money, but Bragg slaved away at hard problems when he was a Nobel Laureate of comfortable means… So often men of genius are hellish to live with, but Bragg was a genial person whose creativity was sustained by a happy home life.

The Molecular Biology Unit originally included only Perutz and Kendrew and their laboratory co-workers, but its staff grew progressively towards some 90 employees. Over the years it came to host an exceptional number of successful scientists, fourteen of whom would eventually receive Nobel Prizes! Before that, many things had happened. One event in particular was the establishment of an independent Laboratory of Molecular Biology (LMB) building in 1962. Already at that time the density of high class scientists — even referred to as prima donnas — was so high that there were concerns about how such an organization could be managed. We will meet some of the most outstanding scientists in the next chapter. The low profile management by Perutz suited the laboratory excellently and he came to chair it for 17 years. He directed most things single-handed, but for major decisions he had formed a board that besides himself included Crick, Kendrew and Sanger — some gathering of Nobel minds! His ambition was to create a working environment facilitating incidental encounters between scientists. This aim of propinquity was furthered by the readily available environments for coffee breaks and for seminars. Max's wife Gisela managed the canteen for more than 20 years. It was truly a family engagement. Ferry uses a whole chapter in her book[8] to describe the impressive atmosphere of the laboratory and its remarkable achievements have been summarized in a separate book[20]. Perutz was often asked what the secret was behind the success of the laboratory. He gave many different answers and the following is just one example:

> Creativity in science, as in arts, cannot be organized. It arises spontaneously from individual talent. Well-run laboratories can foster it, but hierarchical organizations, inflexible, bureaucratic rules, and mountains of futile paperwork can kill it.

At the time of his retirement as head of the laboratory, the Royal Society awarded Perutz its highest honor, the Copley Medal. The citation was:

> In recognition of his distinguished contributions to molecular biology through his studies of the structural and biological activity of haemoglobin, the oxygen-carrying component of the blood.... Under his leadership the Laboratory (of Molecular Biology) has been generally acknowledged as the world's leading centre of research in this subject.

In addition to the Copley medal he received a number of other honors. In 1963 he was appointed Commander of the Order of the British Empire (limited to 24 British citizens), received the Österreichisches Ehrenzeichen für Wissenschaft und Kunst in 1967, the Royal Medal in 1971, the Companions of Honour in 1975 and finally the Order of Merit in 1989.

Perutz also developed his talents as an author. He contributed to the *New York Review of Books* with reviews and essays. Some of these essays were collected in the 1998 book *I Wish I Had Made You Angry Earlier*[14]. Another collection of essays was called *Is Science Necessary?*[21] In the introduction to this book he wrote:

> In science, as in other fields of endeavour, one finds saints and charlatans, warriors and monks, geniuses and cranks, tyrants and slaves, benefactors and misers, but there is one quality that the best of them have in common, one that they share with great writers, musicians and artists: creativity... Imagination comes first, both in artistic and scientific creation — which makes for one culture rather than two — but while the artist is confined only by the prescriptions imposed by himself and the culture surrounding him, the scientist has Nature and his critical colleagues always looking over his shoulder....

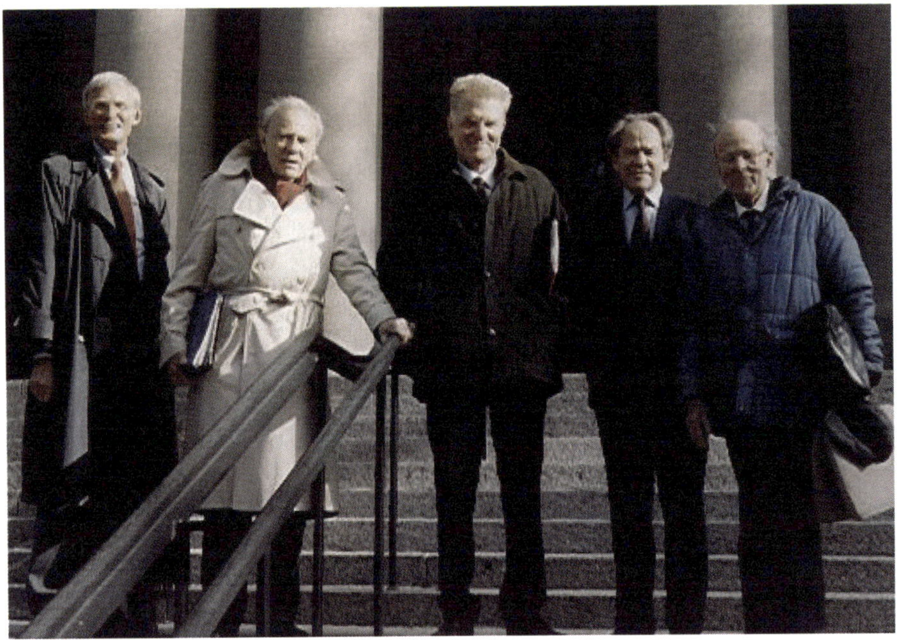

Four of the founding fathers of the International Human Rights Network of Academies and Scholarly Societies; from left: Pieter van Dijk, Francois Jacob, Edoardo Vesentino (not founder; president of the Accademia Nazionale dei Lincei), Torsten Wiesel and Max Perutz. The picture was taken by Carol Corillon of the group on the stairs of the Royal Swedish Academy of Sciences in 1999.

One final commitment to be mentioned reflects Perutz involvement as citizen-humanist. He was a compassionate pragmatist. Like Hodgkin he was a vocal opponent of nuclear weapons, or indeed the use of any weapons. In 1993 Perutz, together with his fellow Nobel laureates the Swedish (at the time US based) neurophysiologist Torsten Wiesel and the French molecular biologist Francois Jacob, joined by the Dutch human rights lawyer Pieter van Dijk founded the International Human Rights Network of Academies and Scholarly Societies. The executive committee of the network had one of its meetings in Stockholm in 1999 at the The Royal Swedish Academy of Sciences hosted by me as its permanent secretary. The Swedish Queen was a special guest of honor. This human rights organization has retained its vitality even after the death of Perutz. It works by accepting cases of academic colleagues who have been incarcerated or harassed in some other way infringing on their human rights. The selective identification of critical cases is made at a secretariat at the U.S. National Academy of Sciences led by Carol Corillon. Individual academies hereafter write letters to heads of states pointing out the injustices in the individual cases. The network's most recent meeting was held in Taipei,

Taiwan in May 2012. I participated in my role as chairman of a human rights committee representing three Swedish Academies, The Royal Swedish Academy of Sciences, The Academy of Letters, History and Antiquity and the Swedish Academy (of Literature). The meeting was able to summarize that during the preceding three years a total of 915 letters had been sent from 20 different academies concerning 52 (occasionally groups of) prisoners in 13 different countries. The result has been the earlier than expected release of 36 of the prisoners in 11 countries. Thus Perutz has left his long-lasting imprints not only as a scientist but also as a humanist. It might be appropriate to finish with one of his favorite citations "In science truth always wins" — and hopefully this does not only — irrefutably, apply to science, but also to other human endeavors. It can be noted in this context that coincidentally the slogan used for Amnesty International when it was founded in 1961 was "Truth shall set you free."

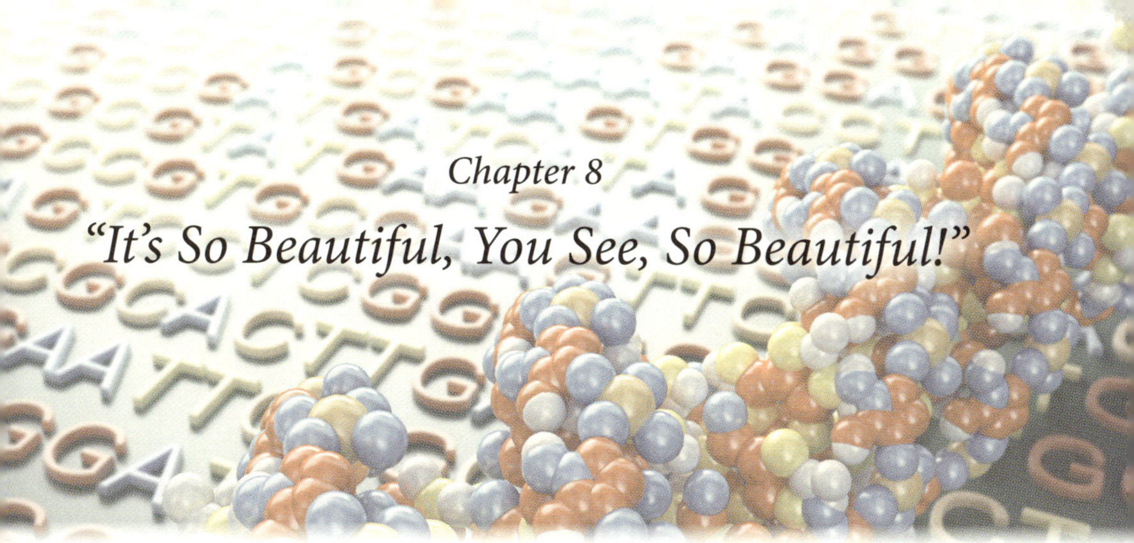

Chapter 8

"It's So Beautiful, You See, So Beautiful!"

The Double Helix
Eternity in a String
Symmetry Well Used

In his personal book *What Mad Pursuit*[1], discussing scientific discovery, Crick has described about an episode when Watson, after having been treated to a good dinner, presented to members of the Hardy Club in Cambridge the discovery of the structure of DNA. He managed reasonably well to give some facts about the double-helix structure, but when it came to summing up he was quite overcome and at loss for words. The best he could manage was "It's so beautiful, you see, so beautiful!" Crick then added, to finish the chapter: "But then, of course, it was." In another place in the same book Crick emphasized that the identification of the double helix was not an ending but a beginning. During the ten years that followed the 1953 discovery there were to be an amazing accumulation of completely new insights into the replication and function of genes and into their roles in protein synthesis.

There is no question about the fact that the discovery of the double-helix structure of DNA represented the largest revolution in biology during the previous century. What makes the order of magnitude of this finding exceptional is not only that it revealed a simple structure that allowed storage of digital information but the additional fact that the genetic language it uses is *universal* and has prevailed since the dawn of life more than three billion years ago. It should have been obvious that this momentous discovery needed to be recognized rapidly by a Nobel Prize either in chemistry or in physiology or medicine. But the Nobel archives at the Royal Swedish Academy of Sciences and at the Karolinska Institute tell a different story. It is a story about the difficulty of changing a major paradigm and about acknowledging that it was nucleic acids and *not* proteins that were the carriers of genetic information. But this was not a difficulty confronting only the committee members; it was also a challenging difficulty to the scientific community at large. Although the principally correct structure of DNA was published in April 1953[2] the first nominations for a Nobel Prize to Watson and Crick, possibly also including Wilkins, were not submitted until 1960!

The Great DNA Discovery

The saga of the discovery of the structure of DNA has been told many times. In fact it is questionable if any paradigmatic finding in biology has been as well examined in its details as the identification of the double-helix structure of DNA held together by hydrogen bonds between matching base pairs. Its climactic phase can be followed almost hour by hour. The two major books describing the events are by Robert Olby[3] and Horace Freeland Judson[4] and in addition the three scientists who eventually received the Nobel Prize, have each told their own story[1,5,6]. Watson's book *The Double Helix* rapidly became famous when it was published in 1968. It is a different kind of book giving an exceptional and radically novel treatment of the "human" side of making science. It started a new era of non-fiction novels. The book is highly subjective and there is no index. Both during the time the book was in the making and also afterwards there has been criticism in particular of how Watson victimized Rosalind Franklin, in the book referred to as "Rosy". The prepublication criticism led Watson to add an epilogue in part paying tribute to her qualities as a scientist. He was also forced to change publisher. We will return to the book later in this chapter.

Biophysics at King's College

As a general introduction to the cataclysmic events of February 1953 it can be noted that the potential to examine the structure of DNA by X-ray crystallography had been appreciated since the 1930s. It was in the middle of this decade that Astbury and Bernal decided to divide the responsibilities for development of the field of structural analysis of large biomolecules. The more amorphous and messy substances were to be studied by Astbury and the more distinctly crystallizing compounds by Bernal. It had been known for a long time that the nucleic acids were high polymers and that solutions of them could be drawn into fine threads. The general view held by chemists was that they were difficult to study due to their heterogeneous nature and were not very exciting objects because of the presence of the four nucleotide bases in equimolar amounts as argued by Phoebus Levene.

By way of recapitulation it should be mentioned that a nucleotide has three components. It is a complex of a nitrogenous base — a pyrimidine or a purine — a five-carbon sugar — either ribose as in polynucleotide RNA or 2-deoxyribose as in the polynucleotide DNA — and phosphate groups. Based on his early crystallographic studies Astbury formulated a hypothesis that the elongated molecule was built by layers of plates of purine and pyrimidine with the attached sugar perpendicular to the fiber axis. He even discussed the possibility that the nucleotides might be arranged in a spiral structure but discarded this idea. One step in developing Astbury's tentative deductions was an important discovery by the Norwegian scientist Sven Furberg. His PhD thesis, developed in Bernal's laboratory at Birkbeck College, in 1949 concerned the pyrimidine cytidine. In X-ray studies, he demonstrated that in chains of cytidine, the pyrimidine and sugar groups were arranged perpendicular to each other and not in the same plane when they formed a part of a single polynucleotide helix. He proposed two possible arrangements for the phosphate groups. Either they were on the outside or on the inside of the single strand helix. When he had finished his thesis he changed the orientation of his research. He continued to use X-ray crystallography but to solve other problems. In 1966 he became professor of theoretical chemistry at the University of Oslo.

Further attempts to examine DNA by X-ray crystallography were initiated by Wilkins when he joined John Randall in moving to King's College London, in 1946 to build a department of biophysics. Wilkins, born in 1916, briefly had the following background[6]. He studied physics at St. John's College, Cambridge, where he learned the fundamentals of crystallography from Bernal, who was regarded as an impressive but casual teacher. Wilkins later became an assistant to the physicist Randall, who was the supervisor of his thesis. Randall in his turn had had Lawrence Bragg as his PhD supervisor.

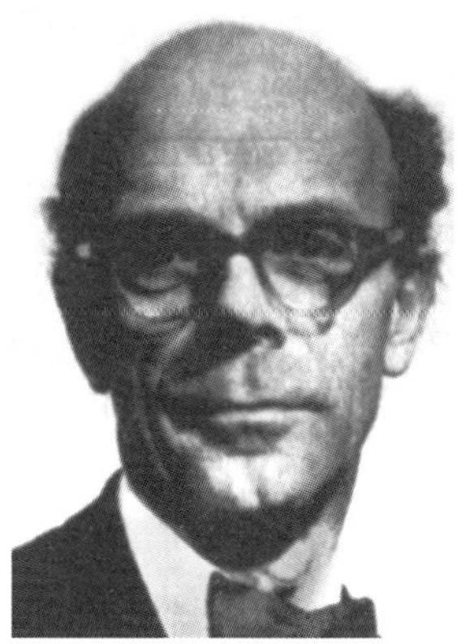

John T. Randall (1905–1984).

During the Second World War Wilkins spent some time in Berkeley, California as one of many scientists engaged in the Manhattan project. Randall had other work commitments in the U.K. at the same time. His research during the war made him famous. He managed to make a radical improvement in the cavity magnetron, which is a critical component of centrimetric wavelength radar. This technical advance turned out to be crucial to the Allies' victory. After the war Randall established a biophysics team at St. Andrews University, Scotland, which included Wilkins. Within a year of its establishment this team moved to King's College London. These developments were supported by the Medical Research Council. This Council also developed a major involvement in another biophysics organization engaged in biological problems at the Cavendish laboratories in Cambridge headed by Randall's PhD supervisor Bragg. By a gentlemen's agreement it was decided that the group in Cambridge would work on the structure of proteins, as described in the previous chapter, whereas the group at King's College should as one major project focus on the structure of nucleic acids.

Soon after he had started at King's College Wilkins had a visit from Crick. Both of them were physicists who had become interested in biological problems, but Crick was still looking for a working environment where he could pursue such an interest. Wilkins suggested to Randall that Crick should be offered a job, but this proposal was not met with enthusiasm. Randall found Crick to be rather boisterous and too talkative. So Crick had to try the Cavendish laboratory, but the two of them, born in the same year, according to Wilkins' biography became firm friends. One might find this a bit surprising considering their divergent personalities.

The possibility of advancing the crystallographic studies of DNA at King's College was dependent on the access to good starting material and also on technical developments and means for mathematical evaluations of the data collected. High quality DNA was generously provided by Rudolph Signer from Berne. He was a student of the great German chemist Hermann Staudinger. Staudinger had pioneered the study of large molecules, later to be called macromolecules, in the 1930s. He received considerable criticism from his fellow chemists for his involvement in this kind of work, but in 1953 his achievements were crowned by a Nobel Prize in chemistry "for his discoveries in the field of macromolecular chemistry". During a conference in London in May 1950 Wilkins met Signer, who generously shared with him vials containing purified DNA. This DNA, prepared from calf thymus glands — in gourmet circles better known as sweetbread — turned out to be of high quality. When

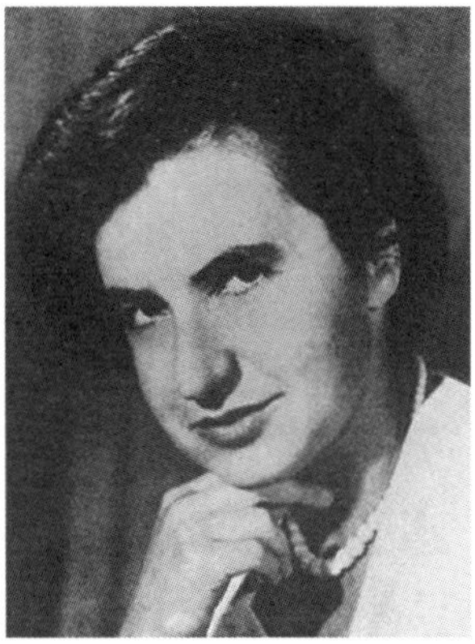
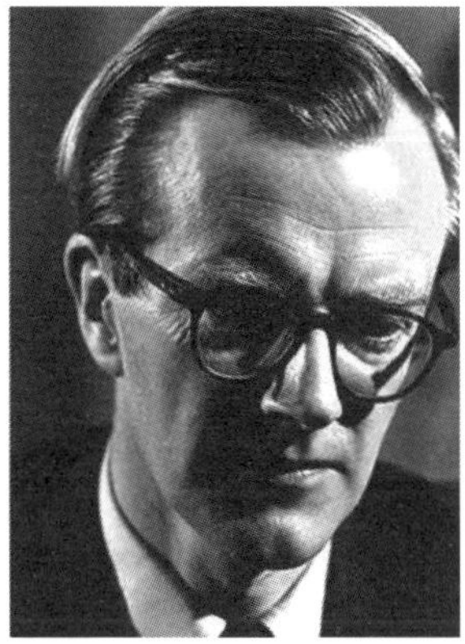

Rosalind E. Franklin (1920–1958) [credit: Jewish Chronicle Archive/Heritage Images] and Maurice H. F. Wilkins (1916–2004) [from *Les Prix Nobel en 1962]*.

moistened Wilkins could draw it into thin threads. Using such material it was possible for him, in collaboration with Raymond Gosling, who knew some X-ray crystallography, to obtain pictures which represented a certain advance compared with those presented earlier by Astbury. Still, progress with the work was relatively slow. This changed when Rosalind E. Franklin joined the team in 1951. Careful examination of DNA molecules at different conditions of hydration revealed that two forms, A and B, could be distinguished. The B form was more hydrated and represented a slender structure. Franklin, together with Gosling, whom she supervised as a PhD student, provided very sharp images, not least of the B form, which turned out to be critical for the later developments.

Watson's Arrival Upsets a Gentlemen's Agreement

It was agreed that the group at the Cavendish laboratories should not get involved in studies of DNA, but this changed when Watson arrived. Watson, born in 1928, had a background from the University of Chicago and did his PhD work with Salvador D. Luria at Indiana University in Bloomington. Luria was one of the leading scientists of the phage school and he was to receive the 1969 Nobel Prize in physiology or medicine together with Alfred D. Hershey and Max Delbrück "for their discoveries concerning the replication mechanism and genetic structure of viruses". Thus Watson learned about phages and the modern genetics of the time. The geneticists Hermann J. Müller, Nobel laureate of 1946 "for the discovery of the production of mutations by means of X-ray irradiation" and Tracy Sonneborn were other inspiring teachers. Watson set as his goal to identify the chemical nature of the genetic material. Reading Erwin Schrödinger's book *What Is Life?*[7] stimulated him in this pursuit and for vague reasons he thought that DNA was the object to examine. Schrödinger's book had already encouraged many physicists, including also Crick and Wilkins, to move into studies of biological problems.

During 1950-51 Watson spent a postdoctoral year in Copenhagen studying phages and the fate of their DNA during infection. In May 1951 he had an opportunity to participate in a conference at the Zoological Station in Naples. On this occasion he met Wilkins for the first time and heard about his X-ray diffraction studies of crystalline DNA. Later during the summer he heard Bragg give a lecture in Copenhagen and he decided to try the Cambridge milieu. Luria arranged a new scholarship for him from the National Foundation for Infantile Paralysis. He was to study under Kendrew. Soon after his arrival at the Cavendish Laboratory he met Crick and they quickly realized that they had a joint interest in DNA. It was a remarkable meeting of minds. Little did they care that the responsibility of the laboratory was not to study DNA but to develop techniques for characterizing large protein molecules.

Crick's life has been presented in a detailed biography by Olby[8]. He had studied physics at University College London, where he also initiated a PhD project. This project was interrupted in 1939 because of the war. During the war he worked at the Admiralty, which he left in 1947 to study biological problems. After a few years at the Strangeways Research Laboratory in Cambridge he joined Perutz's group. In 1950 he restarted a PhD work supervised by Perutz, but according to a frequently cited statement by Bragg "He had a tendency to get involved in solving other people's crosswords." Bragg was in fact concerned about the lack of progress of Crick's PhD work.

Much has been written about the unique partnership of the two highly gifted personalities Watson and Crick stimulating each other by use of their versatile intellects. Watson was only 23 years old whereas Crick was 12 years older. As mentioned he had become delayed in his academic career because of the war. It can be said that the interaction with Watson catapulted Crick, who had a background in physics, into becoming the most pre-eminent biological theoretician of the 20th century. Crick had a particular insight into the general theory of X-ray diffraction by a protein helix, which he had developed together with two co-workers. An important paper on this subject was published in 1952[9].

Watson and Crick set out speculating about the structure of DNA. Based on the limited data they had available they even built a model. It was a triple

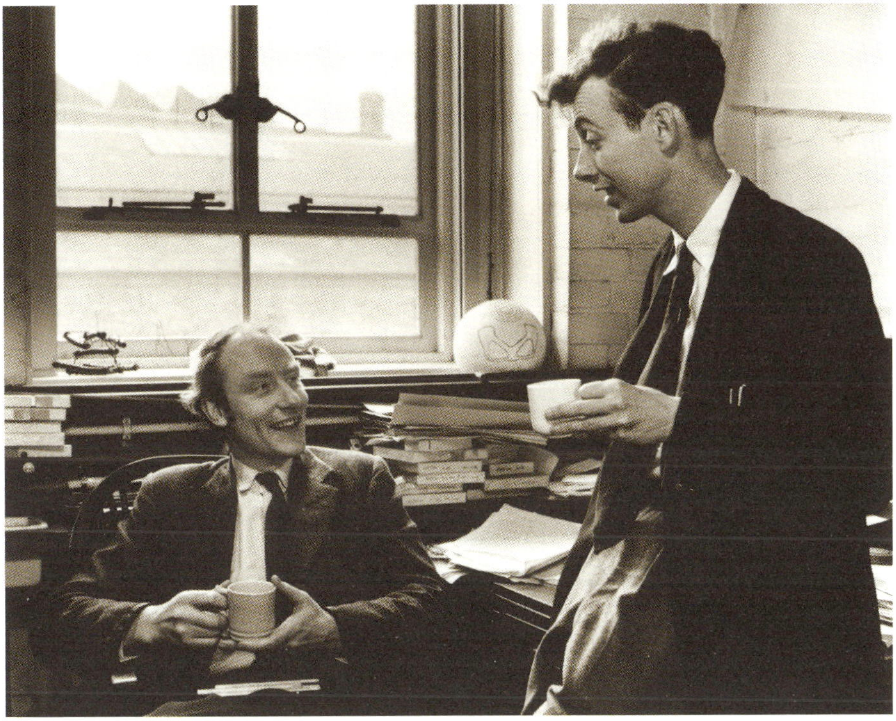

Francis Crick (1916–2004) and Jim Watson at the time of the discovery of the structure of DNA. [Credit: A. Barrington Brown/Photo Researchers.]

helix structure with the phosphates facing its interior and with the nucleotide bases exposed at its surface. When this model was shown to Wilkins and Franklin they quickly pointed out a number of faults in the structure. In particular Franklin was very brusque in her critique. From then on Bragg formally forbade Watson and Crick to continue their engagement in DNA. Watson initiated studies of the protein and RNA representation in TMV using X-ray crystallography and Crick continued his protein studies. Although rarely mentioned Crick did in fact finish a PhD thesis in 1954 entitled "X-ray diffraction: polypeptides and proteins". Before that, however, very important developments had taken place. In parallel with his studies of proteins he continued to think about DNA and in the summer of 1952 as can be seen from his laboratory note book* he also fiddled around with nucleosides of the four bases to see if they had some preferred capacity to interact with each other. No conclusive data were obtained, but in one place it was noted "not too bad".

Thus Watson and Crick, in spite of the moratorium, could not get DNA out of their heads. In the spring of 1952 they met Erwin Chargaff, who was

*Courtesy of J. Craig Venter Institute Archives.

visiting Cambridge. His acerbic statement was: "I never met two men who knew so little and aspired to so much." There was a lot of talk about helices and their pitches. Repeated references were made to Pauling's important protein alpha-helix structure already discussed in the previous chapter. After their conversation Chargaff wrote in a note "Two pitchmen in search of a helix".

In July 1952 Pauling could again travel to Europe after a passport had been denied him for several months because he was accused of having Communist sympathies. After a visit to Paris, where he was greeted as a hero, he continued to an International Phage Colloquium held at the centuries-old Abbey of Royaumont outside Paris. Watson, who was also present at this meeting, knew that Pauling during the year had developed an increasing interest in solving the structure of DNA. Having pioneered the resolution of the building principles of proteins by the demonstration of the alpha helix, Pauling now wanted to uncover the equally important Holy Grail, the structure of DNA. Watson listened attentively. What could he and Crick do to return to the competition for solving the structure?

In the fall of the same year Pauling's second son, 21-year-old Peter arrived in Cambridge to work with Kendrew. A direct hot line between Cambridge and Pasadena — Caltech — was established by the scientists sharing the same office — Watson, Crick, Peter Pauling and in addition another Caltech expatriate Jerry Donohue. Towards the very end of November Linus Pauling seriously started to attack the structure of DNA. The problem was that he had to rely on Astbury's pictures from 1947, which were found later to represent reflections from a mixture of different forms of DNA. Six months earlier in 1952 Franklin had shown Pauling's close collaborator Corey much clearer pictures, but these were not at hand at Caltech. It has been speculated that if Pauling had not been denied a passport for his May travel to the meeting arranged in his honor at the Royal Society he might have had access to a better starting material and hence might have beaten Watson and Crick. Pauling did the best he could with the available material but he was not as careful and meticulous in deducing the final structure as he had been in the case of the protein alpha-helix. Anyhow, a structure was conjectured and on the last day of December Pauling and Corey sent their manuscript entitled "A Proposed Structure for the Nucleic Acids" for publication in the Proceedings of the National Academy of Sciences, USA.

Spirits dropped in Watson's and Crick's office when they heard from Peter that a paper on the structure of DNA was in press. The manuscript did not reach Cambridge until early February. It was approached with great trepidation but to their surprise Watson and Crick quickly realized that the three-helix structure proposed had many similarities with the structure they themselves had been forced to discard about a year earlier. Pauling and Corey had assumed that the phosphate groups were centrally located and that the whole thread-like structure was composed of three helices with the nucleotide bases exposed. It was obvious that the proposed structure was incorrect and the talk of the laboratory was how someone of Pauling's status could have made such mistakes. According to the biography of Pauling[10] the reason was "hubris and haste". Franklin had also received a copy of the manuscript from Randall. Like Watson and Crick she immediately saw the flaws. Being a straightforward person she wrote to Pauling frankly telling the icon of chemistry that he was wrong.

Bragg mused about the fact that his archrival, who had beaten the Cavendish laboratory to the alpha-helix (Chapter 7), had made such a blunder. He agreed to release Watson and Crick from the moratorium. This decision is explained in his foreword to *The Double Helix*.

> It is not easy to be sure whether the crucial new idea is really one's own or has been unconsciously assimilated in talks with others. The realization of this difficulty has led to the establishment of a somewhat vague code amongst scientists which recognizes a claim in a line of research staked out by a colleague — *up to a certain point* (my italics). When competition comes from more than one quarter, there is no need to hold back.

Watson and Crick could go back to their DNA model building. The clock started to tick.

The Rapid Developments of February 1953

Watson communicated Pauling's mistake to Wilkins and again initiated discussions about a possible helical structure of DNA. He then had an unexpected reward. Gosling had shared with Wilkins one of Franklin's most distinct pictures of the B form of DNA, which had in fact been available since several months back. This beautiful negative was referred to as photograh 51. It made Watson dumbstruck. There was no question that the cross pattern on the picture strongly suggested a helical structure of DNA. Watson pressed Wilkins for information on the conjectured helix. One turn was 34.4 Å — 10 times the length between bases, long known as 3.4 Å. Watson took the information back to Crick and ordered new

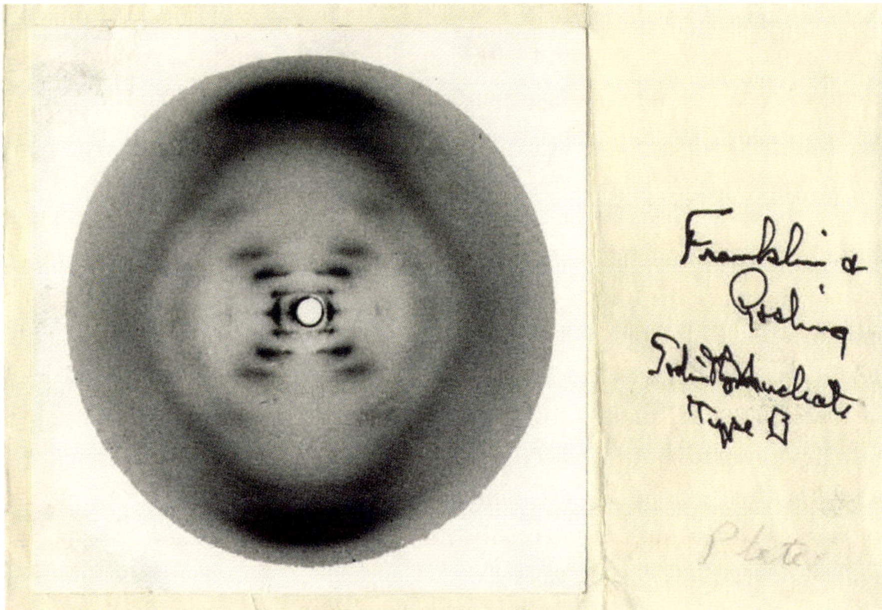

Photograph 51 by Rosalind Franklin and Raymond Gosling. [From archives of the J. Craig Venter Institute.]

metal components from the workshop to resume model-building. This started on February 4. After heated debates they decided to go for a double-helix — an alternative would have been a triple-helix — and to turn the phosphates to the outside of the helices, as proposed earlier in particular by Franklin. It then remained to define in which way the nucleotide bases could hold the molecule together by hydrogen bonds. How could that be done? A few days later Watson and Crick got additional help, this time from Perutz. He agreed to share with them a report to the MRC by its biophysics committee, which it had prepared after its recent December visit to King's College. This sharing of privileged information has not been considered illegal, but it is obvious that the ethics of the disclosure of the (non-confidential) report needed to be deliberated. Perutz himself has explained the basis for his behavior in Science in 1969 by the statement "I was inexperienced and casual in administrative matters and, since the report was not confidential, I saw no reason for withholding it."

When Crick saw the measurements of the "face-centered monoclinic unit cell" ... "with certainty" he could quickly allocate it to a space group called "monoclinic C2". This showed the dyad nature of the structure and that it must be composed of two helices running in an anti-parallel fashion. The two helices must be held together by hydrogen bonds between the nucleotide bases. One problem was that the two purines — adenine (A) and guanine (G) and the two pyrimidine bases — cytosine (C) and thymine (T) were of different sizes. Logically Watson initially tried to match same with same, A-A, G-G etc, but the purine bridges were much longer than the pyrimidine bridges. When he therefore tried A-T and G-C instead, he still had trouble. This was explained in an unexpected way. In what has sometimes been referred to as a serendipitous event[11] there was an intervention by the other Caltech student Donohue working in the same room. He taught Watson that bases could exist in two forms, the enol and the keto form. The Davidson textbook on chemistry predominantly used at the time showed the enol form, which was what Watson had employed. According to Donohue, Watson should instead try the keto form. Watson was still using cardboard cutouts for his model building, since the delivery of the bases prepared from of metal plates had been delayed. Thus he could readily cut out new planar cardboard models of the keto forms of the bases.

Came February 28. When Watson on the morning of that day combined the new models he found to his amazement that adenine joined by hydrogen bonds to thymine gave a shape *congruent with* the pair of cytosine and guanine. Eureka! It must have been an ecstatic feeling for a 24-year-old scientist. The question of the hitherto unexplained fixed ratio between the nucleotides included in each of the two pairs demonstrated by Chargaff was promptly resolved. Why had he — and others — not thought about that before? But not only did the hypothetical structure explain the Chargaff ratios, it also immediately provided elegant answers to two fundamental questions about the "molecule of life". One answer was that the chemical scaffolding created a stable structure that *could replicate itself preserving structure*. Replication of either the one "plus" strand or the other "minus" strand would always lead to a double helix composed of an identical minus and plus strand complex. The original structure would always be preserved. The other answer to a central problem concerned the message (information)-carrying quality of the molecule. The fact that a base pair could occur independently of its neighboring pairs allowed for *combinatorial codes* that could be binary,

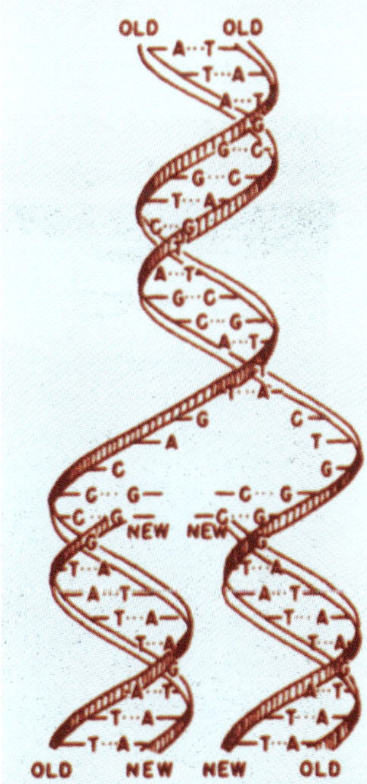

The semi-conservative replication of DNA.

tertiary or quaternary. Rarely has the discovery of a structure provided such important answers to several central questions in one stroke!

When Crick arrived in the office at about 10 o'clock he immediately appreciated the immense breakthrough implicit in Watson's projections on base-pairing. It was time to build the final model. Later during the day it was time for Crick to walk over to his favorite bar the Eagle. On this day the purpose was not only to have a beer but also to tell all the customers that "we have found the secret of life" — or so the myth-making narrative runs[5]. Crick himself did not remember such an event. Nor does his wife Odile remember any particular remarks when he arrived back home that day. He might have expressed some enthusiasm when coming home but that was not an uncommon type of behavior for him. In addition to Crick's brilliant intellect, his boundless vitality and charm, his enthusiasm was an attractive quality. Still, February 28, 1953 was to remain a memorable day. Watson and Crick had set their goals very high and amazingly they had succeeded!

Visitors Were Impressed

A metal-model replica was completed within a few days. Spectators, soon to be amazed, started to arrive. Bragg invited Todd to come and see the model. He confirmed that it was chemically feasible. On March 12, Wilkins, invited by Kendrew (!), arrived. It has emerged that neither Watson nor Crick had the courage to personally invite him. One can only speculate about Wilkins' feelings when he saw the model. The group at King's College had been scooped! Another group of qualified spectators from the chemistry department at Oxford University were Sidney Brenner, Jack D. Dunitz, Hodgkin, Leslie E. Orgel and Beryl M. Oughton. They were all impressed by the model. Later, all of these scientists would make critical contributions to the development of the life sciences.

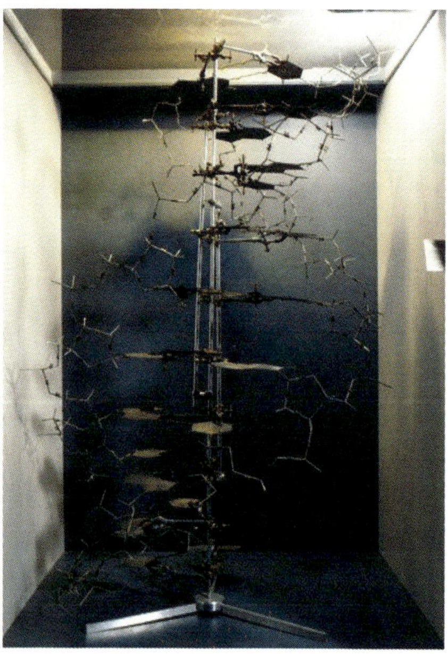

The original Watson–Crick model for DNA.

Brenner became one of Crick's most valuable collaborators and made some immensely important independent contributions. Dunitz became one of the greatest chemical crystallographers developing his career at ETH, Zürich. Hodgkin was introduced in the previous chapter and Oughton was a female crystallographer collaborating with her in important work on antibiotics. Orgel was a chemical evolutionist, who moved to the Salk Institute in La Jolla in 1964. I have met him, Dunitz and Brenner for dinners in the hospitable Arrhenius home in La Jolla.

Franklin and Gosling also came by to see the model and she commented in her poised manner: "It is pretty, but how are they going to prove it?" Her achievements in the field of DNA studies will be further discussed below. One wonders what her true feelings were considering that she herself at the time had already gone a long way towards solving the structure. Was she regretful? Or could it be that she truly and simply accepted the fact that the proper solution had been found and that it only remained to make minor refinements of no great importance. As we shall see Franklin could rise strongly in defense of her own conclusions but she could also in her pursuit of scientific truths elevate herself above subjective considerations and ambitions.

At the beginning of April, Pauling on his way to a Solvay conference in Belgium stopped by in Cambridge, of course to see his son, but in addition and in particular to look at the Watson–Crick model. Pauling generously acknowledged that the model must be correct, but this cannot have been easy for him to do. However, he must have known that his and Corey's efforts had been hurried and not self-critical enough. Pauling's Nobel Prize in chemistry a year later (Chapter 7) should have come as a nice consolation. After all he was the greatest chemist of his generation.

Time to Publish

It was also time for Watson and Crick to rapidly publish the data. There were some discussions about possibly including Wilkins as a co author, presumably at Crick's suggestion because of their longstanding friendship. Wilkins very wisely declined. As he stated in his biography "I would have been embarrassed if the model had been the Watson, Crick and Wilkins model." He was to see the manuscript, however, and took the liberty of making some changes in the last paragraph, perhaps surprisingly somewhat playing down the contributions from King's College. It might have been more appropriate to put forward Franklin

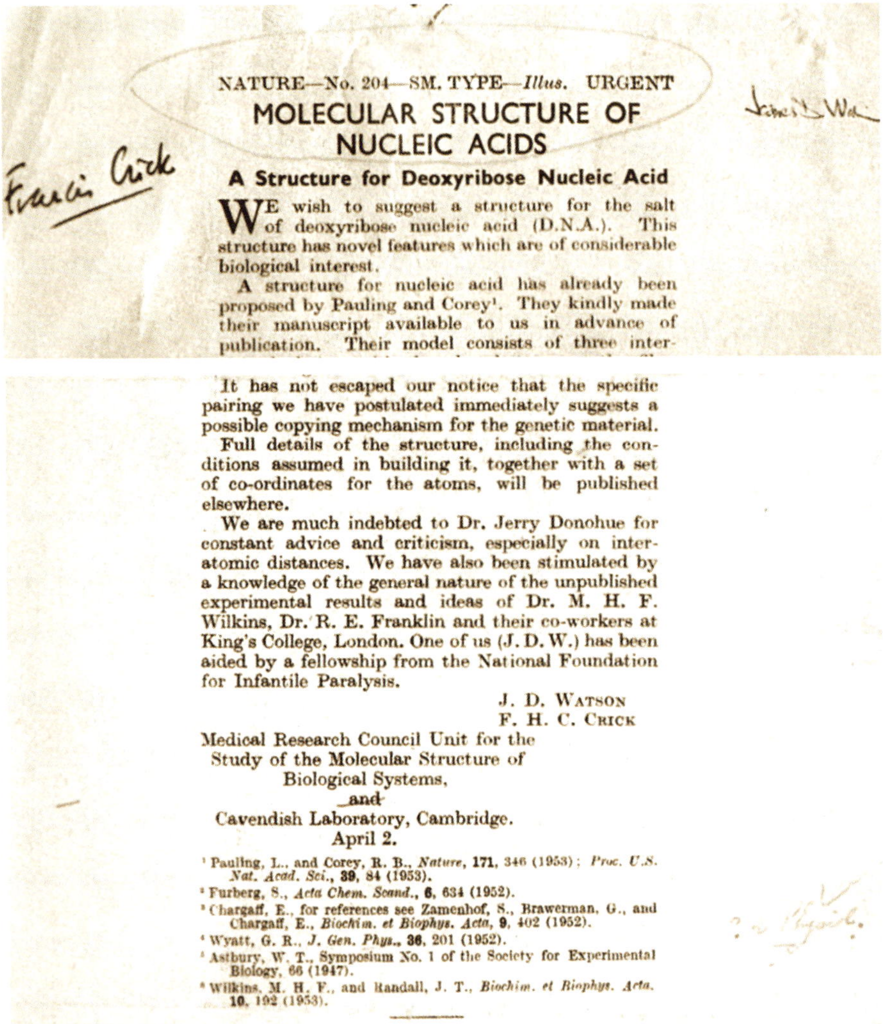

NATURE—No. 204—SM. TYPE—*Illus.* URGENT

MOLECULAR STRUCTURE OF NUCLEIC ACIDS

A Structure for Deoxyribose Nucleic Acid

WE wish to suggest a structure for the salt of deoxyribose nucleic acid (D.N.A.). This structure has novel features which are of considerable biological interest.

A structure for nucleic acid has already been proposed by Pauling and Corey[1]. They kindly made their manuscript available to us in advance of publication. Their model consists of three inter-

It has not escaped our notice that the specific pairing we have postulated immediately suggests a possible copying mechanism for the genetic material.

Full details of the structure, including the conditions assumed in building it, together with a set of co-ordinates for the atoms, will be published elsewhere.

We are much indebted to Dr. Jerry Donohue for constant advice and criticism, especially on inter-atomic distances. We have also been stimulated by a knowledge of the general nature of the unpublished experimental results and ideas of Dr. M. H. F. Wilkins, Dr. R. E. Franklin and their co-workers at King's College, London. One of us (J. D. W.) has been aided by a fellowship from the National Foundation for Infantile Paralysis.

J. D. WATSON
F. H. C. CRICK

Medical Research Council Unit for the Study of the Molecular Structure of Biological Systems,
and
Cavendish Laboratory, Cambridge.
April 2.

[1] Pauling, L., and Corey, R. B., *Nature*, **171**, 346 (1953); *Proc. U.S. Nat. Acad. Sci.*, **39**, 84 (1953).
[2] Furberg, S., *Acta Chem. Scand.*, **6**, 634 (1952).
[3] Chargaff, E., for references see Zamenhof, S., Brawerman, G., and Chargaff, E., *Biochim. et Biophys. Acta*, **9**, 402 (1952).
[4] Wyatt, G. R., *J. Gen. Phys.*, **36**, 201 (1952).
[5] Astbury, W. T., Symposium No. 1 of the Society for Experimental Biology, 66 (1947).
[6] Wilkins, M. H. F., and Randall, J. T., *Biochim. et Biophys. Acta*, **10**, 192 (1953).

The galley proof of the beginning and the end of Watson's and Crick's first publication about DNA in *Nature*. [From archives of the J. Craig Venter Institute.]

instead of Wilkins to be a co-author of the article, but this was never considered.

A first, only 900+ words long article was submitted in early April and published on the 28th of that month in *Nature*[2]. There were almost no changes made in the galley proofs, parts of which are shown in the picture. Certain sections of the text must have been delicate to formulate, in particular the last four paragraphs. In the fourth paragraph from the end a reference was given to the accompanying articles. It said "We were not aware of the details of the results presented there when we devised our structure, which rests mainly though not entirely on published experimental data." What about the MRC report? And how does this tally with the acknowledgement in the last paragraph "We have also been stimulated by experimental results and ideas of Dr M. H. F. Wilkins, Dr R. E. Franklin and co-workers at King's College, London." The acknowledgment paragraph also, in its first part, specified their gratitude to Donohue for his help. It said "We are much indebted to Dr Jerry Donohue for constant advice and criticism, especially on interatomic distances." Although this was a relatively strong expression Donohue was not fully satisfied as he expressed later.

The third paragraph from the end was the frequently cited understatement "It has not escaped our notice that the specific pairing we have postulated immediately suggests a possible copying mechanism for the genetic material." It was then mentioned in the second to last paragraph that more specific information would be published elsewhere. Overall the article provided an example of how brief can be beautiful. Still, of course it is more than twice as long as Thomas Jefferson's Declaration of Independence and three times longer than Abraham Lincoln's Gettysburg Address — texts that defined the new democracy of the USA and for all time changed its own historical development, and hence that of the world. But even scientists can also on rare occasions be brief. Edelman (Chapter 3) once published a paper containing seminal data for the understanding of the composition of immunoglobulin. It was 384 words long!

By agreement the April 28 issue of Nature, following the Watson–Crick article published one article by Wilkins and collaborators[12] and one by Franklin and Gosling[13]. The Wilkins *et al.* publication showed a diffraction diagram from examination of bacterial DNA, but referred to the much sharper picture of the subsequent paper by Franklin. It then went on to discuss the interpretation of the diffraction patterns of helices and referred to unpublished data from Alec Stokes. The latter data showed a considerable agreement with data published in 1952 by the Cavendish group including Crick[9]. The subsequent paper by Franklin and Gosling included the critical picture of the purified B form of DNA from calf thymus — the famous photograph 51 (p. 316). When the plans for publishing two papers from King's College, accompanying the Watson–Crick paper were made, Franklin already had a manuscript ready. All she did was to add the appropriate reference (p. 358).

The biological implications of the double-helix DNA model were discussed by Watson and Crick in Nature a few weeks later[14]. Its capacity to explain the conservation of structure on replication and the potential to store information by varying the sequence of nucleotides were discussed. In fact they even proceeded to speculate prematurely about the relation of the structure to the polypeptide chain. They wrote:

> Our structure, as described, is an open one. There is room between the pair of polynucleotide chains for a polypeptide chain to wind around the helical axis. It may be significant that the distance between adjacent phosphorous atoms, 7.1 Å., is close to the repeat of a fully extended polypeptide chain. We think it probable that in the sperm head and in artificial nucleoproteins, the polypeptide chain occupies this position.

Yes, they did indeed like to speculate, but in this case it would turn out that in the real world relationships were much more complex. Much was to be learnt about how for example the human DNA is wrapped around histone proteins allowing, in total, about two meters of nucleic acid of each individual cell to be packed into the invisible structures of the 24 different kinds of human chromosomes.

There was also to be one more article explaining in much more detail the reasoning behind the hypothesized model by Crick and Watson[15]. Finally Crick was invited to contribute to *Scientific American* describing in a popularizing way the structure of DNA. His article was published in October 1954 and included Franklin's diffraction picture of the B form of DNA. It seems from her contacts with them at that time that there was no obvious disappointment expressed on her side. She seems to have simply accepted the situation as it was. However, at the same time she was probably quite proud of the importance of her photograph.

It would seem that the information about the structure of DNA and the fantastic capacity of the model to explain fundamental aspects of genetics would spread like a bush fire. However, this was not the case. The *Nature* article was sparsely referenced in the beginning, which may serve as a reminder in the present era when citation indexes and impact factors have become a universal method of estimating the progress of science.

In the summer of 1953 Bernal introduced Franklin to Furberg who was visiting Birkbeck College. He was surprised to notice Franklin's interest in his work. Not unexpectedly she asked him what he thought about the Watson–Crick DNA double helix. It turned out that he did not know about their *Nature* article, not to mention that his 1952 publication had been cited as one of only six references in the article.

The Role of Nucleic Acids Finally Appreciated

In my previous book[16], which included studies of archive materials of Nobel Prizes until 1959, the developments in the understanding of nucleic acids as carriers of genetic information were discussed in a chapter entitled *Nobel Prizes and nucleic acids: A drama in five acts*. The most dramatic change of scene occurred over an extended period of several years during the mid 1950s. The various steps in the gradual change towards appreciation of the central role of the nucleic acids, as already mentioned, have been exhaustively described in a number of books[3,4]. In the archives of the Nobel committees of chemistry and of physiology or medicine one can trace the gradual change of attitude.

In 1957 Todd received the Nobel Prize in chemistry "for his work on nucleotides and nucleotide coenzymes" highlighting an interest among nominators and in the committee for the chemistry of nucleic acids. Todd had been nominated for his pioneering work since 1949. Over the years Arne Fredga, one of the many long time members of the committee (1944–1976, chairman 1972–1976; see p. 279), had done four separate reviews. These reviews primarily concerned the development in the understanding of the chemistry of the building stones of nucleic acids, but in the review of 1953 submitted in July one can find a remark that "A number of researchers, among others Pauling, have hastened to make proposals of spiral structures of nucleic acids." One wonders if the reviewer had read Watson's and Crick's April article of the same year. In 1955 the situation had apparently changed. One nominator of Todd stated "… can one fully appreciate the brilliant achievement of his school and himself. They have stimulated a great amount of work outside, and such physical pictures of DNA as Watson and Crick have drawn, rest on the structural theories Todd have developed." Although Todd's laboratory was just across the road of the Cavendish laboratory he had no personal influence on Watson's and Crick's model building of DNA. It was only after the final model had been developed that he was called to see it, at Bragg's request.

In the final review by Fredga of Todd's contributions in 1957, the year of his prize, the following paragraph can be found:

> As is already known, different researchers on the basis of Todd's building principles have developed very interesting theories about the conformation of deoxyribonucleic acids. The most spectacular and perspective-rich model emanates from Watson and Crick (reference), which proposes a double helix, thus two chains with a common axis. The

model explains among other things that certain nitrogen bases appear to be represented in equimolar concentrations (for example adenine/thymidine and guanine/cytosine). This (proposal) makes it possible to explain how a chain molecule of this kind can reproduce. Since the deoxyribonucleic acids have a role in chromosomes one is dealing in this case with very central questions of natural sciences. Todd said in 1955 that it "has passed beyond the state of conjecture"; the following year he says that there can be little doubt that it gives a true picture of the essentials.

There is also other evidence of the fact that in 1957 the chemistry committee accepted that DNA was the carrier of genetic information. This was the previously discussed[16] posthumous evaluation of Oswald T. Avery together with Colin M. MacLeod and Maclyn McCarty. The review was initiated because of a nomination from one of the recipients of the 1946 Nobel Prize in chemistry John H. Northrop, which he had submitted after Avery's death. A paragraph in his letter of nomination read:

> Nucleic acids, then, are the stuff of life, for which so many men have searched for so long. This, I believe, will come to be considered as one of the greatest of all chemical and biological discoveries.

The conclusion of Tiselius who reviewed the nominees was that the discovery that DNA represented the transforming factor of pneumococci bacteria should have been recognized by a prize. But since Avery had already died no prize could be given.

The same development of conceptualized insights, albeit even more slowly, can be followed in the archives of the committee for physiology or medicine as already thoroughly reviewed[16]. After the regrettable failure to recognize the importance of the work by Avery and collaborators the interest in molecular genetics grew rapidly. The 1958 prize to George W. Beadle, Edward L. Tatum and Lederberg (see Chapter 2) clearly highlighted this. Tatum referred in his Nobel lecture[17] to "DNA hereditary changes" and to "The relationships between DNA, RNA and enzymes…" and on the same occasion Lederberg[18], who decided to look forward rather than summarizing his work, commented:

> That genetics should now be recognized is also very timely — for its axial role in the conceptual structure of biology, and for its ripening

yield for the theory and practice of medicine. However, *experimental genetics is reaching its full powers in the coalescence with biochemistry* (my Italics): in principle, each phenotype should eventually be denoted as an exact sequence of amino acids in protein and the genotype as a corresponding sequence of nucleotides in DNA.

Amino Acid Changes Caused by Mutations May Lead to Disease

It had been obvious to scientists only for a short time when Lederberg made his proposal, that the key to genetics was the correlated study of proteins and DNA. Crick, who in the mid-1950s grew to be the dominating theoretician in molecular biology, appreciated this early on and initiated a collaboration with Ingram, whom we met in the previous chapter. Harvey Itano and Pauling had discovered that hemoglobins from normal individuals and from patients with sickle-cell anemia had a different electrophoretic mobility, i.e. they were slightly differently charged. However they could not explain this difference because, by the crude methods available for the analysis, normal and sickle-cell hemoglobins seemed to have the same amino acid composition. Perutz had both of these kinds of hemoglobins available in the laboratory and Ingram examined them by a method developed by Sanger. The method was called "fingerprinting". By this technique a protein was digested by a specific enzyme and the resulting pieces hereafter characterized by electrophoresis. Ingram found that a single amino acid at a specific position in the hemoglobin polypeptide chains had been changed. This *single amino acid change* was the reason for the genetic disease sickle-cell anemia.

Parenthetically it can be mentioned that this genetic disease is rather common in tropical or subtropical areas of the world where malaria infections are prevalent. The reason is that the abnormal gene when occurring harmlessly in a single copy (heterozygotes) provides a higher resistance to the infection, but the prize paid by a population having this collective genetic advantage is that those who have two copies of the gene (the infrequent homozygotes) develop the disease. They have abnormal sickle-shaped red blood cells instead of cells with the normal rounded form. Ingram's finding was the first demonstration that the exchange of a single amino acid — glutamic acid to valine in this case — in a protein could result in a disease. He has therefore subsequently been referred to as "The Father of Molecular Medicine". Ingram was proposed for a Nobel Prize in physiology or medicine in 1960 and the Swedish Nobel laureate

Hugo Theorell made a full investigation. He concluded that the discovery was so important that a prize might be considered. However, since other scientists, in particular Itano, possibly also should be included he recommended the committee to wait and see. In the end Ingram did not receive a Nobel Prize, but the impact of his original discovery remains. The present estimate is that more than 10,000 diseases may be caused by changes in a single gene leading to a dysfunctional single protein. Of course there is an even larger number of diseases that are caused by the added consequences of genetic changes in more than one gene, multigenetic diseases.

A Biochemist with a Particular Influence on the Nobel Work

Tiselius (p. 280) was the main referee when the 1946 Nobel Prize in chemistry was given to Wendell M. Stanley (Ref. 16, Chapter 3). He later grew to be the dominating reviewer of candidates in the emerging field of molecular biology, as we shall see. He therefore deserves to be introduced at greater length. Tiselius was the recipient of the Nobel Prize in chemistry in 1948 "for his research on electrophoresis and adsorption analysis, especially for his discoveries concerning the complex nature of the serum proteins". He was a very likable person and had a major influence on the advance of science in Sweden. He became a member of the Royal Swedish Academy of Sciences in 1939. Over the years Tiselius was to have extensive involvements in the Nobel work. In 1946, 44 years old and professor of biochemistry in Uppsala for eight years, he joined his mentor Svedberg as a member of the Nobel committee for chemistry. He remained a member of this committee until his death in 1971 serving as another pillar in the very stable committee throughout the 1950s and 1960s. In parallel he was also Vice President of the Nobel Foundation since 1947 and its President during 1960–1964. In these many roles he exerted a significant influence.

It has been my privilege to meet Tiselius. One of my first involvements in virus research was to concentrate poliovirus for the purpose of producing an improved inactivated vaccine. One technique tried was the so called two-phase system developed by one of Tiselius' PhD students, Per-Åke Albertsson. An effective concentration was achieved and this led to my first scientific publication, in *Nature*[19]. It was at a dinner following Albertsson's public defense of his thesis in November 1960 that I met Tiselius for the first time. Thus Burnet was not my first personal contact with a Nobel Prize recipient (Chapter 2), but the first laureate from abroad whom I met. Both of them were equally inspiring to encounter for a 23-year-old virologist, who had just entered the field.

Infectious Virus Nucleic Acid

In 1956 there was a nomination for a prize in chemistry to Heinz L. Fraenkel-Conrat and Robley Williams, both at the Virus Laboratory of the University of California at Berkeley, established by Stanley in 1948. Because of his knowledge of the chemistry of tobacco mosaic virus (TMV) from his previous examination of Stanley, Tiselius was selected to be the reviewer. He had learned from earlier Nobel work that viruses were packages of genes that could direct their own synthesis when acting as parasites on cells. The TMV particles were composed mostly of protein but they also contained some nucleic acid. Fraenkel-Conrat and Williams had developed a technique to separate the virus protein and its nucleic acid (RNA) under certain conditions and then allow them to reassemble under different ones. By use of virus strains showing different characteristics it was found that the properties of reassembled particles were determined by the nature of their RNA and not of their protein. In parallel studies in Tübingen by Gerhard Schramm and colleagues, predominantly Alfred Gierer, it was shown that the *isolated* nucleic acid from virus particles was *infectious on its own.* When replicating in cells it gave rise to complete virus particles. Gierer and Schramm had not been nominated for a prize in 1956 and Tiselius therefore recommended a wait and see attitude. His perspective on the state of knowledge at the time is reflected in the following statement: "It may be possible that the ribonucleic acid plays the dominant role for the (infectious) activity and that the protein assists as an accelerator, a specificity-determining factor or only to stabilize the apparently rather instable nucleic acid component."

In 1960 Northrop, an active nominator, made a proposal of a prize to Hershey, Martha Chase, Fraenkel-Conrat, Gierer and Schramm. He wrote:

> I predicted in 1951 that the nucleic acid was the essential part of the virus particle (sic, my remark). This was first confirmed by Hershey and Chase in 1952. They did not actually isolate the nucleic acid, however, and their results, therefore, are not as convincing as those of Fraenkel-Conrat and Gierer and Schramm. The method employed by Gierer and Schramm is of general application, and their paper, therefore, the most important by the three.

At the already mentioned meeting at Royaumond in July 1952 Hershey had given the first presentation of the important experiment he had made together with Martha Chase. In this experiment the separate isotope labeling of the nucleic acid core and of the protein shell of the phage particles strongly indicated that upon infection of a bacterium mainly — or only — the nucleic acid entered the host cell at the start of the infection. This important experiment was discussed in reviews by members of the Nobel committee for physiology or medicine (Ref. 16, Chapter 3) and much later, in 1969, the founding fathers of the phage genetics school, including Hershey were recognized by a Nobel Prize, as mentioned.

Members of the chemistry committee were well aware of the significance of this experiment but in spite of this they did not initiate a review of the proposed candidates in 1960. The committee referred to that it was not allowed to give a prize to more than three people, whereas five had been proposed. It remains to be seen if the chemistry committee ever reviewed the work by Hershey and Chase. Possibly it was considered that the impact of their discovery was more biological than chemical. Still Tiselius referred to their experiment as seen below.

Fraenkel-Conrat, alone, was proposed again in 1961 but this time by Stanley. Tiselius did another review which was extensively cited by the committee in its summary, but prior to discussing that, it is worth citing a short section from the four and a half page long text.

> When judging Fraenkel-Conrat's contribution from the perspective of (Nobel) prize evaluations there are certain circumstances that need to be taken into consideration. At the time of the publication of the discovery (1956) there were already extensive investigations by other researchers which showed that nucleic acids alone could serve as carriers of hereditary traits and had capacity to reproduce. In these cases we are dealing with deoxyribonucleic acid and not ribonucleic acid, but the situation from a general perspective is the same. In the first place one should mention Avery's and later scientists work on bacterial transformation, for example in pneumococci, where (in which system) it was demonstrated already in 1944 that "the transforming factor (English in the original)" was a specific DNA (a reference. See also my (Tiselius) Nobel Prize evaluation concerning Avery in 1957). More recently results have been published, (which are) highly worthy of attention, by A. D. Hershey and collaborators (one paper cited and reference to later

> publications) concerning similar phenomena in bacteriophage T2, in which case a specific DNA again plays the major role as carrier of the genetic information and capacity to reproduce during the infection of the host cell.

Tiselius' careful review was summarized and commented on by the committee in the following way:

> Fraenkel-Conrat was proposed in the year 1956 together with R. C. Williams for the reconstitution of tobacco mosaic virus out of its, as it was believed at the time, inactive components ribonucleic acid and virus protein. Mr Tiselius (no titles are used in the academy; cf. Chapter 5) at the time commented on these publications and recommended, as later turned out correctly, a wait and see attitude to the research in this field. This year he has made a new review of Fraenkel-Conrat, proposed for his work on the infectivity of the nucleic acid isolated in a pure form from the tobacco mosaic virus. The following emerges from his review.
>
> He found that the recognition of the discovery of the role of the ribonucleic acid as carrier of hereditary characters and capacity to reproduce (the multiplication of) tobacco mosaic virus would be possible only under the condition of splitting the prize between Fraenkel-Conrat on the one hand and Schramm and Gierer on the other. The two latter (researchers) have not been proposed this year. In order to consider a prize in chemistry it is of particular importance that the system under consideration belongs to one of the, to a certain degree accessible molecular kinds of viruses, where at present even the structure of the virus protein has been identified in some detail. On the other hand it seems to Mr Tiselius that Hershey's analogous work on the reproduction of bacteriophages and the role that the deoxyribonucleic acid plays in this context is still at present more advanced and significant from a biochemical-genetic point of view. The fundamental discoveries thus also in this case are of an earlier date and, as far as can be judged they have (had) a great influence on both Fraenkel-Conrat's and also on Schramm's and Gierer's work. On the whole it is a matter of an extremely relevant and intensively studied (research) area ("molecular biology"; English in the original, my remark), in which already several researchers have been awarded Nobel Prizes in chemistry or (physiology or) medicine (Todd, Beadle, Tatum, Ochoa, Kornberg, Lederberg) and in which in addition

to Hershey, Fraenkel-Conrat, Gierer and Schramm and further names (for example Crick, Watson, Wilkins) might be considered and where consultations between the chemical and the medical Nobel committees appear to be particularly urgent.

In 1962 Tiselius was called upon to review a proposal that included Gierer. It was the Nobel laureate Northrop, once again, who had nominated Gierer together with K. W. Mundry for their discovery that a chemical change in a nucleic acid could lead to a mutation and a change of characters. It was referred to as *in vitro mutagenesis*. This finding was made in studies of TMV and according to Northrop it was very important because "this discovery finally solves the virus mystery after nearly 60 years". Tiselius made a careful analysis of the *in vitro mutagenesis* findings made by Mundry and Gierer and discussed the further developments in this important field. In the end he did not support the proposal to award Mundry and Gierer and his justification was:

> Thus in spite of the fact that the discovery of the possibility to bring about "*in vitro*" mutations by (introduction of) chemical modifications in nucleic acids is highly important and has given us a new and valuable method to attack central problems in (the field of) protein biosynthesis and in the biochemical genetics, it is difficult for me to share the view of the nominator concerning Gierer's and Mundry's discovery when he writes: "It proves that hereditary characters are determined by the structure of nucleic acid. The classical gene, therefore, may now be defined for the first time as a nucleic acid (English in the original)". However, this (finding) — which without doubt is one of the most important discoveries of our time — is the result of the contributions by many other researchers, and it would seem to me more justified to characterize Gierer's and Mundry's contribution as a natural and anticipated consequence of other discoveries by researchers, who as yet have not been recognized by a Nobel Prize.

In parallel with the examinations of studies of infectious virus nucleic acids by the chemical committee there were evaluations of candidates in this field also by members of the committee of physiology or medicine. In 1959 Fraenkel-Conrat and Schramm were nominated together with Hershey and the year after there was another nomination, but with Gierer instead of Hershey. Two thorough reviews were done by Georg Klein in 1959 (discussed in

Ref. 16) and by Gard in 1960. A section of Gard's review read:

> Like Professor Klein, I am of the opinion that there is no doubt about the prize-worthiness of the discovery. RNA genetics has opened a completely new perspective. The DNA double-helix with its exact complementary halves and the stability that follows from this will hardly allow the chemists to (introduce) calculated and defined changes. The RNA chain in a very different way is accessible to experimentation. If Mundry's, Gierer's and Siegel's observations and interpretations are correct it will be hard to overrate their importance.
>
> In the proposal of the previous year Hershey's name was linked together with Fraenkel-Conrat's and Schramm's. According to my opinion this is not fully adequate. Hershey has demonstrated in an indirect way that the phage DNA contains the genetic information needed for virus synthesis. However it has not been possible for him to exclude the possibility that in addition there is some further component that needs to become introduced into the host cell to allow the process (of replication) to start. On the contrary he has clearly demonstrated that in addition to DNA, protein is also injected at the (initiation of the) infection....
>
> If one were to draw a parallel, it seems to me to be closer at hand to select publications concerning the transforming principle of pneumococci, which provided the first indirect evidence that DNA was the carrier of genetic information. However, after Avery's death these publications cannot be awarded a prize for technical reasons.

Gard's conclusion was that if a prize were to be awarded it should be given jointly to Fraenkel-Conrat, Gierer and Schramm. To ensure that they could be discussed in 1962 he himself submitted a nomination of the three of them on January 31. This was to make sure that Gierer could also be discussed. He could see from the nominations submitted until that date that Schramm had already been proposed by H. Staudinger and also by K. Vosschlte, both from Giessen and in addition by a group of 15 scientists from Mainz. The latter nomination also included Fraenkel-Conrat. Gard carried out a brief review concluding "that the prize-worthiness of the discovery (the infectiousness of free virus RNA) seems to me to become more obvious for every day that passes". However, the discoverers of infectious virus RNA and the possibilities of introducing mutagenic changes into it *in vitro* were never to receive a Nobel Prize. Most likely this was due to the fact that there were so many other major

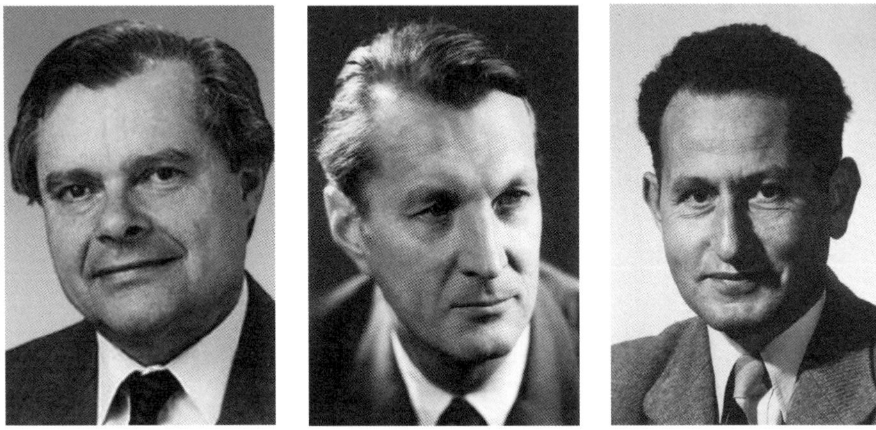

From left: Alfred Gierer, Gerhard Schramm (1910–1969) and Heinz Fraenkel-Conrat (1910–1999). [From Ref. 52.]

advances in the field of molecular genetics competing to be recognized by a prize. Still, Hershey's contributions, proposed for a prize in 1962 by Lederberg but not reviewed that year, were eventually recognized when in 1969 he was awarded a prize in physiology or medicine together with Delbrück and Luria, as mentioned above.

In view of all these developments in the rapidly expanding field of molecular biology in the late 1950s it is very difficult to understand why it would take until 1960 before there were finally nominations for a Nobel Prize to recognize the extreme importance of the discovery of the double-helix structure of DNA with its remarkable base-pairing. Why did the scientific community at large not react to the revolutionary findings and nominate the discoverers?

Bragg Makes Strategic Nominations

Throughout the 1950s and the early 1960s the chairman Westgren (p. 278) presided over a well coordinated chemistry committee composed of members who had been involved in its work for many years, as already discussed in the previous chapter (p. 279). The members included the Nobel laureates Svedberg and Tiselius, Arne Fredga, Karl Myrbäck and the adjunct member Hägg. In 1960 this committee was confronted with particular challenges.

The progress of Perutz's and Kendrew's studies of the structure of large protein molecules prompted Bragg to nominate them for a Nobel Prize in January 1960 as discussed in the previous chapter. In order to be tactical

Table 8.1. Nominations to Nobel Prizes in chemistry and physiology or medicine for the discovery of the structure of DNA.

Year	Chemistry Nominated	Chemistry Nominator	Physiology or Medicine Nominated	Physiology or Medicine Nominator
1960	Watson, Crick, Wilkins	W. Bragg, Cambridge	Crick, Watson Perutz, Crick	M. Stoker, Glasgow E. J. King, London
1961			Watson, Crick Wilkins, Watson, Crick	A. Szent-Gyorgyi, Woods Hole G. Beadle, Pasadena R. M. Herriott, Baltimore
1962	Watson, Crick Watson, Crick, Wilkins	D. H. Campbell, Pasadena W. H. Stein, New York H. C. Urey, La Jolla J. Cockcroft, Cambridge S. Moore, New York J. Monod, Paris	Watson, Crick Watson, Crick, Wilkins Crick, Watson, Wilkins (Benzer, S.), Crick (Benzer, S.), Crick	Gilbert H. Mudge, Baltimore G. Beadle, Pasadena C. H. Stuart-Harris, Sheffield P. J. Gaillard, Leiden F. H. Sobels, Leiden

he decided to nominate these two researchers together with Hodgkin for a prize in physics whereas he nominated Watson, Crick and Wilkins for a prize in chemistry. In the end the chemistry committee was to handle both these proposals. This led to a growing conflict as we shall see. It was decided that Westgren should perform the evaluation also of the DNA work. In his nomination Bragg had mentioned that one might also consider the discovery of the structure of DNA for a prize in physiology or medicine, because of the implications it had for the understanding of genetics. Furthermore Bragg in his nomination had included a supplementary subsidiary nomination of Watson and Crick for their contributions to the understanding of the building principles of virus particles.

The Review by a Crystallographer

Westgren's thorough evaluation covered 14 pages. He had a personal experience of crystallography, but only its application to inorganic material. Although he was not an organic chemist, his involvement in the Nobel committee for many years had most likely broadened his insights to cover chemistry at large, including also organic chemistry. Westgren was a good friend of Hevesy, as discussed in Chapter 5. They liked to take long walks together. This would allow them to exchange thoughts on biology, a discipline in which they had both become heavily involved. Their perspectives were different since they had done their basic training in quite different fields, inorganic chemistry and physics, respectively.

The History of Crystallographic Studies of DNA

A number of key references were given throughout Westgren's extensive text. His evaluation began with a review of the history of crystallographic studies of nucleic acids including the highlights described earlier. Thus he mentioned the early contributions by Astbury and by Furberg and also the model presented by Pauling and Corey in 1953. The strong critique of the latter model was then discussed with particular reference to the identification and characterization of the A and B forms of the sodium salt of DNA by Franklin and Gosling. It was emphasized that these two forms differ in degree of hydration and that the capacity of the salt to absorb water provided evidence for the exposure of the phosphate groups at the surface.

Hereafter Westgren discussed Watson's and Crick's approach to model building in which they, in their final successful attempts, chose to locate the bases inwards in a spiral structure composed of two anti-parallel helices and exposing the phosphates on the outside. In their conjectures they had been inspired by information originally provided by Furberg, but further developed by Franklin. Reference was made to the publication of the February 28 final model in *Nature* two months later[2] and also to the supportive publications by Wilkins's group[12] and by Franklin and Gosling[13]. The reviewer then proceeded to discuss the critical discovery of base pairing and the importance of the Chargaff rules. A brief background to Crick's and Watson's theoretical approach was then given to highlight the fact that their model had not been developed by use of experimental data that they themselves had generated. It relied completely on findings by other research groups, among which were mentioned Wilkins and collaborators and in particular Franklin and Gosling.

Regarding Wilkins's early contributions Westgren cited Bragg's nomination. He noted that Wilkins had devoted considerable work to producing good X-ray pictures and to interpreting these in a critical and skilful way. But he also noted the problem he had in drawing definite conclusions from his data.

The data published by Franklin and Gosling were discussed in more detail with reference to results presented in *Acta Crystallographica* later during the year[20,21] but submitted prior to the demonstration of the Watson-Crick DNA double helix structure (see below). The different measurements were noted to provide support for the hypothetical structure as concerned the number of nucleotides per turn and the pitch of the helical structure. It was mentioned briefly that Franklin in March 1953 had moved from King's college to Bernal's department at Birkbeck College. The follow-up studies during the late 1950s by Wilkins and collaborators providing a deepening of the information about the DNA double helix were then discussed on one page. It was concluded that the additional data gained in essence confirmed the structural model proposed in 1953 by Watson and Crick.

Under a separate heading Westgren discussed the genetic importance of the "molecule of life" discovery made by Watson and Crick. He quoted from material attached to Bragg's nomination, a statement made by Perutz in the *New Scientist* of May 28, 1959. Under the heading *The Molecular Basis of Inheritance* Perutz had written:

> Six years ago two short notes in *Nature* by J. D. Watson and F. H. C. Crick, of the Medical Research Council's Molecular Biology Unit at Cambridge, revolutionized our ideas of inheritance and introduced a new concept into biochemistry.... It is time that we took note of these results and accepted their implications, because they are as fundamental to biology today, as the quantum theory was to physics sixty years ago.

The importance of the model was further discussed in particular in two major contexts. One was the possibility that the sequence of the base pairs can serve as a genetic code and the other that the reproduction of the two chains allowed maintenance of their genetic information. Possibilities for the emergence of mutants were also considered. It was noted that it had been possible to examine some consequences of this kind using the techniques for biological syntheses developed by Ochoa and Kornberg, reviewed for the committee for chemistry by Myrbäck the previous year. Furthermore Westgren discussed the use of isotopes in various kinds of experiments, including the important data generated by Matthew S. Meselson and Franklin W. Stahl[22] documenting the semi-conservative replication of DNA to be further discussed below.

A Detour into the World of Virus Structures

Since Bragg had nominated Watson and Crick not only for their discovery of the structure of DNA, but in addition for their important contributions to the field of virus structure, this work was also reviewed by Westgren at some length. He noted that Watson was remarkably productive during 1953. In parallel with his efforts to resolve the structure of DNA, Watson had also engaged himself in X-ray diffraction studies of TMV. The first pictures of this virus from such studies had been published already in 1941 by Bernal and collaborators. Using a theory developed by Crick and collaborators for X-ray diffraction pictures of helical structures[9] Watson concluded that the elongated virus particle was a large protein helix that in some way surrounded the RNA genetic material of the virus. He postulated that virus-specific protein building stones were used in a repeated regular pattern and proposed a number of such components per turn of the helix and a possible size of the protein. He estimated the molecular weight to be 35,000 which later turned out to be only twice the value eventually found to be the correct one. These data were important for Franklin's more detailed studies of the structure of TMV in the mid-1950s.

When Franklin left King's College for Birkbeck College in March 1953 she switched from studies of DNA to analyses of TMV. Thus she continued her involvement in the examination of biological material by X-ray crystallography, the technique she mastered so well. As will be further discussed below she was remarkably productive during the four years that remained of her life. Publishing some 15 scientific articles about TMV in collaboration with the most prominent scientists in the field she went on to become a central figure in this field of research. Westgren referred to one publication[23] in which she gave experimentally consolidated substance to Watson's speculations on the number of protein components per turn and the pitch of the helix. Thus Watson's and Franklin's different walks in science came to cross several times.

Westgren also discussed the data Franklin had accumulated on the relationship between the virus RNA and the protein helix. Among other contributions he briefly discussed her important collaboration with Schramm and his co-workers analyzing virus particles with and without their nucleic acid defining the position of the latter *inside* the protein helix.

In a joint publication in 1956[24] Crick and Watson had made some very general prophetic predictions on the symmetry of virus particles. These predictions concerned both elongated particles that were formed by helical building arrangements and "spherical" virus particles proposed to represent examples of the use of some kind of cubic symmetry. These were fundamental in future attempts to classify viruses into groups. We will return to this problem later in the present chapter.

Back to the Double Helix

Although Westgren praised the visionary character of Watson's and Crick's predictions concerning virus structures, his concluding discussion quite rightly was devoted to an analysis of the importance of their discovery of the structure of DNA. It deserves to be presented verbatim:

> The research that has been described above has led to advances of epoch-making importance, without doubt highly deserving to be awarded a Nobel Prize. There is a certain difficulty in evaluating the question of a prize because of the many contributors. It is problematic to decide who among the many scientists involved have participated in such a decisive way in the developments that they, in particular, deserve to be recognized. No single research achievement in the field rises in such a definite way above the others and is so mature and cast in one piece that it alone deserves a prize (sic, my remark).
>
> The hypothesis put forward by Watson and Crick concerning the structure of deoxyribonucleic acid and its functions in the genetic doubling process is ingenious. It has played a decisive role in the continued research in the area and has grown to acquire an importance for the theory of genetics that can hardly be overestimated. However the two scientists have not themselves documented the validity of their hypothesis — they have hardly performed any experimental investigations in the field of their own — and the testing (of their hypothesis) has been completely allocated to others.
>
> Those that deserve most credit in this context are on the one hand Wilkins and his large research group, within which he without doubt has a leading role, and on the other hand Franklin and Gosling. A reward to Watson and Crick passing by the researchers who experimentally have confirmed their proposal for a structure would not be worthy of consideration. Among the latter Wilkins without doubt is in a class by himself. Those who come next are Rosalind Franklin and Gosling, among whom the first mentioned is deceased. If she had survived *she*

could well have had claims to receive her part of the prize (my italics). Bragg, who closely followed the research in the field, did not include Gosling in his proposal and it is therefore likely that his contribution has not been of decisive importance in the work by the research duo Franklin and Gosling.

There are *no reasons to question the well-founded opinion of Bragg* (my italics), that if a prize should be considered to award the research discussed, it should be split between Watson, Crick and Wilkins.

Bragg considers in his proposal whether the award should be in the field of chemistry or in (physiology or) medicine. Obviously a prize in chemistry would be fully motivated in this context; the important identifications of structures are without doubt of importance in chemistry. However the major importance of the achievements made is within the field of genetics and a prize in physiology or medicine therefore seems to be most appealing.

Hereafter followed the discussion, already alluded to in the previous chapter that the prize in chemistry needed to first recognize Perutz' and Kendrew's work before it could recognize the discovery by Watson, Crick and Wilkins.

Pauling Reflects on Nominations for the Discovery of the Structure of DNA

Surprisingly there was no nomination for a prize in chemistry for the discovery of the DNA double-helix structure and base pairing in 1961 (Table 8.1, p. 333). However, Pauling (p. 271) had received copies of Bragg's nominations in 1960 for prizes to the protein crystallographers and Hodgkin and to Watson, Crick and Wilkins in physics and chemistry, respectively. This had prompted Pauling to make a nomination of Perutz and Kendrew for half the prize and Corey for the other half, as discussed in the previous chapter. In a separate letter he made some uncalled for comments on the proposal to award a prize to Watson, Crick and Wilkins. A part of the letter reads:

> The hydrogen-bonded double-helix for DNA proposed by Watson and Crick has had a very great influence on the thinking of geneticists and other biologists, and I believe that their idea is a valuable one. It is my opinion that there is little doubt that nucleic acid molecules have a

> complementary structure resembling in its general nature that proposed by Watson and Crick, and that the complementariness is determined by the formation of hydrogen bonds. The detailed nature of the structure of DNA is, I think, still uncertain to some extent, however, whereas that of polypeptide chains in proteins is now certain.
>
> The first detailed structure to be proposed for the nucleic acids was a triple-helix structure, with hydrogen bonds between the phosphate groups rather than between the nitrogen bases. This structure was proposed by Professor Robert B. Corey and me in *Proc. Natl. Acad. Sci.*, 39:84–97. Watson and Crick had a manuscript of this paper before publication, and may to some extent have been stimulated by this proposal to formulate their double-helix structure, as well as by the X-ray photographs of Wilkins.

Pauling then continued by discussing alternative forms of hydrogen bonds between the bases. Hereafter he reiterated his nomination of Corey for his protein work. The letter then continued:

> On the other hand, I think that it might well be premature (in 1961! My remark) to make an award of a Prize to Watson and Crick, because of existing uncertainty about the detailed structure of nucleic acid. I myself feel that it is likely that the general nature of the Watson-Crick structure is correct, but that there is doubt about details.
>
> With respect to Wilkins, I may say that I recognize his virtuosity in having grown better fibers of DNA than any that had been grown before (the DNA used came from an external source; my remark) and in having obtained b(y)etter x-ray photographs than were available before, but I doubt that this work represents a sufficient contribution to chemistry to permit him to be included among recipients of a Nobel Prize.

The Temperature Rises and a Powerful Nomination

In 1962 there were — eventually — several brief nominations for a prize to Watson and Crick and one comprehensive nomination by Jacques Monod from the Pasteur Institute in Paris (Table 8.1, p. 333). Only the latter nomination also included Wilkins. Monod was the next scientist in line to be recognized by a Nobel Prize for contributions in molecular genetics after the 1962 award. In

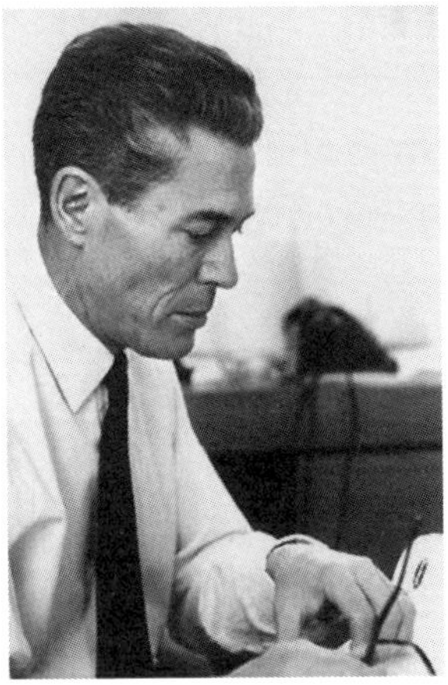

Jacques Monod (1910–1976).
[From *Les Prix Nobel en 1965*.]

1965 he was awarded a Nobel Prize in physiology or medicine together with Francois Jacob and André Lwoff "for their discoveries concerning genetic control of enzyme and virus synthesis".

It has been well documented that Monod corresponded with Crick to get advice about which scientists he should include in his nomination. *En passant* it might be mentioned that Monod's nomination was given in flawless English although at the time French scientists in official functions were expected to use their rich and euphonious native language. Tiselius was given the responsibility of conducting another review of the three candidates. Whereas Westgren gave his opinions with a background as a crystallographer studying inorganic compounds, Tiselius was an organic chemist lacking experience in crystallography. Thus he could provide a broader picture applying a chemical as well as a biological perspective. Against the background of the extensive nomination by Monod and the evaluation by Tiselius the following 1962 perspective on the discovery of DNA and its consequences can be given. First some extracts from Monod's nomination.

The concept of the DNA double-helix had been consolidated both by extended structural studies and by a range of different functional studies. Monod first referred to the two papers by Watson and Crick supported by the accompanying *Nature* papers, one by Wilkins and collaborators and two (see below) by Franklin and Gosling. The knowledge at the time of Watson's and Crick's discovery was summarized as follows:

1. The formula of the bases and the nature of the backbone had been well established. The linkage of the base to the sugar was assumed to be of the beta kind as communicated privately to Watson and Crick by Todd.
2. The most likely tautomeric form of the bases had not been established. The forms illustrated in textbooks at the time were often incorrect. Donohue's knowledge of the proper (keto) form shared in in-houses contacts was indispensible.
3. No one at the time had drawn the proper conclusions from Chargaff's finding of equimolar concentrations of adenine and thymidine as well as guanidine and cytosine.

4. The titration curves for DNA showed hysteresis. This suggested that the bases formed hydrogen bonds in the structure.
5. The initial X-ray studies by Astbury were interpreted to show that the bases were stacked one upon the other.
6. Important studies using X-ray crystallography of the nucleotide cytidine had been made by Furberg defining the correct relationship between the base and the sugar.

Monod hereafter wrote:

> The only serious X-ray work on DNA up to 1953 was carried out by Wilkins and his colleagues and by Franklin and Gosling, both in the same laboratory at King's College, London. The work had been initiated by Wilkins and it was carried on in part by Franklin when she joined the laboratory. In 1953, Franklin joined Bernal's laboratory at Birkbeck, and the subsequent work was carried out almost entirely by Wilkins and collaborators (ten references).

Monod then discussed the interpretation of the X-ray pictures taken at King's College. Density considerations made it unlikely that there would be only one strand — two or three were more likely numbers. The incorrect triple structure proposed by Pauling and Corey and its dismissal was referred to. Further on Monod deliberated on the incitement to examine helical structures. He did not believe that it derived from the demonstration of the alpha-helix by Pauling and Corey although, as acknowledged by Crick, it served as an object-lesson of great value. Monod then made an intermission summary:

> There appears to be no doubt, and indeed there has never been any dispute about it, that the double-helix (duplex) base-paired structure of DNA, was profoundly original and novel theoretical discovery directly based upon, and justified by, the experimental (X-ray) work of *Wilkins and his associates* (my italics).
>
> Although the extreme importance of Crick, Watson and Wilkins' contribution was immediately realized (true? My remark) by workers in the field of macromolecular structures, as well as by biologists, many years were to elapse until the chemical validity of the proposed structure was finally confirmed by a variety of methods. Simultaneously the extreme importance of the structure for biochemical and genetic theory

became more and more apparent, until today, when it is accepted as *one of the essential keys to the chemical interpretation of life.*

A little further on Monod wrote:

> The most original and at once the most profoundly significant feature of the Watson–Crick structure, evidently is the specific pairing of the bases, through hydrogen bonds, in the "duplex molecule". At the time the structure was first published, this feature appeared as a brilliant guess. All the recent developments have proved this guess not only to have been correct, but to have shown immense heuristic value, emphasizing the profound chemical and biological insight shown by the authors of the structure. These developments and confirmations may be classified as follows:
>
> a. Direct (physical chemical) tests of the "specific duplex" state of native DNA molecules.
> b. Biochemical evidence relating to the mode of replication of DNA.
> c. Evidence concerning chemical functioning of DNA in the cell.

The nomination then cited some experiments confirming the duplex nature of DNA. These include Julius Marmur's and Paul Doty's denaturation and renaturation studies, Kornberg's and Ochoa's nucleic acid replication studies, the brilliant Meselson and Stahl experiment, already briefly alluded to above, and finally the early advances in identifying the genetic code with critical contributions by Crick and others. Monod also discussed the correlation between nucleotide sequence and the primary structure of proteins and the consequential relations between a change in a single base-pair and the exchange of one amino acid for another. A reference was made to Ingram's work on hemoglobin (p. 325).

Not surprisingly Monod emphasized the transcription phenomenon and the role of messenger RNA and ribosomes, a field in which he and his colleagues had made seminal early discoveries.

The concluding two paragraphs of the nomination expressed French wittiness and deserve to be quoted in full:

> I would like to state my conviction that, with all these recent developments, we are now witnessing the most fundamental advances that have ever been made into the chemical structure and interpretation of living

> beings. And although it is always difficult to trace such a far reaching scientific advances to a single person or group, there is no doubt that the elucidation of the DNA structure by Crick, Watson and Wilkins has been not only the starting point and the main incentive, but actually and directly the basis and immediate condition for all these new developments, which have at once demonstrated the validity of their work, and its immense importance.
>
> It is my warmest hope, therefore, that the Nobel Committee will find it possible to bestow their universally respected award upon the authors of this discovery; and I would venture also to express my feeling, that all the scientists engaged in this fundamental field would gratefully accept such a decision, not only as well earned by the recipients, but as a token of the success and value of their collective effort.

It must have been hard for the committee for chemistry to resist such a nomination. The quandary in which the committee found itself when it had to chose between the protein work by Perutz and Kendrew, discussed in the previous chapter, and the discovery of the DNA double-helix became a major issue in the concluding part of Tiselius' nine-page-long evaluation.

Tiselius' Final Analysis

Tiselius first summarized the different nominations that the committee had received emphasizing in particular the elaborate proposal by Monod. He then picked up where Westgren's previous evaluation ended. In particular he examined the most recent three publications by Wilkins and his collaborators and also referred to a lecture that Wilkins had given in Stockholm at a symposium on "Biological Structure and Function" in September 1960. The conclusion was that these publications were important for the biochemical verification of the double-helix model proposed by Watson and Crick.

Tiselius then discussed the accumulated evidence verifying the phenomenon of specific base-pairing. The demonstration of dissociation and re-association between nucleic acid strands of different origins and specificity as examined by Marmur and Doty was described in some detail. The importance of the regaining of biological activity of for example "transforming factor" after careful re-naturation was mentioned. Re-naturation (hybridization) had been found to be a phenomenon that could only occur between genetic materials from organisms that were genetically and taxonomically closely related. The discovery that a synthetic double helix DNA could be produced by the mixing of polyadenylic acid and polyuridylic acid was also mentioned. Tiselius then went on to discuss the synthesis of new DNA from a single-stranded primer DNA using the Kornberg enzyme illustrating the dependence on base-pairing.

A particular paragraph was devoted to the by then already classical Meselson–Stahl experiment[22]. The density of DNA was followed in *Escherichia coli* bacteria grown in the presence of the (non-radioactive) isotope of nitrogen ^{15}N, which is heavier than its normal isotope ^{14}N. DNA labeled by either of these isotopes had different densities and could therefore be separated by equilibrium density gradient ultracentrifugation. Hence it was possible to follow how after replication for one generation the density of offspring DNA had increased and was in between the density of DNA from bacteria propagated in regular ^{14}N medium and the "heavy" ^{15}N medium, respectively. The conclusion was that one strand of DNA in a duplex was exchanged at a time. There was in fact a small slip in Tiselius' presentation. He referred to the fact that replicating bacteriophages and not bacteria were the object of the study. However it is bacteria and other cellular organisms, but not viruses, that multiply by binary division and in which the combination of one labeled and one unlabeled strand of DNA potentially can be detected.

Tiselius went on to discuss the controlling role that DNA has on protein synthesis in the cell. He wrote:

> Thus the function of DNA is not only duplication of itself, but it determines in a way that as yet is not known the specific sequence of amino acids that is the signature of every protein. The insight into this goes back to the investigations in the 1940s by Caspersson and Brachet (sic, my remark) but it was first by a series of studies by among others Avery, Hershey, Fraenkel-Conrat, Schramm and others that the absolutely decisive and very specific importance became apparent.

The review then alluded to the intensity of research devoted to the coding problem and introduced the importance of ribosomes and of messenger RNA, but Tiselius did not refer directly to the central dogma — DNA gives RNA gives protein. However he did discuss the possible existence of a triplet non-overlapping code. A reference was given to the very fresh and spectacular data from Marshall Nirenberg's laboratory showing that poly-U RNA gave a protein polymer composed only of phenylalanine.

Towards the end of the review Tiselius reflected on a particular problem. That was that the rapid developments in the field might very likely soon lead to the emergence of new important candidates for a prize. It is therefore important to recognize the discovery of the DNA double helix *as soon as possible*. Tiselius stated: "I believe, and in this context I can also refer to the nominators (only Monod, my remark), that a prize to Watson, Crick and Wilkins would cause general satisfaction and, at least in my opinion, none of these three (candidates) can be passed by if we wish to award a prize in one of the most fruitful areas, rich in results, within the natural sciences and medicine."

In the last paragraph Tiselius introduced the major dilemma of the committee that arose from the fact that it also had to seriously consider Kendrew and Perutz. As mentioned in the previous chapter the chemists felt that they first had to recognize these two scientists although the impact of their work was not at all as great as that of the discovery of the structure of DNA. Tiselius, the man who probably at the time had the largest influence on the Nobel system resorted to politics and concluded:

> Thus the situation is complicated. It would be particularly attractive to award a prize to these candidates in the same year — something which in addition would be very suitable (to do) since the contributions have a certain connection to each other. I would therefore like to propose: if the chemical Nobel committee this year, after having taken part of Mr Hägg's evaluation, find that Kendrew and Perutz belong among those who should be considered in the first place, one (the chemistry committee) inquires about the possibility that the medical Nobel committee considers a proposal to award a prize to Watson, Crick and Wilkins in this year, and that the medical Nobel committee is provided with the evaluations and (documents of) discussions on these matters. All things considered it is my view that Watson, Crick and Wilkins to a very high degree deserve a prize and that they apparently are among the leading candidates to be considered at present.

It would seem that after this authoritative statement the prize recipients in chemistry and in physiology or medicine in 1962 should be a given.

The Karolinska Institute — A Slow Starter that Won the Trophy

The first time Watson and Crick were nominated for a prize in physiology or medicine was in 1960 (Table 8.1, p. 333). The nominator was Michael G. P. Stoker professor of virology at the University of Glasgow since 1958, incidentally the first chair in this discipline in Great Britain. Stoker was highly regarded as a scientist studying mainly tumor viruses. There was also another nomination by E. J. King in London for a prize to Crick together with Perutz for "their work on X-ray crystallography, and their experimental evidence educed in favor of the helix structure of deoxyribonucleic acid and of proteins, e.g. myoglobin…". The committee considered these nominations to be important, but decided not to conduct a review of its own but instead to collect information from the evaluation made by the chemistry committee. Watson and Crick were not mentioned in the document summarizing the work of the committee at the Karolinska Institute in 1960!

In 1961 there were three nominations for the discovery of the DNA double helix. Two of them, by the Nobel laureates George W. Beadle and Albert N. Szent-Györgyi, proposed Watson and Crick but the third by Roger Herriott, a phage geneticist at John Hopkins University, also included Wilkins. The nomination by Herriott is somewhat misleading since it stated "Dr Wilkins and his colleagues then made the tedious but precise X-ray diffraction measurements of DNA and found that molecules of this substance consisted of double stranded helices (two references)". The two references are the 1953 *Nature* article by Wilkins *et al.*[12] attached to the Watson and Crick article describing the discovery of the structure of DNA and a 1956 article in *Cold Spring Harbor Symposia*. There is no reference to Franklin's and Gosling's articles. Further on the nomination discussed the Watson–Crick model.

The committee asked Arne Engström, professor of medical physics to make an evaluation. Engström had been trained by Caspersson at the Department of Cell Research, Karolinska Institute, a Mecca for technique developments in the field at the time. Engström presented his thesis in 1946. It was entitled "Quantitative micro and histochemical elementary analysis by roentgen absorption spectroscopy". The thesis introduced a number of pioneering techniques. 50 years later Engström was terminally ill and therefore I, in my capacity as a Dean of the medical faculty of the Institute, arranged a special academic ceremony at the hospice where he was staying. In an event to confer his doctor's degree he was created "Jubilee Doctor" (one who has held a doctorate for 50 years) and two months later he was dead.

In 1952, aged only 32 Engström had become a professor at the Karolinska Institute. The subject area of his professorship was originally called physical cell research, but four years later this was changed to medical physics. In 1961 he was the organizer of the First International Congress of Biophysics in Stockholm. At this meeting he got to know four of the five Nobel Prize recipients in 1962, including Wilkins. According to material left behind, kindly made available by Engström's son, Wilhelm, himself a cell biology researcher, the father had had contacts with Wilkins since 1956 and had met him on a number of occasions. Together with other new professors at the Institute, like Klein and Bergström, Engström contributed to increasing the intensity and freshness of the Nobel work.

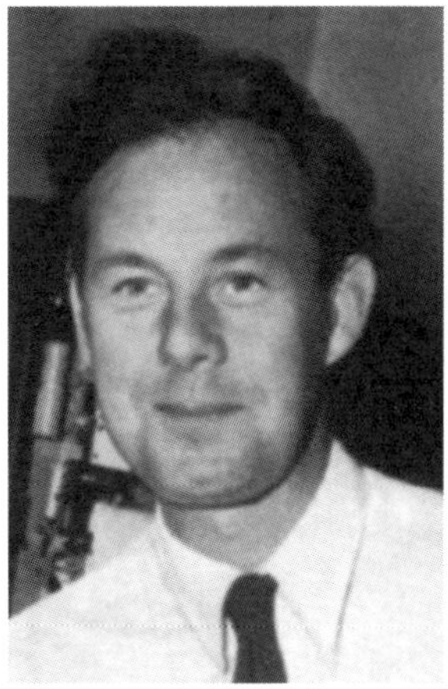

Arne Engström (1920–1996). [Courtesy of the Karolinska Institute.]

The First Review of the Discovery of the Structure of DNA

Engström's review extended over 16 pages. He briefly mentioned Friedrich Mischer's original discovery of DNA and the development of knowledge about the chemistry of the two forms of nucleic acids over many decades. He then commented:

> However, one might, without exaggeration, make the statement that when the journal *Nature* in 1953 in a composite of contributions brought into force a new model of the molecular structure of DNA by Crick and Watson and also Wilkins and collaborators (note that Franklin was not mentioned, my remark), the whole field of nucleic acid research received such a strong injection (stimulus) that the consequences came too include a large number of disciplines; genetics, virology, immunology, information theory, cell biology, to mention only a few.

Prior to presenting the state of knowledge of the structure of DNA Engström emphasized that

> The possibility of representing a living molecule (?, my question mark), which to a large extent is responsible for the transmission of hereditary

> characters, according to the principles of information theory, has had and will continue to have an extraordinarily great importance in the drive to establish a quantitative biology and medicine.

He cited the advances presented by the recent Nobel laureates Beadle, Kornberg and Ochoa and then briefly alluded to the Meselson and Stahl experiment presented above. Rewriting history he then added, as a tribute to his mentor:

> ...viewed in retrospect it is with the highest admiration and esteem that one can now acknowledge that the general ideas about the role of nucleic acids in the production of protein, which were proposed by Caspersson in 1939–1945, in general terms are correct, as verified in several ways.

Caspersson could have made such a proposal but the sad thing is that he never fully understood the significance of his findings, according to Klein one of the largest blunders in studies of biological phenomena — but probably not unique. Incidentally it could be mentioned that Caspersson was nominated many times for a Nobel Prize, as described earlier[16]. He was nominated again in 1962, this time also for a prize in chemistry, and Tiselius carried out an evaluation of him together with Brachet and Alfred Mirsky. The final paragraph of his review read:

> After a certain hesitation — with reference to the long time that has passed since the discoveries were made, which in the first place should be considered as recognized — I find that the contributions by Caspersson and Brachet could be considered for recognition by a prize. However I can imagine that the intensive developments in the field during the last decade have led to other candidates being much closer to a prize, even with consideration taken to the pioneering nature of Caspersson's and Brachet's contributions.

Engström continued his review by discussing the emerging knowledge about the structure of DNA with a brief mention of contributions by Astbury and Bell, Furberg and the incorrect model published by Pauling and Corey.

In the remaining part of his presentation of the 1953 discovery by Watson and Crick, Engström gave a remarkable emphasis to the importance of Wilkins' work. His name is cited 50% more often than the names of Watson and Crick in the whole review. Engström misinterpreted Franklin's seminal contributions and continuously referred to her as a member of Wilkins' group. However he did state "In particular Rosalind Franklin's extraordinary beautiful publications should be mentioned." He referred at length to the late 1950s publications by Wilkins and collaborators which confirmed the correctness of the Watson-Crick double helix structure of DNA. It could be added that, although valuable, these studies did not add any new dimension to the original discovery. They provided confirmation of the correctness of the hypothesis. In view of his particular respect for Wilkins' contributions and with reference to "Because of my personal knowledge about the developments at the time of the work...", he proposed that the model should be called the Wilkins-Watson-Crick model. This is precisely what Wilkins in his biography had stated should *not* be the case! It is likely that the source of his, and probably also Tiselius's insights were contacts with Wilkins himself and possibly also with Bragg. Engström also noted that in 1960 the Lasker Award was conferred on all three scientists.

Engström then presented the distinction between the A and B forms of DNA, without emphasizing that the understanding of their nature was primarily based on Franklin's work. When describing the characteristics of the Watson–Crick model he referred instead to the fact that it was deduced from X-ray diffraction data generated by Wilkins. In the presentation of the developments that led to the final structure proposed by Watson and Crick there were a number of statements which might be debated in the light of later findings. It was explained that the proposed structure was deduced from the diffraction pattern of the B form of DNA — Franklin's picture (!) — using ten bases per turn and with a repetition period of 34 Å. The idea of a helix structure was referred to as having been derived from Wilkins' work during 1952–1953. On more than two pages the formal background to X-ray diffraction patterns of spiral structures was discussed departing from the 1952 article by Cochran, Crick and Vand[9]. It was summarized that because of the limitations of the diffraction patterns of biological substances, additional information on stereochemical conditions were important. Insights into the three-dimensional orientation of molecules were the basis for the discovery of the alpha helix structure in proteins by Pauling and Corey. Engström then continued: "in parenthesis it can be added that the existence of the alpha helix in a protein was fully proved first when Kendrew had described the molecular structure of myoglobin", a doubtful statement. In the running text the model progressively became Wilkins' model and three pages of the review were devoted to the late 1950s follow-up studies.

The review then evaluated the importance of synthetic polynucleotides used by Ochoa and collaborators. The formation of a double helix by combining poly-A and poly-U was mentioned and also Alex Rich's (p. 383) studies of complexes of synthetic poly-A and poly-I (inosinic acid), which gave a diffraction pattern, similar to the B form of DNA. Under the heading *Biological consequences of the double helix structure of DNA* Engström discussed the replication of the structure. Meselson's and Stahl's studies using isotopes of nitrogen and their results providing strong evidence for a double helix structure were praised, again. In the same section Engström also discussed the significance of the discovery for the interpretation of the organization of the gene. He wrote:

> The progress of modern genetics with the construction of genetic fine structure maps has led to the demonstration of units that can mutate, which are positioned at distances corresponding to the distance between the bases in a DNA molecule. The identification of these conditions has led to a rational formulation of the gene concept and solving (reading) the genetic code will be (an) analyses of the sequence of bases in a certain area. One can therefore be optimistic that one will find the Rosetta stone of genetics that is translating the A-T-G-C-hieroglyphs to the language of protein structures.
>
> Finally it can be stated, although it is beyond the primary task of this investigation, that the fact that the virus nucleic acid by itself is infectious, not antigenic and resistant towards all antibodies against the whole virus opens new and fascinating aspects and research areas within the (discipline of) clinical virology and the knowledge of diseases in general.

In his concluding paragraph Engström stated:

> It is apparent to me that Wilkins, Watson and Crick (this is the name order used; my comment) by their work in mapping the molecular structure of deoxyribonucleic acid have provided a splendid scientific contribution to the understanding of the most fundamental processes of life. M. H. F. Wilkins', J. D. Watson's and F. H. C. Crick's formulation of the structure of deoxyribonucleic acid is exceptionally worthy of a prize.

The faculty of professors finally decided in 1961 to give the prize to Békésy as described in Chapter 6.

The Critical Year

In 1962 there were three nominations for Watson and Crick and two additional proposals for Crick alone combined with Seymour Benzer for a prize in physiology or medicine (Table 8.1, p. 333). Benzer was a very influential scientist in the field of molecular biology, but he would never receive a Nobel Prize. In the late 1950s he mapped the fine structure of a gene by studies of T-even bacteriophages. There were two nominators from Leiden who proposed to combine him with Crick, referring to his pioneering contributions during the late 1950s to defining the triplet code in collaboration with Brenner and others. Out of the remaining three nominations concerning the discovery of the structure of DNA two also included Wilkins. No particular motivations were given in the latter two nominations for the inclusion of him. Beadle's nomination contained an interesting remark. "I'm afraid the Chemistry Committee will regard DNA structure as Biology (Physiol. Med) and that you may regard it as Chemistry. I have no doubt myself that this discovery (the structure of DNA) is one of the most important in *Biology* of this century."

Engström was asked to conduct a supplementary review of the three candidates. It was brief, only five pages long and it only supplied a limited amount of new information. Firstly it took note that cracking the genetic code was currently the main focus of the field. Then it discussed if the double-helix structure of DNA also could be applied to RNA. With reference to some preliminary data from Wilkins and collaborators in studies of crystals of crude preparations of transfer RNA, published in 1962 it was deduced that double-helix formation might represent a general kind of structure in the case of RNA too. As later became apparent the situation turned out to be much more complex than what was understood at the time. It is certainly true that RNA can form helix structures, but in the case of transfer-RNA it was later shown to have a "clover-leaf" structure only in parts double-helical. In the world of viruses all possible variations have been found; single-stranded RNA (in most cases); double-stranded RNA; single-stranded DNA and of course double-stranded DNA.

Engström also referred to the early studies of nucleic acids by electron microscopy. He mentioned that the diameter of the structure tallied with the expected dimensions of the Wilkins–Watson–Crick (again, my remark) model. The review finished by a reference to the pioneering contributions by Crick and collaborators in defining a degenerative code using triplets. In conclusion it was stated:

> Concerning the priority for identification of the structure of DNA there is no doubt, as was already argued in the investigation of the previous year that it belongs to Crick, Watson and Wilkins. The research group of the latter included and had as coauthors on the first publications a number of persons, for example Stokes, Gosling and Franklin (Franklin never published a paper with Wilkins; my remark). Miss Franklin is deceased and concerning the first two mentioned, they participated in the work under Wilkins' leadership.

The three candidates were concluded to be exceptionally deserving of a prize.

The committee submitted its summary conclusions to the College of Teachers *without* a recommendation for a prize on September 24. The reason must have been that it wanted to wait for the outcome of the deliberations by the Royal Swedish Academy of Sciences on the Nobel Prize in chemistry. The decision by the Academy to select Kendrew and Perutz was taken on October 11. Afterwards the committee for physiology or medicine proposed Crick, Watson and Wilkins when the Faculty of the Karolinska Institute met on October 17. Whereas in the previous two years there had been a strong minority and a majority, respectively, of the committee members recommending a prize to Eccles, which however was overruled by the Faculty (Chapters 2 and 6), this was not a situation repeated in 1962. The committee was unanimous in its final recommendation of Crick, Watson and Wilkins. Eccles had to wait one more year.

Honest Jim and the Double Helix

When the manuscript of what came to be *The Double Helix* was in the making Watson circulated copies of it to a number of scientists with whom he had personal contacts and for whom he had a certain respect. According to his own words he had set his goals high also in this life project of his. Using science as his point of departure, and by the way science is a human pursuit, he wanted to create a non-fiction novel on a par with *The Great Gatsby* by Scott Fitzgerald. The title of the original draft of the text was *Honest Jim*. This catchy working title had the following origin. It referred to a comment that Watson had overheard on a walking tour in the Swiss Alps. In this setting he once met one of Wilkins' collaborators who sarcastically alluded to him as "honest Jim", referring to the fact that Watson and Crick had used data obtained by others, without their knowledge, when making their monumental discovery.

The reactions of Watson's colleagues to his manuscript varied, but in many cases they were highly critical. In particular Crick's and Wilkins' reactions were strong. Wilkins' copy of the manuscript with all his markings in the margin as well as the summary of his critique expressed in letters to Watson is preserved in the Norman collection at the J. Craig Venter Institute in Rockville, MD. It is a fascinating read. A specific critique to different sections of the text was given on eleven full pages attached to a letter dated July 25, 1966. Amusingly there was a handwritten note on the top of the carbon copy of the letter saying "Juvenile, we know him." Wilkins's letter ended "Concerning Rosalind, is there any mention in your book that she died?" The original critique was followed up by a letter of October 6, sent 11 days later. The first paragraph of this letter ended "It (the book) is, in my opinion, unfair to me, and this has made it more difficult to sort out my thoughts." Later on the letter read "Most top scientists are fairly civilized, but your book, though you may not intend it, would give many people an impression of Francis as a feather-brained hyperthyroid, me as an overgentlemanly mug and you as an immature exhibitionist!" Who said that Wilkins did not have a sense of humor?

The original plan was to have Watson's book published by Harvard University Press. Due to the criticism and the threats of Watson being sued for libel the publisher decided not to go ahead with printing the book — and lost a best-seller. As already mentioned, in the final book Watson added an epilogue in which he partially resurrected Franklin as a scientist.

The Short Life of a Devoted Scientist

On March, 1953 Wilkins wrote to Crick "I think you will be interested to know that our dark lady leaves us next week.... At last the decks are clear and we can put all hands to the pumps!" There is an element of irony in the fact that when this was written, unbeknown to Wilkins, it was all over. The proposed model of the DNA structure was available to be seen by Wilkins on Kendrew's invitation. The expression "The dark lady of DNA" was later used as a subtitle by Brenda Maddox in her book *Rosalind Franklin*, which was published in 2002[25]. This book gives an excellent description of Franklin's life and it provides an opportunity, together with a book published 27 years earlier by Franklin's friend Anne Sayre, to obtain an insight into Franklin's complex personality. Sayre's book was called *Rosalind Franklin and DNA*[26]. Her husband, a crystallographer, had worked in the same laboratory as Franklin in Paris in the late 1940s. Franklin's friendship with the Sayre family developed in connection with travelling to crystallography congresses, such as the one in Stockholm in 1951. In connection with Franklin's two long trips in the US in the mid-1950s she stayed for some time with the Sayre family, who at the time had settled in that country. One purpose of Sayre's book was to give a presentation of Franklin that could serve as a contrast to the less favorable description of her in *The Double Helix*. The course of Franklin's life can briefly be summarized as follows.

The Background

Franklin was born into an affluent and influential British Jewish family in 1920. Already early in her life she showed an excellent scholastic capacity and also an independence of mind, choosing to adopt a non traditional secular attitude to life. She had decided to choose a career as a scientist already at the age of 15 and entered Newnham College, Cambridge in 1938. This was not in the tradition of the Franklin family. Women of that well-to-do family were generally engaged in commendable philanthropic activities. Although not a

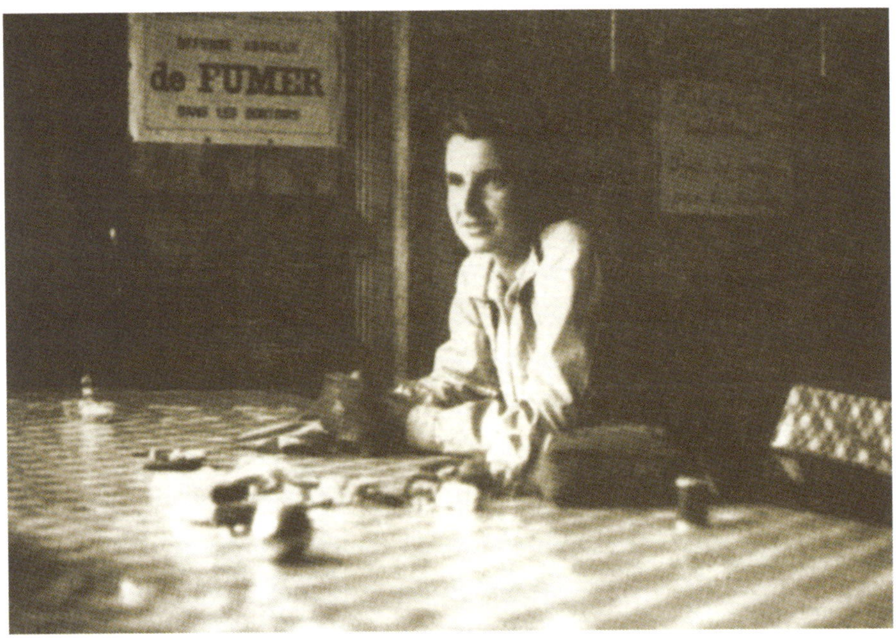

Rosalind Franklin. [Photograph by Vittorio Luzzati in 1950, National Portrait Gallery.]

practicing Jew she remained close to her family.

After three years at Newnham she had produced material equivalent to the requirements for a bachelor's degree. Women were not conferred such degrees in Cambridge until 1947, but at this later time they were awarded retroactively. It might be noted that due to the war, many of the male teachers at the university were absent because of involvement in different kinds of special missions. After graduation Franklin received a research scholarship and worked for one year in the laboratory of Ronald G. W. Norrish, a recipient of the shared 1967 Nobel Prize in Chemistry for his studies of extremely fast chemical reactions, and then at the British Coal Utilisation Research Association (BCURA). This association was formed at the beginning of the war to stimulate nonprofit interactions between industrial companies. Franklin did well at BCURA and was able to present her PhD thesis dealing with organic coal compounds at Cambridge in 1945.

Paris — Good Science and Good Life

Her increasingly expertise on the subject of coal led her to Paris to work at the Laboratoire Central des Services Chimiques de l'Etat. At this laboratory she developed a fruitful collaboration with Jacques Mering, who taught her many aspects of working with amorphous coal-containing substances. She established a particularly warm personal relationship with Vittorio Luzzati, a colleague in the laboratory, and his wife Denise. Franklin had a very productive time in Paris, a city she came to love because of its culture and people. Many scientific publications were produced. Still, she felt that she needed to get back to London to be near her family. She had developed an impressive skill in using X-ray crystallography and therefore she applied to Randall at the MRC's Biophysics Unit at King's College. A Turner and Newall Research Fellowship for three years allowed her to pay her own way. Although it was originally planned for her to work on proteins and lipids in solution, this was changed at the time of her arrival.

From Coal to DNA

Randall realized Franklin's qualities as a crystallographer and set her to work on fibers of DNA. He gave her responsibility for Gosling as a graduate student.

He was the only researcher who previously had been practically involved in crystallographic work at King's College. When in January 1951 Franklin started her work in Randall's laboratory he had given her the impression that she should have independent responsibility for pursuing the DNA project. She had not been informed that the reason Randall had changed the direction of her starting project — Wilkins later argued that it was his idea — was results presented during the preceding year by Wilkins and Gosling. They had obtained markedly improved diffraction pictures of DNA, compared to those originally produced by Astbury. Franklin immediately took the lead in the continued work on the X-ray analysis of DNA. This for obvious reasons led to major frictions with Wilkins, amplified by their markedly different personalities. The sources of the frictions that developed and their consequences have been analyzed at length and many adjectives have been used in describing Wilkins' and Franklin's contrasting personalities. These adjectives will not be repeated here, but it needs simply to be noted that no collaboration between the two was ever established. Suffice to recognize that Franklin successfully managed to further improve markedly the DNA diffraction patterns and in particular to elucidate the importance of two forms of DNA depending on the conditions of humidity. There were what had been called the A and the B forms. The A form was a dryer short and thick structure of the molecule, whereas the wetter B form was long and thin. High quality diffraction patterns were recorded and in the case of the B form there was no question about its helical structure. The famous photograph 51, already alluded to above (p. 316), was a beautiful example of the quality of her work. The photograph was used by Franklin in the *Nature* article by herself and Gosling[13] accompanying the April 1953 original article by Watson and Crick and then reused by Crick just over a year later in his review of the structure of DNA in *Scientific American*, as mentioned. She was proud of this but did not seem to show any regrets.

Randall certainly did not create an environment of propinquity for DNA research at King's College. In order to dampen the rising tensions between Wilkins and Franklin, he stated categorically that Franklin in her continued work should only study the A form, whereas Wilkins should focus on the B form. It was probably Franklin's own choice to continue her struggle with the A form, but one wonders what would have happened if instead she had focused on the B form. Randall's decision prevented Wilkins from making headway, since Franklin was the only one to use the high quality Signer DNA, whereas Wilkins had to satisfy himself with DNA obtained from Chargaff. The latter material turned out to be of inferior quality and it was not useful for Wilkins purposes. His work stalled. One wonders who decided the allocation in the use of available DNA at King's College.

Because of the tensions of the working environment at King's College Franklin decided to leave and she eventually had an offer from Bernal to join him at Birkbeck College. Her original plan was to move there in January 1953, but for various reasons she stayed an additional three months, making her total sojourn at King's College last for 27 months — but what 27 months of human turmoil and scientific creativity!

She Came So Close

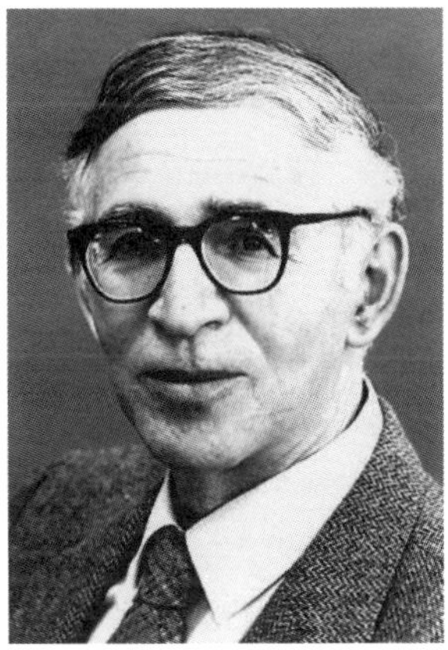

Aaron Klug. [From *Les Prix Nobel en 1982.*]

Thanks to Aaron Klug's careful analyses of Franklin's notebooks and his distillation of her five publications on DNA it is possible to track her stepwise conceptualization of the structure of DNA[27,28]. Klug became Franklin's close collaborator and also her particular friend during the last years of her all too short life. He received a Nobel Prize in chemistry in 1982 "for his development of crystallographic electron microscopy and his structural elucidation of biologically important nucleic acid-protein complexes", as briefly presented in my previous book[16]. When Franklin took over the DNA project her introductory stepping stone was the improved pictures that Gosling and Wilkins had obtained with the oriented fine fibers of the high quality Signer DNA. Her first major contribution was to evaluate carefully the importance of humidity on the structure of DNA. She could demonstrate the change from the crystalline structure A to the wet para-crystalline state B and the reversibility of this change. Already at the start the B form was interpreted to be helical — it showed beautifully in the X-ray diffraction picture what later came to be called the "helical cross" (p. 316) — but there were questions about the number of helices. In March 1953 she favored two helices. Klug had discovered a manuscript dated March 17, the day before she saw the Watson–Crick Model specifying this conclusion. It took minor changes to modify this manuscript to accompany the original Watson and Crick paper in *Nature*. She simply inserted "Thus our general ideas are consistent with the model proposed by Crick and Watson."

Thus, while we do not attempt to offer a complete interpretation of the fibre-diagram of structure B, we may state the following conclusions. The structure is probably helical. The phosphate groups lie on the outside of the structural unit, on a helix of diameter about 20A. The structural unit probably consists of two co-axial molecules which are not equally spaced along the fibre axis, their mutual displacement being such as to account for the variation of observed intensities of the innermost maxima on the layer-lines; if one molecule is displaced from the other by about 3/8 of the fibre-axis period this would account for the absence of the 4th layer-line maxima and the weakness of the 6th. These general ideas are consistent with the model proposed by Crick and Watson.

The conclusion that the phosphate groups lie on the outside of the structural unit has been reached previously by quite other reasoning[1]. Two principal lines of argument were invoked. The first derives from the work of Gulland and his collaborators[6] who showed that even in aqueous solution the -CO and $-NH_2$ groups of the bases are inaccessible and cannot be titrated, whereas the phosphate groups are fully accessible. The second is based on our own observations[1] on the way in which the structural units in structures A and B are progressively separated by an excess of water, the process being a continuous one which leads to the formation first of a gel and ultimately to a solution. The hygroscopic part of the molecule may be presumed to lie in the phosphate groups $(C_2H_5O)_2PO_2Na$ and $(C_3H_7O)_2PO_2Na$ are highly hygroscopic[7] and the simplest explanation of the above process is that these groups lie on the outside of the structural units. Moreover, the ready availability of the phosphate groups for interaction with proteins can most easily be explained in this way.

Acknowledgments

The authors are grateful to Professor J.T. Randall, F.R.S., for his interest and to F.H.C. Crick, A.R. Stokes and M.H.F. Wilkins for discussion.

One of us (R.E.F.) acknowledges the award of a Turner and Newall Fellowship.

References

1. Franklin, R.E. and Gosling, R.G. (in press)
2. Cochran, W., Crick, F.H.C. and Vand, V., Acta Cryst. 5, 501 (1952)
3. Pauling, L., Corey, R.B. and Branson, H.R., Proc. Nat. Acad. Sci. Wash., 37, 205 (1951)
4. Pauling, L., and Corey, R.B., Proc. Nat. Acad. Sci. Wash., 39, 84, (1953)
5. Franklin, R.E. and Gosling, R.G. (To be published)
6. Gulland, J.M. and Jordan, D.O., Cold Spring Harbour Symp.on Quant. Biology., p.5 (1947)

The typed manuscript with an inserted handwritten sentence of Franklin's and Gosling's first publication in *Nature*. [From archives of the J. Craig Venter Institute.]

Throughout the second half of 1952 Franklin's and Gosling's main efforts concerned the A form. Alternative structures were considered and it was not apparent to the researchers what the relationships between the B and the A forms might be. It is regrettable that they did not speculate on the possibility that they were two variants of the same helical structure. Eventually the data obtained were summarized into two manuscripts submitted to *Acta Crystallographica* on March 6, 1953[20,21], i.e. before the Watson–Crick model had become public. The first paper described the identification of the distinct A and B forms, and defined the helical structure of the B form containing, most likely, two helices. Beautiful diffraction pictures were presented. At the time of submitting the manuscripts Franklin had done some model building leading to the conclusion that there were two chains also in the A structure, but their helical structure was not deduced at the time. However, in an often overlooked second publication in *Nature* in 1953[29] it was shown conclusively that the A form too contained two-chain helical molecules. The fifth and last paper in the series published in 1954 provided some supplementary observations on the A structure[30], but Franklin herself was not fully satisfied with this contribution.

Franklin and Gosling had spent many hours well into the late evening making calculations to work out the space group — the shape of the unit cell — in their crystals. In this work the tables of X-ray patterns compiled by Astbury and the female crystallographer Kathleen Lonsdale, mentioned in Chapter 7, were of great importance. It should be noted that at the time no computers were available so Franklin's slide rule was extensively used.

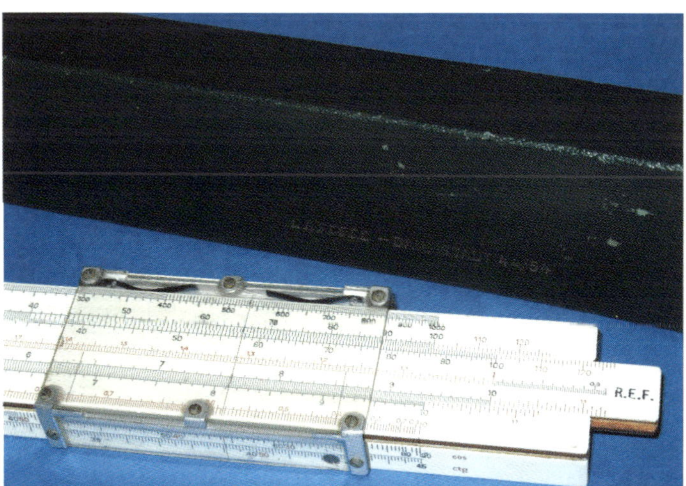

Rosalind Franklin's slide rule with her initials R.E.F.
[From archives of the J. Craig Venter Institute.]

A major limitation in her analyses of the B form was that she did not understand that it belonged in a space group called C2. Importantly this was identified by Crick, but in the case of Franklin, Klug stated: "… she was not enough of a formally trained crystallographer". Because Franklin did not appreciate the C2 characteristics she did not identify the perpendicular dyads, specifying the existence of two anti-parallel helices. She had, however, some indications that this might be the case for form A. If Franklin had known that the B form was anti-parallel, she would have been much closer to the final solution. But there was one more very important conceptual leap to take and this concerned the base pairing. She understood that the phosphates were on the outside and the bases were on the inside connected by hydrogen bonds. She also noted that the two purines or the two pyrimidines were interchangeable within the pairs, but it was a long way from there to recognizing the possibility of the formation of purine-pyrimidine pairs. The Chargaff ratios were recorded in her notebooks but to take the final step would have required access to the proper tautomeric forms of bases, which she did not have. And finally, she was not a biologist and one may ask without ever being able to find the answer to what extent she might have reflected on the chemistry of the gene and the information storage problem.

The Attraction of Virus Structures

When Franklin moved to Birkbeck College she was forbidden by Randall to continue working on DNA. Being a devoted scientist of high integrity Franklin of course did not follow this edict. She kept in contact with Gosling and mentored him throughout his whole thesis work. Once settled in at Birkbeck, Franklin started what came to develop into a pioneering work on TMV.

Contradicting leading virologists in the field, she claimed in print that TMV particles had a uniform length. Arguing for this she contested the main authority in the field, Norman W. Pirie. Together with Frederick C. Bawden he had made the important finding in 1936 that TMV contained a substantial amount of RNA[16]. Pirie not only believed that the TMV particles could have varying lengths, but also that its nucleic acid only had some subordinate importance. One might say that he acted like a Caspersson of virology, because he hesitated to the last moment to accept that the nucleic acid played some major role. When Crick asked him point blank at a meeting in the mid-1950s if he believed that the TMV protein was infectious, he hedged and referred to some possible interaction between the protein and the nucleic acid. Such an answer was probably representative of the attitude of many scientists at the time.

Franklin managed to get high quality X-ray photographs of TMV and when, sometime after her arrival at Birkbeck College, she showed these to Klug "his fate was sealed" according to his own words[31]. The work on TMV developed in an excellent way and additional scientists were brought into the group. Franklin rapidly became a world authority in the field and established a number of important international collaborations. They included Fraenkel-Conrat and Schramm and their co-workers. Her influential role in studies of TMV can be seen from the Nobel review on Fraenkel-Conrat, Gierer and Schramm that Gard wrote in 1960. He stated:

> Finally Rosalind Franklin (two references from 1957 and 1958) by use of X-ray crystallographic and absorption measurements could give an in all probability most definite and exact picture of the structure of the virus particle. According to her the particle represents a hollow cylinder in the form of a double helix, in which an uninterrupted chain of nucleic acid is embedded in a protein helix; in every turn of this there are 16⅓ protein units. The inner and outer diameters are 20 Å and 75 Å, respectively, and the nucleic acid spiral is located at the axis distance of 40 Å.

At this time Franklin knew how to resolve helical structures! It was an important discovery that the nucleic acid was not located in isolation in the center of the rod-like particle but embedded in its protein structure. The work

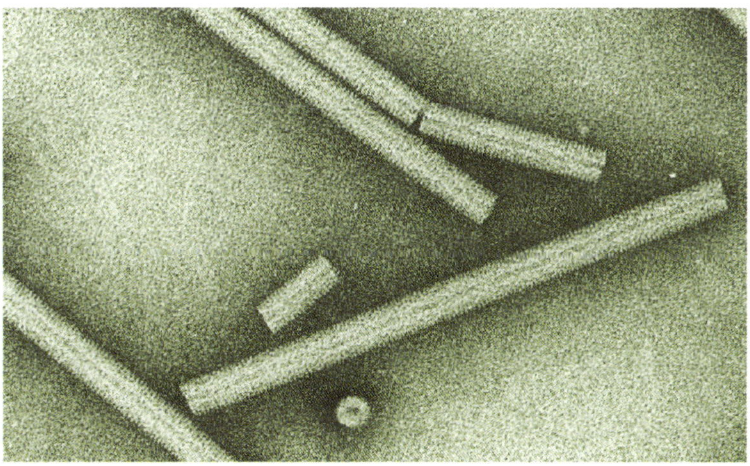

Electron microscopic picture of TMV. [From Ref. 52.]

was performed in collaboration with an American scientist Don Caspar, who together with Klug and others contributed in an important way to Franklin's advances in her work on TMV. As discussed above, the Nobel committees regarded Gierer's and Schramm's discovery of the fully infectious nature of RNA isolated from TMV as a major achievement. It was an important extension of Avery's uniquely pioneering discovery. Had their discovery been selected for a prize, one could speculate about also including Franklin, in a contra factual perspective, in such a prize.

Because the money for the research group that Franklin built at Birkbeck College originally came from the Agricultural Research Council (ARC) it was referred to as the ARC group at Birkbeck. Later on she also received money from the US. Bragg respected the advances she had made in her research and helped her to receive support for her work and also invited her to submit models of the viruses she was studying at an International Exhibition in Brussels in 1958. In a letter of June 1956, extending the invitation to her, Bragg wrote "My young people were much impressed by your models when I showed them in my lectures recently." Her scientific life was up and running. Her research group started to develop their work to also include studies of spherical plant viruses. In mid-1957 she also initiated a collaborative project to examine the fine structure of poliovirus, a spherical animal virus. She received an offer of virus material from Berkeley and for safety reasons the samples, when they had arrived, were stored at the neighboring London School of Hygiene and Tropical Medicine. Franklin never got an opportunity to start generating data and one wonders how far she might have taken this project. Klug managed to obtain some preliminary structural data[32], but it was not until the beginning of the early 1980s that the molecular structures of the capsid proteins of poliovirus were eventually described[33]. At that time the technology for ultrastructural studies by X-ray crystallography had advanced enormously and the computer power to resolve complicated structures had been amplified many times over.

International Contacts

Franklin loved travelling and the developments of her science gave her several opportunities to meet colleagues abroad at conferences or at seminars. In June 1951 she travelled to Stockholm to participate in the Second International Conference of Crystallography. On her way to Stockholm she shared a ship's cabin with the foremost female crystallographer, Hodgkin. Sadly the latter was severely seasick and the opportunities for developing a deeper contact were missed. However, they were to meet on a number of occasions later. A particular situation developed when Franklin had received her first clear diffraction pictures of DNA. She took some selected photographs to Oxford to show Hodgkin, who praised their high quality.

Crystals are classified by their symmetry expressed as space groups determined by their unit cell, as already mentioned, and Franklin had concluded that her pictures might be interpreted as one of three space groups. Hodgkin pointed out that only one of these could be the correct one since the two other had to be excluded for reasons that Franklin had overlooked. Dunitz, who was also present, then explained to Franklin why the right- and left-handedness of the sugars limited the number of alternatives to one. She was constantly learning how to become a fully-fledged crystallographer.

At the Stockholm conference Franklin was able to listen to Pauling who provided the fresh data on the alpha-helix structure that he had just discovered and also to Bernal who gave a speculative lecture on the possibilities in applying X-ray diffraction analysis to complex protein structures. Gradually Franklin became acquainted with biological problems. She also had an opportunity

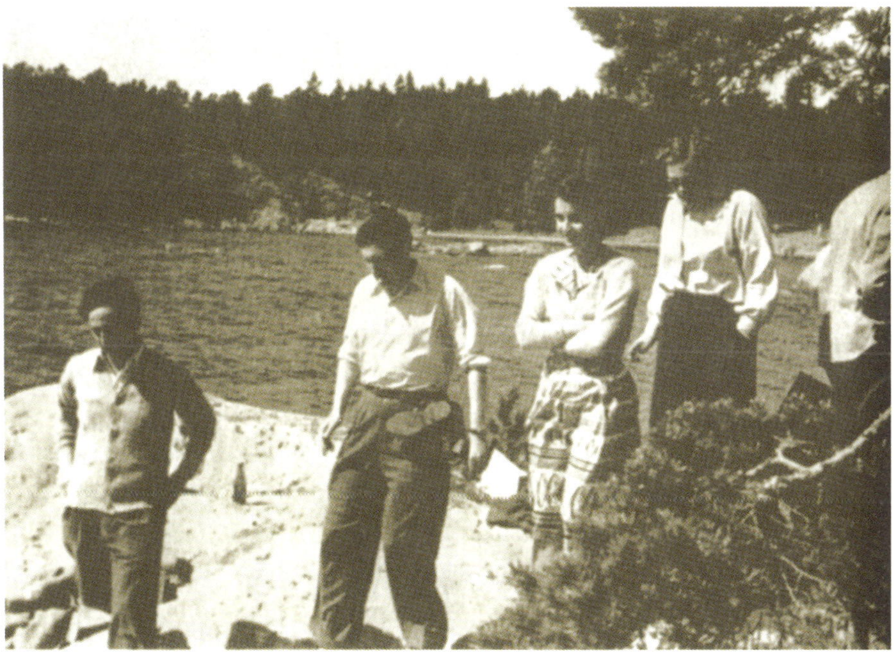

Rosalind Franklin in the Stockholm archipelago on the occasion of the 1951 International Union of Crystallography conference in 1951. [From American Society for Microbiology Archives, Anne Sayre Collection of Rosalind Franklin materials.]

to meet her good friends Luzzati and the Sayres in an outing in the beautiful archipelago of Stockholm.

It was the authority she had developed in her coal research, and not her contribution to DNA research that brought her on her first travel to the US in 1954. She was invited to participate in a Gordon Research Conference in New Hampshire in a session on coals and related substances. She extended her stay and managed also to visit many other places on the American east coast. In Boston she was hosted by Rich and his wife. They generously arranged for her to stay with Mrs Rich's mother. This kind of arrangement is not uncommon among fellow scientists. There often develops a special camaraderie among them. The scientists are driven by their curiosity and obsession and meet colleagues who share this attitude. The exchange of professional ideas frequently develops into a friendship including various aspects of the private spheres of life. Thus it is rather common, in particular in the US and Canada that a visiting scientist is invited into the homes of the host scientist, where there is an opportunity to meet the members of the family. Such encounters then frequently develop into shared enjoyments of non-professional activities too, like active or passive sporting or cultural pursuits. The contacts may evolve into a special friendship between selected scientists. From this perspective their often very demanding work can be seen as a vocation. Franklin, although described as a person not to be readily approached, encountered many examples of the richness of the camaraderie of science during her travels. In the final paragraph of what was probably her last handwritten letter in life Franklin wrote on March 16, 1958 to Caspar "I certainly hope to see your mother and sister when they are over here — let me know when to expect them."

She also had an opportunity to visit California during her first US trip, to a considerable extent thanks to efforts by Watson and Crick. In fact Watson, whom she met at Woods Hole, even offered to let her join him and Brenner in travelling across the US by car, but her schedule did not allow her to accept this offer. She had many interesting contacts throughout the country and visits on the west coast included Pauling at Caltech and Stanley and Fraenkel-Conrat in Berkeley. The latter contact was important for the future TMV work. She wrote weekly letters to her parents. These letters show a very curious and inquisitive visitor first somewhat skeptical about her experiences in general and about her new country, but gradually becoming more enthusiastic and impressed not least by the academic environments she encountered. There is a touch of Alexis de Tocqueville in the reflections contained in her correspondence.

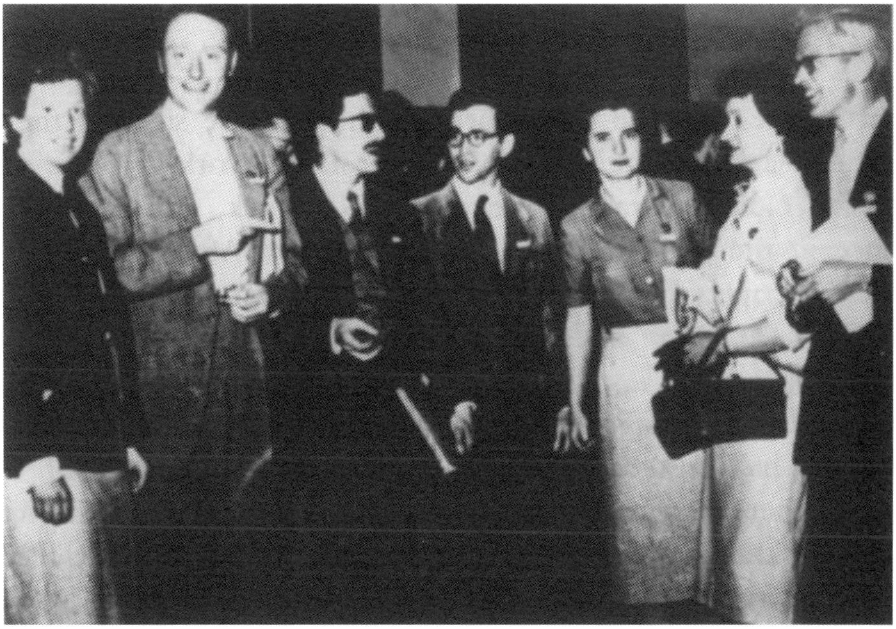

Rosalind Franklin at the International Union of Crystallography symposium in Madrid 1956. [Courtesy of Dr D. L. D. Caspar.]

By 1956 her work had developed to the point where she was able to report new data from her group at a number of conferences. In London she joined in a Ciba Foundation meeting on "The biophysics and biochemistry of viruses". She was the only female participant. A few weeks later she travelled to Spain. Previously she had avoided meetings in Spain out of contempt for the Franco regime, but this time the high caliber of the meeting overrode her antipathies. Full of confidence in her science and among many good friends she enjoyed life. The picture illustrates Franklin in a group with Ann Kennedy (*née* Cullis), another female crystallographer working with Perutz, Crick, Caspar, Klug, Franklin, Odile Crick and Kendrew. Franklin's life was at a zenith and she joined the Crick family for a tour of southern Spain after the meeting.

Later in 1956 she was able to make her second trip to the US By this time her reputation had grown and there was no problem in finding travel money. The Rockefeller Foundation was willing to pay her way not only to a Gordon Conference on nucleic acids but also to tour American laboratories afterwards. She had a productive and enjoyable time on both the east and the west coast of the US, again carefully and regularly reporting her experiences and impressions to her parents. During her trip she had the pleasure of revisiting many laboratories in California. Among other places she gave a seminar at Caltech. In connection with this visit she enjoyed immensely an invitation from Dulbecco (see Chapter 3) and some friends of his to visit Mount Whitney, the highest peak in the US outside Alaska. The outing, involving climbing to a high plateau of the mountain and to staying overnight in a tent, was very much to her liking. This was the world she loved, good science and friendship in challenging outdoor settings.

During the last week of her trip, before departing for home from the US east coast, she noticed some trouble in zipping up her skirt. She needed to see a doctor, but postponed this until she had arrived back in England.

The Tragic End

Just as Franklin's scientific work was accelerating and she felt a harmony in her research, clouds started to mount in the sky. She had always had excellent health and was an outdoor person, who relished mountain climbing. However, during the extended business trip in the US in 1956 she noticed the first symptoms of an impending illness, as mentioned. An operation in September the same year revealed two tumors in her abdomen originating from one of the ovaries. The tumors were removed but the relentless nature of the cancer soon became apparent. She managed her disease in a courageous and stoic way. She kept her concerns to herself and continued with focus and discipline to manage her high quality scientific work. As mentioned previously, Crick and his wife opened their home for her during parts of her convalescence. Watson too showed his empathy. In a short letter of November 13, 1956 to Klug he expressed — in a surprisingly legible handwriting — "I have heard that Rosalind (not Rosie, my remark) was not well and I hope that she recovers soon. Please convey to her my best wishes." And towards the end he repeated his concerns "With best wishes to your wife and again my wishes for Rosalind's speedy recovery."

Rosalind's group published seven papers in 1956 and six more in 1957. In January 1958 Franklin for the first time in her life obtained a career academic position as Research Associate in Biophysics. In a typed business letter of March 25, 1958 she thanked a Dr Leonard Karel at the National Institute of Allergy and Infectious Diseases for his approval of a request to use a part of her research grant to support a trip by herself and Klug to the Congress of Biochemistry in Vienna in September. She would never get there since she died on April 16. A few of her papers were published posthumously.

Classification of Viruses

The work on viruses that Franklin pursued during the short time allotted her at Birkbeck was to have major consequences for the development of virology in general. Already during her leadership of the group its work had expanded to include not only rod-shaped but also spherical viruses. Some years after her death Klug and his collaborators John Finch and Kenneth Holmes, originally a graduate student supervised by Franklin, in 1962 moved to the Laboratory of Molecular Biology in Cambridge, where the discovery of DNA had taken place nine years earlier. In the same year Caspar and Klug published what came to be the breakthrough paper on the principles of virus structure and the symmetries that regulate this[34]. This paper which became a citation classic in fact built on the theoretical work that Crick and Watson published in 1956[24]. Since this work was also reviewed by Westgren in 1960 it is worth revisiting.

In the joint 1956 publication Watson and Crick had made some very prophetic predictions concerning the symmetry of virus particles. They postulated that the shell surrounding the genetic material of virus particles was constructed by one or more identical protein subunits. These subunits were proposed to be arranged in a helical fashion in elongated particles and by some kind of cubic symmetry aggregation in "spherical" particles. The Platonic

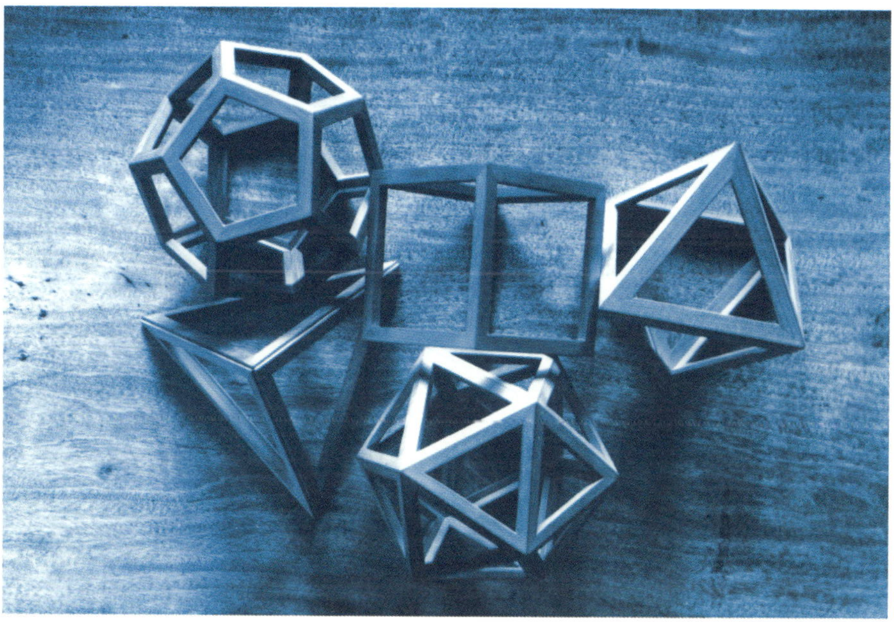

Models of the five Platonic bodies.

bodies are examples of regular three-dimensional building arrangements using cubic symmetry. There are five kinds of such bodies displaying different number of facets; the tetraeder — 4, the cube — 6, the octaeder — 8, the dodecaeder — 12 and the icosaeder — 20. The icosaeder is the symmetrical structure which most closely resembles the sphere, providing the largest possible volume for the surface material used. The numbers of building stones in an icosaheder may vary extensively and they can also be of many different kinds. However they always represent a multiple of 60. It has since been discovered that all spherical viruses use some kind of icosahedral symmetry employing varying numbers of one or more building stones. For example an adenovirus particle has a shell — a *capsid* — containing 252 morphological units, the *capsomeres*.

During the more than 50 years that have passed since the original publication of Watson's and Crick's predictions of virus structure it has been possible to reveal a remarkably detailed three-dimensional structure of the three surface building stones — different proteins — and their interaction in this virus by use of X-ray crystallography. There are 240 non-vertex capsomeres each one built by three proteins — not six as could also have been an alternative. At the 12 corners there are complexes of five proteins. Finally there are projections extending from the corner complexes. I discovered these

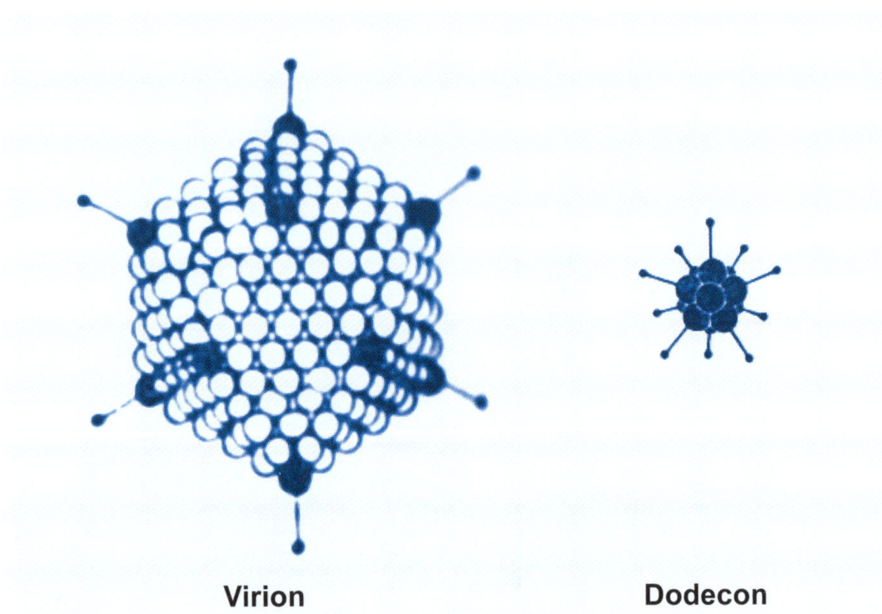

Schematic presentation of an adenovirus particle and of a separate hemagglutinin formed by 12 vertex capsomers carrying projections.

so-called *fibers* in 1965[35] because the vertex capsomers could form a separate particle, the dodecon, and in the electron microscope the short projections were readily visible in this small structure. These structures had not been observed previously in the much larger intact virus particle of the type of adenovirus studied. Simultaneously a much longer kind of fibers were also discovered in studies of another type of adenovirus by Helio Pereira and Robin Valentine at the National Institute of Medical Research at Mill Hill, London. It is not uncommon that discoveries unknowingly are made simultaneously in two different laboratories. The time may have become right for their fulfillment. Later crystallographic studies of the fibers have demonstrated that they are trimers of a specific protein. The total number of building stones in the adenovirus capsid, not including the fibers thus is $240 \times 3 + 12 \times 5$, an even multiple of 60 as predicted by Watson and Crick.

In the classical 1962 follow-up publication by Caspar and Klug the concept of icosahedral symmetry was expanded further[34]. With reference to Buckminster Fuller's geodetic dome designs they elaborated on the theme of construction of spherical shells for viruses and they also deduced the mathematical rules for a series of structures using an increasing number of capsomers. In addition they were able to define possibilities for skewed arrangement of surface components providing some sufficiently stable quasi-equivalent icosahedral capsids protecting the internal nucleic acid.

Watson's and Crick's original identification of principles for the structure of virus particles as well as Caspar's and Klug's further extensions of these principles were to have a major impact. It was decided to derive a system for classification of viruses by use of the structural characteristics of virus particles. Although this system, like the Linnaean system for classification of plants, was not a genetically based system it has served its purpose well. It was codified by the establishment of the International Committee on Nomenclature of Viruses in Moscow in 1966, a name later modified to the International Committee on Taxonomy of Viruses (ICTV). The hierarchical classification employs the levels Orders, Families (Subfamilies), Genera and Species. The definition of a species has since a long time been a matter of controversy, but in 1991 virologists agreed on a pragmatic way of describing a species. In this definition reference is made to the concept "polythetic class" meaning that the definition uses more than one property and that no single property is essential or necessary.

In 2011 ICTV published its ninth report[36] which listed 2,284 virus species distributed amongst 349 genera, 19 subfamilies, 87 families and 6 orders — and the numbers are growing fast. In spite of the expanding efforts of ICTV to recognize and classify viruses it is still only scratching the surface of the problem of achieving a total inventory of all viruses present in nature. Viruses are ubiquitous and as emphasized earlier[16], wherever there are cells there are viruses. Water in oceans and lakes contains 10 million virus particles per milliliter which multiplied with their total volume gives a total number of virus particle of 10^{24}, ten times more than the stars in the universe! At present the number of different species they may represent is anyone's guess.

It is now high time to get back to the structure of DNA and the possible third ticket besides Watson and Crick, for the 1962 Nobel Prize in physiology or medicine.

Wilkins or Franklin?

Since Franklin died untimely in 1958 she was never nominated for a Nobel Prize and hence never directly discussed as a potential candidate. As mentioned the first nominations for the discovery of the structure of DNA were not submitted until 1960. Let me, nevertheless, discuss hypothetically what might have happened if Franklin would had been alive in 1962. Since the maximum number of prize recipients is limited to three, the committees would have had to make a choice between Wilkins, Franklin or neither of the two. As can be seen from Table 8.1 (p.333) the majority — nine — nominations only proposed Watson and Crick, the two who have their name on the critical *Nature* paper, but there were five nominations that also included Wilkins. One of them was the critical nomination by Bragg.

Bragg if anyone should have had a good insight into the sequence of events and the role of different actors in the discovery. He of course knew that Watson and Crick would never had found the final solution if they had not had access to information from the scientists at King's College. It was this information that told them that the scaffold of the molecule most likely was an anti-parallel double helix. Bragg also knew that there was a gentlemen's agreement that DNA work should not be pursued at the Cavendish laboratory and he had specifically banned Watson and Crick from pursuing their DNA work after their first failed attempt. However, when he read the manuscript from Pauling describing another failed attempt to conjecture the structure he released the moratorium. He motivated his behavior in the Foreword to Watson's book as already cited. This citation concluded "… there is no need to hold back." After this the text continued "This dilemma comes out clearly in the DNA story. It is a source of deep satisfaction to all intimately concerned that, in the award of the Nobel prize in 1962, due recognition was given to the long, patient investigation by Wilkins at King's College (London) as well as to the brilliant and rapid final solution by Crick and Watson at Cambridge."

The motivation for including Wilkins in Bragg's nomination for a prize in chemistry submitted in 1960, eight years before he wrote the Foreword to *The Double Helix* ran as follows:

> The very thorough analysis of the fine diffraction pictures of DNA obtained by Wilkins and his collaborators at King's College, London, refined and somewhat modified their (Watson's and Crick's, my remark) structure, while amply confirming its general correctness.

Is this a sufficient motivation for a Nobel Prize? A prize in physiology or medicine can only be given for a discovery and the question is which discovery did Wilkins make? Furthermore in the case of multiple prize recipients the unofficial rule is that each recipient shall be qualified enough to carry the prize on his own. Since Franklin's data were crucial to the discovery, one additional question concerns why Bragg did not mention her significant contributions. According to his biographer[37] it could simply be that he was not well informed about the major conflicts between scientists pursuing the critical X-ray studies of DNA at King's College. He might well have been unwilling to listen to gossip and slander involving scientists in that environment. To Bragg there might have been no conflict in talking about Wilkins' collaborators as a homogenous group. By including Wilkins he satisfied his and the Cavendish Laboratory's bad conscience about the fact that Watson's and Crick's immense breakthrough was only possible because they had access to data from King's College. But his conscience should primarily have bothered him regarding data accessed *prior* to the discovery and not Wilkins's follow-up studies mentioned in his nomination. It could be added that during the mid-1950s Bragg had closer contacts with Franklin and helped and encouraged her work at Birkbeck College. It is also clear that at that time he had developed a considerable respect for her as a scientist, as mentioned.

Wilkins was included in the extensive nomination by Monod in 1962. When Monod received the invitation to nominate for a Nobel Prize in chemistry for this year he contacted Crick. It was Crick who in his letter of response advised him to include Wilkins in the nomination. Monod properly cited the two papers in *Nature* by Watson and Crick and the three supporting papers, the one by Wilkins *et al.* and the two by Franklin and Gosling. Two pages later in his long motivation he made a plea for Wilkins, as follows:

> It is sometimes believed that the helical structure for DNA, proposed by Pauling and Corey, was the origin of the assumption that DNA is helical. Actually, to my knowledge, this is not so. The first person to realize that DNA was probably helical appears to have been Wilkins, and the work by Cochran, Crick and Vand (1952) (reference x) where the general formula for the diffraction of helical structures was worked out, was indeed, in part, a result of his suggestions. It would be more correct to say that the remarkable success of Pauling and Corey in solving the protein alpha-helix was a great incentive to pursue along similar general lines, and that the tactics followed by Pauling and Corey in this work was an object-lesson which greatly helped Watson and Crick, as clearly acknowledged by Crick himself (1954 (reference)).
>
> To summarize: there appears to be no doubt, and indeed there has never been any dispute about it, that the double-helix (duplex) base-paired structure of DNA was a profoundly original and novel theoretical discovery based upon, and justified by, the experimental (X-ray) work of Wilkins and his associates.

This reminds me of Winston Churchill's note in the margin of the notes to one of his speeches — "weak point, shout." Apparently Monod was not well informed about developments of DNA diffraction studies at King's College and of Franklin's central role in them. It should be recalled that it was when Wilkins showed Franklin's diffraction picture of the B form of DNA that Watson's clock started to tick.

Wilkins had several opportunities to make his research known to members of the Nobel Committees. Tiselius mentioned in his review in 1962 that Wilkins had been in Stockholm in September 1960 to give a lecture in a symposium on "Biological structure and function" and it is also appears that he participated in the First Biophysics Conference in Stockholm arranged by Engström in 1961. In addition he had several contacts with Engström over the years. One can only speculate on the possible importance of these personal contacts between a critical candidate and his judges in the committees. Wilkins certainly could blow his own trumpet. It is also likely that Bragg had several contacts with critical persons in the committees, like Tiselius, for many years (see previous chapter).

It is striking that Tiselius in his 1962 review never mentioned Franklin. By way of contrast the crystallographer Westgren gave a much more balanced perspective in his 1960 review. He correctly stated that it was Franklin who clarified the distinguishing characteristics of the two important forms of DNA, A and B. She described how they were related and the importance of relative moisture. In his summary Westgren referred to the Watson–Crick model as a hypothesis and recommended that someone contributing critical experimental data should be included. He mentioned Wilkins, Franklin and Gosling as names to discuss. Franklin's role as mentor of Gosling was noted. Finally, to repeat, taking into consideration that Franklin was dead he stated "If she had still been alive, she might well have had claims on receiving her fair part of a prize."

To this could be added that it is only during more recent times that reviewers of Nobel Prize candidates are requested to declare their challengeability. Before this, it has been the responsibility of a selected reviewer to use their own conscience to decide whether they might be disqualified from evaluating a particular colleague, because they know him too well. In my opinion this has generally worked very well, perhaps due to the particular ethics prevailing in a small previously Lutheran, now secularized, country in the far corner of Europe. Everyone involved in the work of committees is well aware of the seriousness of their responsibility. They strive, as far as is possible within the framework of an individual human being, to the uttermost to be objective in their evaluations. Still there is a great value in continuous discussions of the pristine nature and objectivity of Nobel Prize reviews.

As we shall see, Wilkins was the only prize recipient who spoke about DNA in his Nobel lecture[38]. One wonders what his feelings were on this occasion and later, since after all he remained the eternal third man. He presented his perspective of the development of the X-ray crystallography studies of DNA. One would expect that being in an exalted situation he would have shown a magnanimous and generous attitude. However all he said was simply "Rosalind Franklin (who died some years later at the peak of her career) made valuable contributions to the X ray analysis". In the acknowledgment he added: "my late colleague Rosalind Franklin who, with great ability and experience of X-ray diffraction, so much helped the initial investigations of DNA." Of course winners take all and they also write the history. But in this case history caught up with the unfair overemphasis on Wilkins' work and the underrating of Franklin's important contributions. A few years later Randall wrote to Gosling "I have always felt that Maurice's Nobel lecture did rather less than justice to this setting (Randall's biophysics laboratory at King's College) and particularly to the contribution of yourself and Rosalind." Some 20 years later the tone was different. Klug stated in his Nobel lecture[39]:

> In seeking to understand how proteins and nucleic acids interact, one has to begin with a particular problem, and I can claim no credit for the choice of my first subject, tobacco mosaic virus. It was the late Rosalind Franklin who introduced me to the study of viruses and whom I was lucky to meet when I joined J. D. Bernal's department in London in 1954. She had just switched from studying DNA to tobacco mosaic virus, X-ray studies of which had been begun by Bernal in 1936. It was Rosalind Franklin who set me the example of tackling large and difficult problems. Had her life not been cut tragically short, *she might well have stood in this place on an earlier occasion* (my italics).

Finally parts of a paragraph of Engström's presentation of the three prize recipients at the ceremony in the Concert Hall of Stockholm deserve to be mentioned in this context[40]. It read:

> Wilkins' X-ray crystallographic recordings indicated that the very long molecular chains of deoxyribonucleic acid were arranged in the form of a double helix. Watson and Crick showed that the organic bases were paired in a specific manner in the two intertwined helices and showed the importance of this arrangement.

In hindsight, this appears to be a rather subjective interpretation of history. Franklin of course was not mentioned in his speech.

In my mind there is no question about the fact that if the Nobel committees in a contra factual situation had had to make a choice between Wilkins and Franklin, they should have chosen Franklin. It was Franklin's progress in her work in 1952 which gave the high quality data that kicked off the process leading to a speedy discovery of the structure of DNA. Thus it is very tempting to make a plea for Franklin in a hypothetical situation of having to choose between her and Wilkins. However, more penetrating reading of critical archive material turned out to temper this temptation. The rich and important material of the Norman Collection at the archives of the J. Craig Venter Institute provided a widening of insights.

Crick and Klug Discuss Franklin's Qualifications as a Scientist

In September 1979 Crick published an article entitled *How to live with a golden helix*[41]. On this occasion it was Crick's turn to be harsh in his description of Franklin. One wonders what the basis for his reaction might have been. Could it have been the current attempts to describe Franklin as a victim of her time and conditions of work? He was obviously concerned about the iconogenetic initiatives to make her a hero for improper reasons, including references to her sex. Crick started with a speculative but completely unfounded comment on the importance of her family background:

> The major opposition Rosalind Franklin had to cope with was not from King's College, London (an Anglican foundation, it should be noted, and therefore inherently biased against women), but from her affluent, educated and sympathetic family who felt that scientific research was not the proper thing for a normal girl.

He then continued:

> Rosalind's difficulties and her failures were mainly of her own making. Underneath her brisk manner she was oversensitive and, ironically, too determined to be scientifically sound and to avoid shortcuts. She was rather too set on succeeding all by herself and rather too stubborn to accept advice easily from others when it ran counter to her own ideas. She was proffered help but she would not take it.

Not unexpectedly this description elicited criticism. One strong reaction came from Charlotte Friend, a famous tumor virus researcher at the Mount Sinai Medical Center, New York. She expressed criticism in particular of the expression "too determined to be scientifically sound". In his response to her Crick tried to explain what he had meant by his formulation and he added "Rosalind would have been the first person to object to this misguided movement to make her a martyr."

The discussion of Franklin's research personality was continued by an exchange of letters between Crick and Klug. The seriousness of the matter is apparent from the fact that the letters are marked "Not for publication". Still one can extract from the discussion a certain agreement between the two on the strength and weaknesses of Franklin's research personality. She was a first rate scientist, but not of the class of Eigen, Bragg or Pauling or for that matter Hodgkin. She was also an excellent experimentalist and a good analyst, better than average in her processing of theoretical crystallography data. To this should be added that she was a cautious kind of scientist, although she could take risks by tackling larger and difficult problems. However, the problem of determining the structure of DNA was given to her by others. On the critical side it was also agreed that she to a certain degree lacked flexibility and in addition possibly was not highly imaginative. She did not take inductive leaps. Instead she wanted to have all data available before she started model building. But science is not always from design and planning. Instead there is a considerable room for maximum tinkering and for recognizing opportunities as they arise and this was Watson's and Crick's, but not Franklin's strength. As a truism it can be noted in conclusion that personalities of all human beings are a composite of strengths and weaknesses, and obviously this applies also to Watson, Crick and Franklin as well as to all the rest of us.

When it comes to the issue of being a female scientist it is worth noting that the field of crystallography developed to a considerable extent because of qualified contributions by women. In the previous chapter we met Lonsdale, who together with Astbury was one of the pioneers in the field and the first woman to be elected to the Royal Society. We also met in addition Hodgkin, perhaps the most impressive scientist of them all, Oughton and Cullis (Kennedy). Both Bernal and Randall had a very positive attitude towards engaging female scientists. For a period 8 out of 31 scientists in Randall's group were women.

It should be noted that Crick and in particular Klug were among Franklin's best friends. Crick and his wife Odile were very hospitable towards Franklin, not the least during phases of her severe illness, as mentioned. She stayed with them for many weeks, but she was even closer to the Klug family. Aaron Klug was the primary beneficiary of her will of December 2, 1957.

Following the exchange of thoughts on Franklin's performance with Klug, Crick wrote a letter to the editor of the journal The Sciences in October 1979. He wanted to explain the meaning of his sentence "She was … too determined to be scientifically sound and to avoid short cuts." He specified that he meant that "she was determined to follow a conservative, X-ray analytical course and not allow other considerations to enter," but he *did not intend to express* that her approach was *not scientifically sound*. It is not known to me if the journal published Crick's supplementary comments.

Three or Two?

Although the committees acted in good faith it is apparent that Wilkins became included as a token to satisfy the guilt felt by the Cavendish group towards that at King's College. The honorable British tradition of gentlemanly behavior looms in the background. It was a considerable relief to Bragg and to Watson and Crick when they learned that he was included, but is guilt resolution a sound base for a Nobel Prize? As mentioned there is a rule in the Nobel work which says that if there are several prize recipients, each one of them should be capable of carrying the prize on his own. It is a good rule even though it may not have been applied categorically. In a comparison between Wilkins and Franklin it was concluded above that Franklin was clearly the stronger candidate, but would it have been appropriate to have included her had she been alive at the time of the prize? Could she have carried the prize on her own?

It is very easy to build up a considerable sympathy for this brave woman. Like a heroine in a Greek tragedy Franklin's personality seems to have contained an impressive number of contradictory qualifications which became apparent during her too short life, but probably also many others that her reserved and very private nature may not have allowed the identification of. She had a brilliant mind and also a remarkable manual dexterity displayed when solving practical technical problems connected to the devices used to collect X-ray diffraction data. She was also very focused and energetic. This strong-willed and uncompromising scientist managed to leave her mark in whichever field of science she embarked on. Her carbon studies in the late 1940s were pioneering and when entering the field of biophysics she excelled in her DNA studies and in her studies of virus structure. A paragraph in the obituary in *The Times* read:

> Her life is an example of single-minded devotion to scientific research. A woman of great intelligence and wide culture, her main interest lay in discovering the evermore complex and significant patterns underlying the processes of nature. In this pursuit she was above all personal considerations and ambitions, she never sought or missed academic honours. Reserved in her relations with her colleagues outside her own circle she was not as well-known as a person as she should have been and inspired more respect than familiarity.

Klug who has played a major role in securing Franklin her proper place in the history of science finished a eulogy of her with a quote. The citation was taken from Samuel Johnson's epitaph on Oliver Goldsmith, a famous 18th century Anglo-Irish writer. It read:

> Olivarii Goldsmith, Poetae, Physici, Historici, Que nullum fere scribendi genus non tetigit —Nullum quod tetigit non ornavit

The latter part of the citation means in translation, *What she touched she adorned.* These are beautiful words coming from a person who had excellent prerequisites to judge her scientific greatness. Thus it is no doubt very tempting to conjecture an association of Franklin and the two discoverers of the double helix, Watson and Crick, for a Nobel Prize, had she been alive. But I think this would have been wrong and I do not believe that she, being a woman of principles, would have accepted this. It should be noted that the majority of nominators naturally recommended only Watson and Crick. There were a few nominators with a personal direct or indirect appreciation of the guilt that the MRC group at Cavendish Laboratories felt towards the MRC group at King's College in the case of DNA studies, that also nominated Wilkins.

Disregarding this aspect of the matters it is easy to argue for a prize only to Watson and Crick. What is wrong in using data of others and re-interpreting them in a visionary and unanticipated way leading to a new insight of paradigmatic proportions? No one has denied that they had an absolute reliance on the indispensable but solitary information from Donohue, but there was no suggestion to include him as a co-author. Furthermore no one has denied that they were categorically dependent on the pictures and calculations by the group at King's college, but this group at the time did not have the final synthesis within reach. The openness of scientific pursuit is very important but one wonders how categorically Sayre's formulation "candor is the chastity of scientists" in her book about Franklin[26] should be applied.

The Watson and Crick "hypothesis" did not only give the basically correct structure of the scaffolding parts of the molecule, the anti-parallel helical strands kept together by hydrogen bonds between the mutually complementary nucleotide bases. It also gave a dramatic insight into how the molecule might serve as a carrier of information, the language of life, and how it might replicate. It would have sufficed many times over to refer to the central discovery that concerned base paring to justify a prize to them alone. Base pairing was the Gordian knot to cut. It was after all the largest discovery in biology or probably also in science in general in the 20th century.

A metaphorical parallel can be drawn with the search for the correct structure of DNA. In the end it turned out that all triple helix models were wrong. The correct structure was a double helix — one strand Watson and one strand Crick.

Days of Festivities in December 1962

It was a colorful gathering of Nobel Prize recipients that met in Stockholm in the dark December of 1962 (Chapter 7, p. 298). The recipient of the prize in physics Lev D. Landau, could not be present in person because of a serious car accident. The two protein crystallographers Perutz and Kendrew, who had pioneered a foray into resolving large and convoluted molecular structures; the discoverers of the DNA structure, Watson and Crick, who had aimed high and to the surprise of the scientific community found the most remarkable molecule of life, and Wilkins providing X-ray crystallographic information confirming, in essence, the correctness of the proposed double

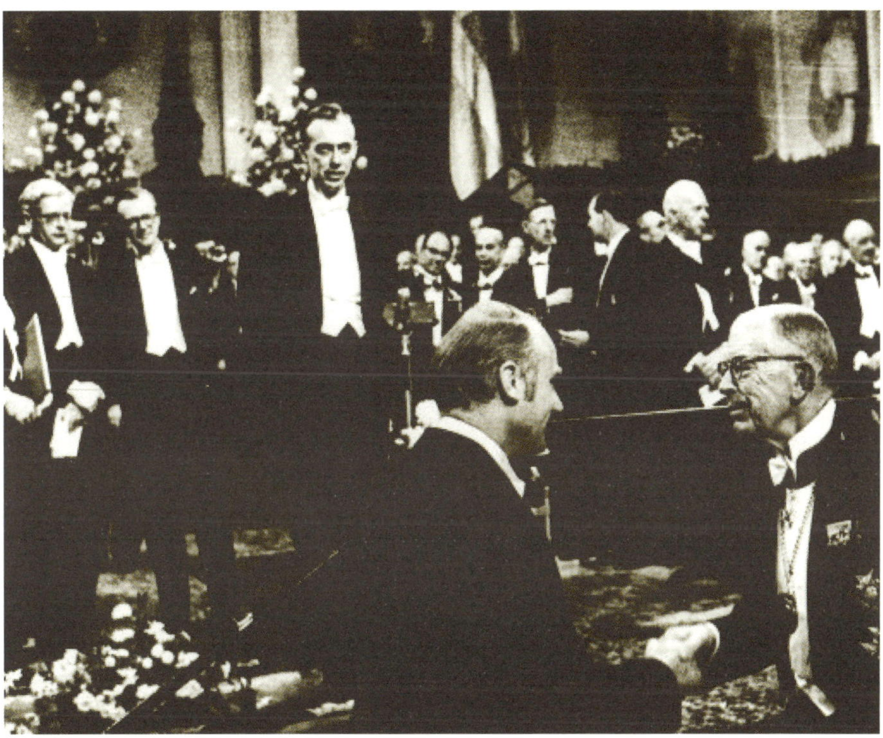

Crick receiving his Nobel Prize. [© Scanpix Sweden AB.]

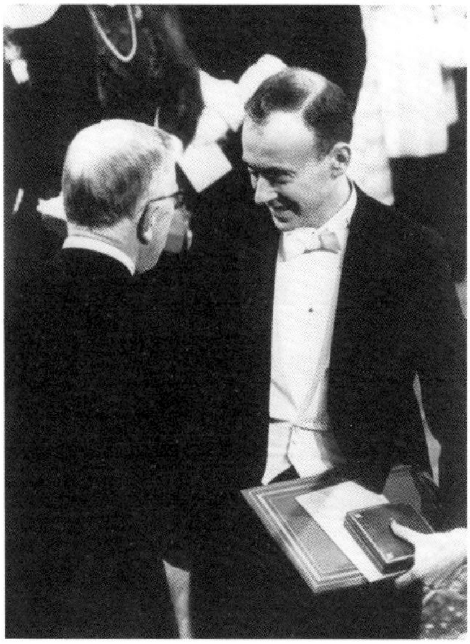

Watson and His Majesty King Gustaf VI Adolf. [© Scanpix Sweden AB.]

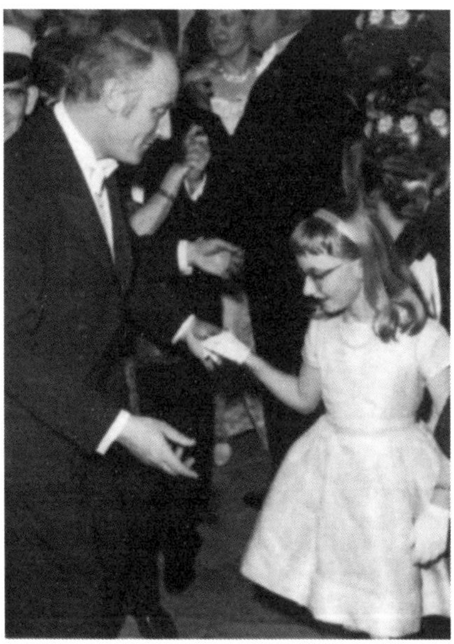

Crick dancing with daughter Gabrielle. [© Scanpix Sweden AB.]

helix structure, all had gathered for the event. This quintet was complemented by the colorful writer John Steinbeck, to be further presented in Chapter 9 (p. 408), in a discussion of Ramel's travails while serving as his escort. At the prize ceremony the diplomas and other insignia were presented by His Majesty the King to the discoverers of the structure of DNA in alphabetical order with Crick receiving his prize first and Watson second. For the first time the diploma did not carry the signatures of all members of the College of Teachers, but only of the chairman and secretary of the Nobel Committee and also the head of administration at the Karolinska Institute.

The children of the laureates gave color to the feast. The Cricks brought along his son Michael from a previous marriage and their eight- and eleven-year-old daughters Gabrielle and Jacqueline. Wilkins, who had married his second wife Patricia Chidgey in 1958, was accompanied by two small children. As can be seen from the picture Crick's daughters literally "had a ball".

Watson was still a bachelor learning about the complexity of interaction with the opposite sex. His ambition to aim high was encouraged by a telegram congratulating him on the prize. The telegram was from Richard Feynman, a richly colorful figure in the world of science, who was to receive a shared Nobel Prize in physics in 1965. The telegram was signed gly for glycine, the name Feynman had as one of the 20 highly selected members of the RNA tie club to be further described below.

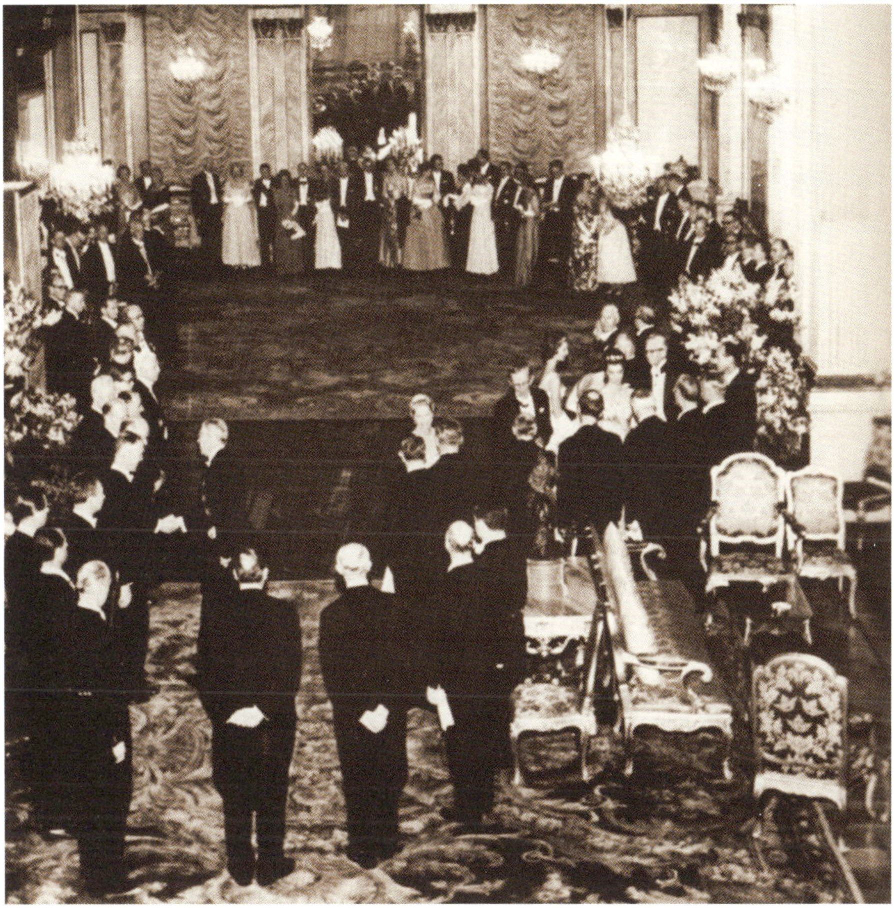

The King and his family, including the princesses greeting the guests at the Royal dinner on December 11 walking by the receiving line. [From Ref. 53.]

The text of the telegram was "And there he met the beautiful princess and they lived happily ever after." Watson did indeed meet princesses. There were four of them Margareta, Birgitta, Désirée and Christina ranging in age from 19 to 28 years, sisters of the present Swedish King Carl XVI Gustaf, born in 1946. Some of them were represented in the moving reception line at the Royal dinner the day after the prize ceremony (see also Chapter 6). No romance was spurned but years later Watson met the youngest Princess Christina when she studied in Boston[42].

The lectures by the five natural scientists marked the remarkable advance of molecular life sciences. Of course Watson and Crick who had become major contributors to the impressive further advances in this field, did not speak on the subject of the structure of DNA. Instead Crick spoke about the advancing insight into the genetic code which already at this time was interpreted to be a three letter code in a redundant way specifying the 20 different amino acids[43]. Watson spoke about the role of RNA in the synthesis of proteins[44]. He first mentioned his studies initiated in 1952 of the interaction between RNA and proteins in TMV examined by X-ray crystallography, the findings that Franklin brought to a beautiful conclusion a few years later. Already early on he speculated that RNA when interacting with protein could acquire a regular structure. This idea was of importance when he later, in 1956, together with Crick, formulated some general principles on viral structures[24], as already presented above. Watson also discussed the state of knowledge of functions of different kinds of RNA in the various steps of the central dogma — DNA gives RNA gives protein. Only Wilkins spoke on the crystallographic studies of DNA presenting both a brief history and also the post-1953 data that he and his group had generated. These data provided a validation of the Watson–Crick double helix model[38].

The Tallest Beacon among Molecular Biologists

As repeatedly emphasized by Crick the discovery of the structure of DNA became the starting point of an exceptional development within molecular life sciences. He was critically stimulated by his interaction with Watson into becoming the dominant theoretician in this field. Of course many other great experimentalists and thinkers also became involved in the developments as excellently described in a number of books[3,4]. In my previous book on Nobel Prizes[16] a chapter entitled "Nobel Prizes and nucleic acids: A drama in five acts" gives a condensed presentation of key scientists and the developments, including the rich opportunities to read and also write the books of life. It is fair to say that throughout the early fundamental developments of molecular biology Crick remained the tallest beacon among molecular biologists. He had a unique position among the theoreticians. In particular he had a particular capacity to ask the right and the important questions. There is a truth in his statement "If you ask big questions, you get big answers."

The Johnson citation used by Klug to describe Franklin could just as well have been applied to describe Crick. In 1953 Crick started to ponder the structure of collagen. Again he was entering hostile territory since examination of the structure of collagen was one of the major projects at King's College. In the first days of 1954 he circulated his first proposal for the structure of the

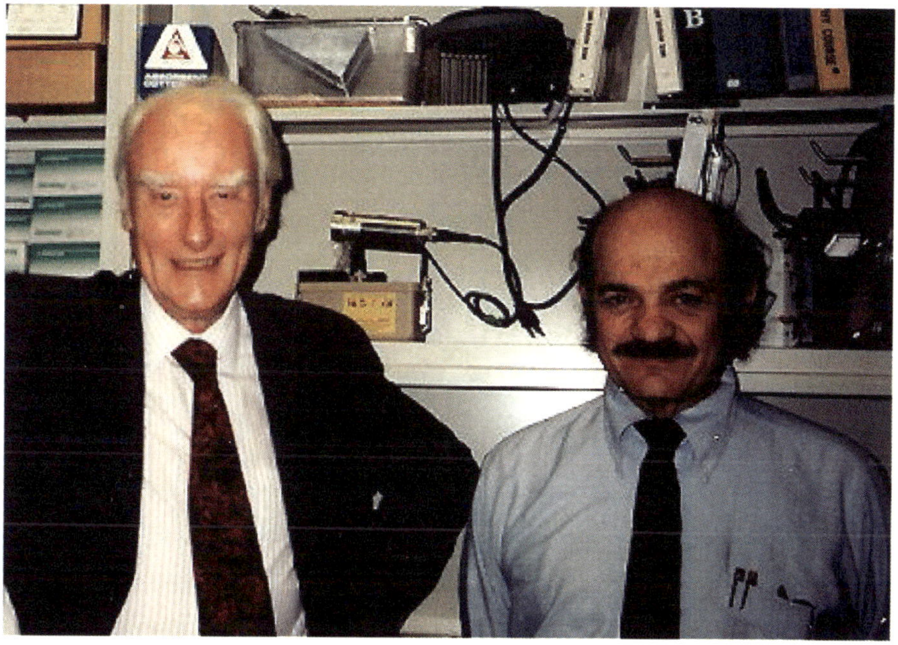

Crick and Alex Rich in the early 1990s. [Courtesy of Shuguang Zhang, MIT, Mass.]

substance. When the data reached Randall he was very upset. Crick had done it again! The model structure consisted of two anti-parallel strands just as in DNA. However the conjectured structure turned out to be completely wrong as pointed out by Pauling and others. Diffraction data on collagen from King's College that were available in a conference proceeding attracted the interest not only of Crick but also of other scientists. V. N. Ramachandran and G. Kartha in Madras developed a model that came close to being the correct one. It turned out to be a triple helix and not a double helix! In 1955 Rich came to Cambridge to work for a month, which developed into six months. This was the start of a friendship that was to last a lifetime. During Rich's stay in Cambridge he and Crick together managed to find the ultimate right solution. Again they made headway using information collected by others. Crick has referred to the fact that this contribution in principle had the same character as the discovery of the structure of DNA[1]. However no-one has written a book on *The Race for the Triple Helix.* Obviously the subject under study was of considerable interest. Collagen is certainly of importance in our bodies, where, as in other mammals, it represents about one third of all proteins. But it does not occur in plants and it certainly cannot compete with DNA when it comes to generality of importance. DNA is ubiquitous, whereas collagen is not. Crick quipped: "It is the molecule which has the glamour, not the scientists."

In 1954 Crick developed a collaboration with Ingram which later on led to his success in demonstrating for the first time a specific amino acid change caused by a mutation in DNA, already presented above. It was the first example of a molecular genetic disease. When Watson later came back to Cambridge he interacted with Crick to formulate the building principles of viruses in 1956 as repeatedly mentioned. Crick's greatness, however, has become most visible in his numerous contributions to the development and consolidation of the central dogma. He laid the foundation for understanding the nature of the genetic code, facilitated the conceptualization of the existence of messenger-RNA and postulated the existence of adaptor RNA molecules, later referred to as transfer RNA. Throughout the evolution of new insights he found critical intellectual sparring partners, among whom should be mentioned in particular Sidney Brenner, who took over after Watson in the late 1950s (Ref.16, pp. 227–229).

According to Crick[1] it was Brenner who, at a Good Friday session in Crick's home on account of a visit by Jacob, conceptualized the existence of a separate class of RNA molecules, later to be named messenger-RNA. It seems that overall the generous hospitality of Francis and Odile Crick in their home fostered important intellectual discourses, but also a means for developing the emotional qualities of human affairs.

Crick's involvement in cracking the genetic code began as early as in late 1953 at which time he had moved with his family to the US to work at the Polytechnic Institute of New York University located in Brooklyn. His task was to elucidate the structure of ribonuclease by use of X-ray crystallography analyses. He shared an office with Luzzati, Franklin's good friend from Paris. At the institute Crick met for the first time George Gamow, a colorful Russian-born American physicist. He was the first to develop a language by which the DNA base sequence could be translated into an amino acid sequence. Soon his proposal turned out to be way off the mark, which however did not discourage him from further involvement. Already in 1953, in correspondence with Gamow, Watson and Crick had declared for the first time that the number of amino acids to consider in developing a genetic code should be 20. There were many steps of development before the final triplet code was defined and the state of the art in 1962 was presented in Crick's Nobel lecture[43].

Gamow was a burlesque scientist who liked practical jokes. His contributions to the great decade of development of quantum theory were relatively marginal. The most important paper of his was from 1948 and dealt with the Big Bang. The name of his co-worker was Ralph Alpher. He therefore asked his friend the physicist Hans Bethe if he would agree to lend his name to the paper. He did, and therefore the list of authors became Alpher, Bethe and Gamow, the Latinized ABC of physics!

Gamow always spurned new ideas and in 1956 he founded an organization called the RNA Tie Club. The focus of this club was to encourage exchange of information between its members to understand the structure of RNA and to deduce how it directed the formation of proteins. Originally it had 16 members, a number of whom were physicists and by the addition of another four, including Crick and Watson, there were finally 20 members. Each member was addressed by his amino acid three letter designation. Crick was Tyr for tyrosine. Each member had a club pin that carried the three letter abbreviation. And of course there was a tie designed by Gamow to include sugar-phosphate chains in green and purines and pyrimidines in yellow embroidered in silk against a black background. Orgel arranged for the ties to be produced by a haberdasher in Oxford. The club even had its own letter head with the slogan "Do or die, or don't try" formulated by Delbrück. The letterhead also listed the different officers — Geo Gamow, Synthesizer, Jim Watson, Optimist, Francis Crick, Pessimist (intellectual realist?, my question), Martynas Ycas (biologist and friend of Gamow's), Archivist, Alex Rich, Lord Privy Seal. It is not clear how intense and important the interactions between members of the club were, but one paper contributed by Crick was of first-rate significance in the development of thoughts about the triplet code. However, what can be deduced is that the members enjoyed the fun of the pranks and craziness associated with the virtual club.

It is important to have fun in serious academic intercourse. There is a need for release of the intellectual and emotional intensity connected with ground breaking academic endeavor. And there is a need for cheering-up activities, since most experiments are failures or may lead into blind alleys. Many successful scientists have a good sense of humor, which also helps them to keep a distance from their own role in the critical developments. One rarely had an encounter with Crick without a good laugh. Personally I only had a few contacts with him and in my previous book[16] the meetings of the Thursday Club in La Jolla were mentioned. My first encounter with Crick, however, was in the early 1980s when Richard Lerner, the future President of the Scripps Research Institute arranged a catered dinner in a house at Princess Street in La Jolla where our family was temporarily housed. Francis and Odile Crick were the guests of honor and they shared their rich personalities in a very generous and happy way. Crick's laugh was readily heard.

The fundamental advances in molecular biology were soon to be recognized by Nobel Prizes in physiology or medicine, but not for some time in chemistry. In 1965 a prize was awarded to Jacob, Lwoff and Monod as mentioned above. In 1968 the prize recognized Robert W. Holley, H. Gobind Khorana and Marshall W. Nirenberg "for their discoveries concerning the interpretation of the genetic code and its function in protein synthesis" and finally the following year the founders of phage genetics, Delbrück, Hershey and Luria eventually received awards, as also already mentioned. It was Luria who had arranged support for Watson's premature and intense early scientific activities in Copenhagen and in Cambridge.

In the mid-1960s Crick and Brenner thought it was time to move on and selected the field of embryonic development. Brenner chose the nematode worm, *Caenorhabditis elegans*, as a model system. He was never to be recognized by a Nobel Prize for his critical contributions to clarifying phenomena connected to the central dogma, but eventually in 2002 Brenner received his — long overdue — prize (shared) "for their discoveries concerning genetic regulation of organ development and programmed cell death".

In 1977 Crick left Cambridge for a professorship at the Salk Institute. He had taken a sabbatical year at the institute earlier and liked the living conditions in Southern California. He did not only change his academic environment but also switched his research field to neurobiology with a particular focus on consciousness. By his insightful thinking he came to have an important influence on the development of this field too. He remained a scientist to the bitter end, correcting a manuscript on his death bed.

After his death in 2004 Crick was cremated. There was not to be a brain for later analyses by curious scientists. Being a true humanist he wanted no grave or headstone. His ashes were scattered on the Pacific Ocean and memorial services, one private and one general, were held allowing his large circle of friends, including many of the world's first rate scientists to reflect on a uniquely endowed colleague.

Living for 60 Years with the Golden Helix

Watson hitherto is the third youngest among recipients of Nobel Prizes in physiology or medicine. He revisited Stockholm and the Nobel festivities in December 2012 to celebrate the 50th anniversary of his prize, a very rare experience which he shared with Bragg (p. 301). In this year the Nobel Media, affiliated with the Nobel Foundation took a new initiative. In order to celebrate the 50th anniversary a full day Nobel Week Dialogue entitled "The Genetic

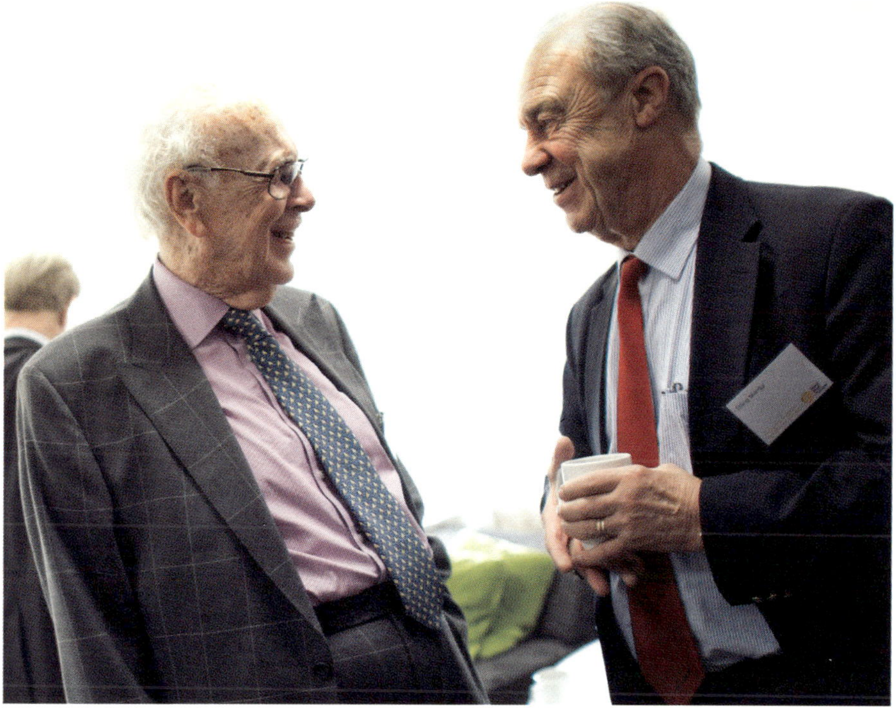

Watson and the author on December 9, 2012. [© Nobel Media AB. Photo by Alexander Mahmoud.]

Revolution and its Impact on Society" was arranged the day before the prize ceremony. Several Nobel laureates, including Watson, were represented among the 15 or so speakers. In an interview with Matt Ridley, Watson revisited among other things the morning of February 28, 1953.

Watson never managed to engage the Swedish Princesses. He had to wait another six years for his own "princess". In the year in which The *Double Helix* was published he married Elisabeth Lewis. They have two sons and together they have developed a rich and eventful life. The title of one of Watson's books *Avoid Boring People*[42] is indicative. Their home at Cold Spring Harbor is a hospitable milieu that has been enjoyed by a large number of visiting scientists over the years.

Carrying the nimbus of being the father of the golden helix, Watson has remained impressively active during the 60 years since its discovery. Like Crick he was heavily involved in the consequential developments from the discovery to the maturation of the central dogma identifying the critical molecular actors. Together with Crick he outlined the building principles for viruses[24], praised in a Nobel Prize review, and he was also one of the leaders in the search for mRNA. Furthermore he has been and is a very productive author. Already before publishing his best-seller *The Double Helix: A personal account* in 1968[5], he had produced a very popular textbook *The Molecular Biology of the Gene*. This was first published in 1965 and has since been printed in several new editions. Other books are *A Passion for DNA: Genes, Genomes and Society*[45], *Genes, Girls, and Gamow: After the Double Helix*[46] and *Avoid Boring People. Lessons from a Life in Science*[42]. Apparently like Crick, Watson was fascinated by Gamow and included him in an alliterative title with genes and girls. A more recent book by Watson (together with Andrew Barry) is *DNA. The Secret of Life*[47], dedicated to Crick. Several books by other authors deal with Watson and his life as a scientist, one of which is *The DNA Doctor: Candid Conversations with James D. Watson*[48].

Besides being a qualified developer of his science and publishing important books Watson has also made major contributions as leader of academic institutions. He began a tenured position at Harvard in 1956 which he kept until 1976. During this time he built a strong representation of molecular biological research at the university's Biological Laboratories. In parallel he became the Director of the Cold Spring Harbor Laboratories (CSHL) on Long Island in 1968. This institution which originally had a tainted history because of its involvement in racial hygiene studies was resurrected by Delbrück, who turned it into a Mecca for studies and discussions of molecular biology. As its director, Watson became the architect of further dynamic changes of this institution. He had the leadership of this remarkable science and conference center until 2007 serving consecutively as its President since 1994 and Chancellor since 2004.

There is something very special about the atmosphere of CSHL and I have had the privilege to experience it personally over more than ten years of involvement in conferences about vaccines, originally as a participant and later as organizer for several years. The first years of these high quality conferences were held in the original complexes of houses. There were very simple dormitories and hygiene conditions were shared. Doors were never locked. The conference presentations and discussions were held in a room of moderate size but with a large black board. One could almost feel the discovery discussions of historical dimensions that had taken place in this room. There were a lot of opportunities for incidental encounters in the seductive environment at the waterfront. Among my favorite memories are the early mornings jogging on some of the trails in the surroundings of the grounds. Later on Watson raised money to build a modern conference center, the Grace Hall, and also more convenient lodgings. Most of the original atmosphere remained, but it was not quite the same.

The Third Man Remained the Third Man

Wilkins enjoyed the limelight of being a Nobel laureate, but he always remained "the third man". His studies of DNA were finally concluded in 1967 and after this he made some attempts to study nerve membranes using X-ray crystallography. There were no further breakthroughs and essentially Wilkins enjoyed life in a harmonious family setting and with widening interests in political issues; the responsibility of scientists, nuclear arms, world poverty, etc. In the 1960s he became involved in an organization of a decade long temporary existence, The British Society for Social Responsibility of Science. It had very broad, perhaps too broad parameters, like the relations of science and the arts. Wilkins died in 2004.

Franklin's Posthumous Recognition

In time the posthumous recognition of Franklin's contributions to science has progressively grown. The books written about her[25,26] and several articles not least from Klug's hand,[27,28] have made it clear that she belongs in the Hall of Fame of Science. It was Franklin's and Gosling's development of the crystallographic work at King's College that led to the sharp diffraction patterns of the B form of DNA. It was pictures of this pattern which unbeknown to her sparked Watson into a renewed, and this time successful attack on the structure of DNA, as repeatedly emphasized in this chapter. Photograph 51 over time has become emblematic of Franklin's achievements. In more recent times *Photograph 51* has been used as the title of a play by Anna Ziegler. It has been presented in highly-praised performances in many theaters in the US. The play has been cited to present and discuss "ambition, isolation and the race for greatness" in science. In 2011 the play was performed at the World Science Festival in New York. After the performance a panel including Watson, Caspar and Gosling discussed its content.

Several initiatives have been taken to mark the emerging posthumous recognition of Franklin. A bust of her was placed in the Garden of Newnham College of which she was an alumna. Two years later the School of Crystallography at Birkbeck College, University of London opened the Rosalind Franklin Laboratory. One year later, significantly, the UK National Portrait Gallery added a photograph of Rosalind Franklin next to those of Crick, Watson and

Wilkins. King's College also honored her by naming a newly-opened laboratory the Franklin–Wilkins building. Watson participated in the inauguration ceremony. Further on, the Finch University of Health Sciences/The Chicago Medical School changed its name to the Rosalind Franklin University of Medicine and Science. There were also awards named after her; the Rosalind E. Franklin Award for Women in Science established by the American National Cancer Institute and the Rosalind Franklin award established by the Royal Society for outstanding contributions to any area of natural sciences, engineering or technology. Finally can be mentioned a DNA sculpture placed outside Clare College's Thirkill Court in Cambridge College donated by Watson. On the helices there is the following inscription: "The structure of DNA was discovered in 1953 by Francis Crick and James Watson while Watson lived here in Clare" and the inscription on the base states: "The double helix model was supported by the work of Rosalind Franklin and Maurice Wilkins."

What Is a Gene?

As a conclusion of this chapter some reflections will be presented on how the understanding of the chemistry of the gene has influenced our definition of this concept. One would think that knowledge about structure would simplify understanding of function. This is of course fundamentally true, but as far as the question of the structure of a gene is concerned, characterizations of the whole genomes of different species have revealed a remarkable complexity. Paradoxically this has led to the concept of a gene becoming more diffuse and poorly defined. It seems that the more we learn the more nebulous and ephemeral the concept appears. In my previous book[16] the remarkable developments of the reading and writing of the books of life and also the new insights into the complex mechanisms of expressions of genes were briefly outlined. The impressive advances made will not be revisited here but it is worth adding that the Encyclopedia of DNA Elements (ENCODE) has recently published another impressive progress report[49]. A large international consortium of more than 400 scientists have characterized the human genome in its details and examined different functional parts in various kinds of tests in a wide array of human cell lines. The summary conclusion was that as much as 80% of the genome serves some function in at least one of the cell lines used to identify the activities of human DNA. And still only somewhat more than 1% represents protein-coding sequences. A major part of the genome apparently is dedicated to regulation of the scattered genes. However, the high value of 80% has become severely criticized by a number of scientists. They believe that the true value should be less than 10%. Thus on this fundamental matter the jury is still out.

At first sight it seemed that identification of the central dogma would answer the fundamental questions of the nature of the gene. It was understood how the coded message in DNA led to the production of a protein with a specified amino acid sequence. DNA was transcribed into RNA which directly in prokaryotes or after transport to the cytoplasm in eukaryotes, could be translated to proteins. The persistence of the lineage of DNA ever since the origin of life some 3.8 billion years ago and the universal nature of the genetic code were fundamental to the understanding of gene functions. But very soon it became appreciated that it was not as simple as if a gene equalled a continuous piece of DNA which in turn equalled a polypeptide. It was found that the intermediary RNA extended beyond its coding parts. Various parts and sometimes very large parts of the RNA turned out to be engaged in regulatory functions. The need for a program of gene expression was originally identified by Jacob and Monod. The insight into the diversity and complexity of an ensemble of signals harbored by messenger-RNA grew with time and a proposal to designate this program a *genon* has even been made[50]. It was proposed that this be used to conceptualize the existence of various parts of DNA engaged in the expression of a particular gene, leading to the eventual expression of a specific messenger-RNA in the appropriate time and place. Expressed in another way a gene is not a single unit. It is a coordinated modality — a consortium of functions. Thus there is a wide-ranging program resulting in the phenotypic change of for example one color to another in a flower.

A major blow to the projected general *co-linearity* of a stretch of a messenger RNA and a polypeptide was the discovery of *splicing*. This surprising finding was recognized by a Nobel Prize in physiology or medicine to Richard J. Roberts and Phillip A. Sharp in 1993. Thus a single stretch of DNA transcribed into a corresponding stretch of RNA could be edited. Pieces of the RNA were specifically removed. A single "gene" in DNA could be edited in multiple ways resulting in the production of more than one protein. The historical one gene — one enzyme concept originally formulated by Beadle and Tatum had to be modified. The human genome has 20,000–22,000 protein-coding regions, but can produce about 100,000 different proteins. All the proteins produced may be separated into two broad categories, *structural* and *controlling (regulatory)* entities, but there is no sharp dividing line between the two. The structural proteins may have functions as building stones, like cytoskeleton proteins — collagen is one example —, but often they also carry other functions, such as an enzymatic or a signaling activity.

Separate from the protein-coding genes there are genes producing RNA molecules, which are *not* translated — the triplet code is not used — but instead carry their own independent functions. The fundamental finding that RNA, in addition to serving as messenger-RNA, on its own may carry enzymatic as well as structural properties has also been recognized by a Nobel Prize. The prize in chemistry in 1989 was awarded to Sidney Altman and Thomas R. Cech "for their discovery of the catalytic properties of RNA." However the total function of the whole genome is even more complex. The extended examination of not least the human genome has revealed that in addition there exist a large number of RNA products of different categories that neither have the above-mentioned messenger-RNA functions nor carry the independent structural-functional properties of isolated RNA[51]. The properties of these additional categories of RNA have only been partially mapped.

Hence in a simplified way one can distinguish four categories of genes — *structural and regulatory protein genes and structural and regulatory RNA genes*. But this dissection of gene functions as yet does not allow a full understanding of the different factors that in the end decide whether a certain stretch or stretches of DNA determines particular properties in a species, such as the particular color of a butterfly or a particular trait in humans. In order to grasp this it will be necessary to continue mapping the total cascade of regulation of the complex expression of a certain stretch of DNA. Several important discoveries — potentially to be recognized by Nobel Prizes — remain to be made. Described in a sketchy outline the sequential critical steps in protein formation, as understood at the present time, can be summarized as (a) chromatin modification and activation, (b) transcription and formation of RNA-protein complexes, (c) processing, transport (in eukaryotes) and modifications to formation of the functional messenger-RNA and (d) activation or repression of the messenger-RNA for the final translation.

Paradoxically our expanding knowledge of the mechanisms of expressing the information carried by DNA has blurred our specification of what we mean by a gene. The concept has become more poorly defined. One alternative way of solving the problem is to state that any stretch of DNA that, when mutated e.g. by a nucleotide change leads to a change of phenotype, is a gene (Darnell, personal communication and Ref. 51). But such a general definition leaves a number of problems unresolved. The outcome of the discussion depends on what emphasis is laid on the phenotypic expression, the selected character for examination, or on information storage and mechanisms of expression. At this stage there needs to be a greater focus on the latter issues. Further advance of science by application of the remarkable human creativity will allow this field to develop. The source of this creativity can be searched in the remarkably rich Nobel archives but future discoveries by definition will be unpredictable and unexpected. Nature still has many surprises — fortuitous solutions to challenges of the environment — for us to reveal.

Chapter 9
Coda

CREATIVITY
AN ENIGMATIC CONCEPT
HOW INSPIRING

Both in classical music and in improvised jazz a coda is occasionally used to bring a piece of music to an end. The word has its origin in the Latin *cauda*, meaning tail. In the mid-1950s I was extensively engaged as a member of a Dixieland band called *Les Saints Bleux*. Our idol was Louis Armstrong and we used the same set of instruments as he had in his all star sextet. It was my responsibility to play the piano, which was managed with an autodidact background using harmonies. To finish the performance of a certain tune we sometimes extracted a few bars of harmonies or a longer cadence of one of the leading musical themes and repeated these in a coda.

Jazz is a cultural development of the 20th century originating in a meeting between African-American and European musical traditions and has evolved through many different forms into the present time. A common trait is improvisation using a given set of harmonies originally formed to carry a leading theme. The keywords in jazz are *spontaneity*, *vitality* and *swing* emerging from a close interaction in the band. Thus parallels can be drawn between jazz and science in that a scientist breaking new ground needs to be flexible and to take inductive leaps, as mentioned on p. 376. To improvise and think out of the box is important in scientific performance as will be further discussed. A successful performance by a scientist is often furthered by good interaction with fellow scientists in the research group, as is the case in a band of musicians playing jazz. The importance of creating an environment of propinquity was discussed in the presentation of the Medical Research Council Unit of Molecular Biology in Cambridge in Chapter 7. However, of course the analogy only carries a certain distance. Jazz is a recent cultural phenomenon, whereas science has deep cultural roots and accumulation of organized knowledge started at the dawn of human civilizations. Incidentally, it might also be added that so far the representation of African-Americans among successful scientists is dismally small. Hopefully we will see a much larger multi-ethnic involvement in the future evolution of hypothetical-deductive (post-Galilean) science from its original cradle in Europe.

This final chapter highlights a series of interconnected themes that were originally associated with the preceding eight chapters, but which had a tendency to take on a life of their own. Thus the term coda used in the musical context, based on repeats, is not a full analogy to the content of this last chapter, but it was selected as a better alternative than "All That Jazz", which was a temporary candidate title. The first issue to be considered will be the changing science and the potential opportunities for future paradigmatic discoveries.

Paradigmatic Discoveries

At the dawn of the emergence of a new branch of science one can find that a very simple but ingenious experiment may break open a whole new field of research. Many examples can be given. At the turn of the previous century it was believed that all communication between one part of our body and another was by the nerves. This dogma, originally formulated by the old Greeks, was supported by the authoritative physiologist Ivan P. Pavlov, who received the 1904 Nobel Prize in physiology or medicine "in recognition of his work on the physiology of digestion". This dogma was overturned by a clever intuitive experiment in a small laboratory at University College in London in 1902.

By a comparatively simple arrangement it was demonstrated that stimulation of the small intestine of a dog with a weak solution of hydrochloric acid led to a production of new chemical substances in the fluid that was collected from the pancreatic gland. This secretion was proven to take place also when all the nerve contacts between the intestine and the gland were eliminated. This was the first documentation of the existence of chemical "messengers" in addition to the nerve signals. The substance that had been discovered was named *secretin* and it was the first among the large group(s) of chemical substances acting (signalling) on distance — later called hormones — to be identified. This discovery of the first hormone was made by William M. Bayliss and Ernest H. Starling. Over the years there were multiple nominations of these two scientists, in particular Starling, but regrettably the Nobel Committee for Physiology or Medicine missed this opportunity to award a major primary discovery.

Later on a similar paradigmatic discovery was made by Otto Loewi, but this was identified by the Committee and he received a Nobel Prize in physiology or medicine in 1936 together with Dale (see Chapter 1) "for their discoveries relating to chemical transmission of nerve impulses". There were many similarities between Bayliss-Starling's and Loewi's discoveries. The latter departed from the observation that electricity stimulated contraction of muscles, an observation that dated back all the way to the 1790s when the Italian Luigi Galvani demonstrated this phenomenon in experiments with frogs. At the time of Loewi's critical experiment in 1921 there were vague ideas that the electrical impulses should act directly on the muscle cells, without any comprehension of how this might work. The idea for a new kind of experiment came to Loewi in a dream — perhaps this state of mind released him from his traditional "galvanized" thinking . He worked with heart tissues with or without connection to their regulatory nerve. After stimulation of a heart tissue via the nerve the fluid surrounding the tissue was collected. This fluid was then transferred and mixed with fluid surrounding another piece of heart tissue *not* connected any longer to its nerve. What Loewi found was that fluid from a heart, stimulated to increase its heart rate, also caused an increase of the heart rate of the second denervated heart. Conversely, if the first heart tissue showed a decreased rate of contraction this effect could also be transferred by the surrounding fluid to the second organ. These experiments demonstrated for the first time that the nerve impulses cause a release of some chemical substance that in its turn causes the muscle cells to contract. A new field of science was born and since then our knowledge of a multitude of *neurotransmitters* has expanded enormously.

A third example, closer to home, concerns the group of substances called *prostaglandins*. This name was introduced by Ulf von Euler (see Chapter 2, p. 76), engaged as ordinary or associate member of the committee for physiology or medicine in the late 1950s and early 1960s and its secretary 1961–1962. He received a Nobel Prize in 1970. However von Euler did not get his shared prize for his identification of prostaglandins, but for his later work on neurotransmitters. It was in the early 1930s that von Euler, following the practice of physiologists at the time, made a phenomenological observation by extracting tissues and testing the extracts in different systems with the aim of identifying different chemical messengers. He observed that in semen and in extracts of prostate or vesicular glands of different animals there was some factor which decreased blood pressure and stimulated smooth muscles. He gave this lipid-soluble factor the name *prostaglandin*. When the committee was preparing to award the 1982 Nobel Prize in physiology or medicine to K. Sune Bergström, Bengt I. Samuelsson and John R. Vane "for their discoveries concerning prostaglandins and related biologically active substances" we had long discussions as to whether von Euler, the father of these compounds should not be included among the three recipients of the prize. In the end we decided that this was not necessary. He had recognized the existence of prostaglandins, but had left it to others to unravel their chemistry and multitude of different functions as well as their potential for use as pharmaceutical compounds.

One final example might be added to emphasize the importance of the introduction of new techniques. It was Tiselius (p. 326) who developed a method to separate proteins on the basis of their different charges. This was recognized by a Nobel Prize in chemistry in 1948 as mentioned in the previous chapter. He could separate the major serum proteins into three fractions referred to as alpha, beta and gamma. The latter fraction, gamma globulins was found to play a central role in the immune functions, as already discussed in Chapter 3. It contained antibodies that protect us against infections and serve many other functions.

Following these examples it would be appropriate to ask if, at the present time, it is still possible to make discoveries that may have a general fundamental impact. The various qualities of scientific pursuits have been discussed extensively in particular after the publication of Thomas S. Kuhn's book *Structure of Scientific Revolutions*[1]. Kuhn made a distinction between the everyday (validating, "horizontal") science solving defined problems by use of already established techniques, and (revolutionary, "vertical") research leading to discoveries creating completely new vistas and possibilities for previously unanticipated approaches to science. The latter form of breakthrough he called *paradigmatic shifts*, a term reserved only for rare and dramatic changes in science. Thus the question is if it has become more and more difficult to make paradigmatic discoveries for example in the life sciences when this field has advanced into more and more detailed problem-solving. Is the development such that by definition we are only capable of analyzing the finer and finer details of various particular predefined phenomena?

Peter Reichard is a highly qualified biochemist with whom I had the privilege to work for a considerable number of years in the Nobel Committee at the Karolinska Institute, also during a time when he was its chairman. He frequently expressed the view that "eventually everything becomes biochemistry". In the end of course it will depend on which perspective is applied.

The formulation by Alfred Nobel in his final will is ingenious. The five prizes represent a progression from physics, the study of matter in its finest details, to chemistry, the art of characterizing all the different complexes of elements represented by the periodic table (Chapter 5), many of which — the organic molecules — have importance in the conundrums of life. Thereafter comes physiology or medicine which deals with the interplay of these organic molecules in various forms of life of different complexity. The two last-mentioned prizes, the ones in literature and peace, concern behavioral sciences, where nature and nurture are in full play with the advancing human cultures as their sounding board. If we consider an increased resolution as the main tenet in the advance of sciences, a physicist might pick an argument with Reichard and say that in the end everything becomes physics. But it is probably better when it comes to physiology or medicine to stay at the level of resolution that allows us to answer the complex and seemingly enigmatic questions about the origin of the harmonious homeostatic functions rather than being paralyzed by the "uncertainty principle" and determinism.

There have indeed been fantastic recent advances in the field of life sciences. And still in our present time it is — and also in the future it will be — possible to make very fundamental discoveries that go to the heart of biological phenomena. As examples of recent paradigmatic findings can be mentioned the discovery of catalytic RNA, rewarded by a Nobel Prize in chemistry in 1989 to Altman and Cech; the identification of the strange infectious agents called prions recognized by the prizes in physiology or medicine in 1976 and 1997 (Ref. 2, Chapter 8); and the discovery of RNA interference — gene silencing by double-stranded RNA by Andrew Z. Fire and Craig C. Mello, awarded the same prize in 2006. It is a reliable forecast to state that we will continue to see paradigmatic discoveries and that much remains to be learned from Nature.

The availability of advanced modern techniques implies a change in the way in which most scientists approach the problem they have selected for scrutiny. Many of these techniques allow and depend on the harvesting of a large or even huge amount of information which can then be stored and analyzed by use of impressive computer facilities. Without these techniques it would not have been possible to unravel, by use of refined crystallographic studies, the detailed complex molecular mechanisms underlying for example the transcription of messenger-RNA from DNA and the translation of messenger-RNA into a polypeptide chain, recognized by the Nobel Prizes in chemistry in 2006 and 2009. These new possibilities of harvesting large amounts of information also lead to new approaches, to a lesser extent incited by the formulation of specific hypotheses. This approach is sometimes referred to as "data mining".

Once all the data on, for example, the complexity of nucleotide sequences of a selected genome, sometimes including billions of nucleotide bases, has been retrieved it is possible to evaluate the information by bioinformatics analysis. It is very critical how this is approached. If it is carried out in a skilful way it might be possible that an unexpected pattern would emerge to be recognized and that this may lead to insights into new, previously unrecognized, fundamental mechanisms. Scientists have become progressively more dependent on the processing and interpretation of the hidden patterns of huge volumes of data. And still, in the end, it is the responsibility of a unique human brain to select the right question to ask and to make the final interpretation of the accumulated experimental data. It has long been recognized that sometimes one can formulate competing theories that make exactly the same predictions. In such a situation the Ockham razor, formulated by William of Ockham in the 14th century should be used. It states that the simpler a theory is the more likely it is to be true — *entia non sunt multiplicanda praeter necessitatem* (entities are not to be multiplied beyond necessity).

Genius Is a Fire that Lights Itself

It follows from the reasoning in many of the previous chapters that there will always be room for the unique intellectual analysis and intuition of anointed scientists. When scientists of such qualities are presented it is tempting to use the word genius, but in Swedish it is generally easier to use this word as an adjective — *genial* — than as a noun. In English the word genial with time has taken on an altered meaning — kindly in disposition, imparting comfort. The word genius has its etymological root in a Latin word meaning tutelary spirit (*gen* — stem of *gignere* "beget"). A genius is protected by some spirit or deity, who has endowed him or her with exalted intellectual power capable of operating independently of tuition and training, and marked by an extraordinary faculty for original creation, invention, discovery, expression, etc. To be a genius means to be endowed with an incomprehensible and mysterious force animating only highly selected human beings. A genius has a capacity to see profundity in simple facts. The German mathematician Hermann Weyl has expressed the unique force of thinking of geniuses in the following way "Theories permit consciousness to jump over its own shadow, to leave behind the given, to represent the transcendent, yet, as is self-evident, only in symbols." Thus the term indicates some special inherent trait that goes beyond the particular talent of even the deep and wide-ranging capacity of a polymath, a *l'homme universelle*. Hence the word genius needs to be reserved for use only in selected circumstances, also in the case of Nobel laureates.

Richard Feynman was one of the most remarkable scientists in the field of physics. *Genius. The Life and Science of Richard Feynman*[3], the title used for James Gleick's book, is probably therefore acceptable. Feynman was a fascinating person. Together with Murray Gell-Mann, the Nobel laureate of physics of 1969 he revolutionized our insight into elementary particle physics. On the side he was a master of breaking the codes of locks and managing syncope using drums synchronizing a 12-beat and a 13-beat. One enjoyable way of getting an insight into this remarkable person is to read his books, for example *Surely You're Joking, Mr Feynman*[4].

Feynman's colleague Gell-Mann is also a polymath as well as a genius, who has developed his deep insights on projects at the Santa Fe Institute during the last few decades. Once when he was changing offices he was helped by two younger scientific colleagues in the moving of his many books. Gell-Mann expressed his gratitude and received the anticipated courtesy remark "It is just a pleasure to help someone like you." To which Gell-Mann responded "But there is no one like me!" — end of anecdote.

In Gleick's book on Feynman a reference is given to William Duff, the Scottish minister who in the 18th century aimed at providing a description of the meaning of the word "genius". He reflected on the fact that geniuses have "enlightened, penetrating and capacious minds" and referred to their "god-like power of invention, of creation of what has previously not been seen". But he also noted their "rambling and volatile power" frequently leading to their ending up in the direction of erring. Geniuses like Newton and Einstein and Mozart are often referred to as wizards, meaning in the case of scientists someone with a unique capacity to tease from nature its hidden secrets and for the gifted artist to create a deep and persisting emotional engagement in us.

The question of what makes geniuses see further has been the subject of endless discussions[5]. How relevant is their personalized use of sensorial information and how important is their intuition — another nebulous concept? As mentioned in Chapter 7, Feynman used to say that what he could not see (construct) he could not understand. However, by this statement he probably meant something more than "visualizing". In his monumental 1781 book *The Critique of Pure Reason*, Immanuel Kant distinguished intuition from sensation. But it is hard to judge the nuances, since in German intuition is translated as *Anschauung* which can also mean visualization. And the question remains if there are some other forms of higher cognitions that transcend direct sensory perceptions. It remains to deepen our understanding of how perceptions of qualitatively different parts are integrated into a comprehensible full picture. This problem has been the particular focus of the theory of mind formulated in *Gestalt* psychology. The key question is how we interpret a picture, how we can accentuate the relevant features and suppress the irrelevant aspects of the two-dimensional information. Too close attention to details or too deep engagements in some of them, due to a biased, dogma-directed interpretation, may obscure an understanding of the whole. The computer picture of our three children presented below may illustrate this problem. When a part of the picture is viewed at a larger magnification it appears to convey no meaningful information, but at a lower resolution the features of our offspring become apparent. The picture was taken at Newmarket, Philadelphia in 1978 and was kindly given to us by our good friend Maurice Hilleman (Ref. 2, p. 118) with the dedication "to our favorite Vikings". Sometimes it is not a matter of

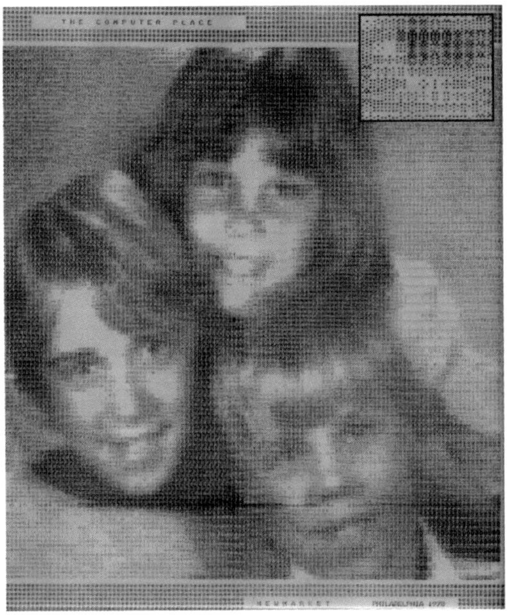

Computer picture of the author's three children taken in 1978 at Newmarket, Philadelphia. A part of one of our daughter's eyes has been enlarged (top right corner) and the pattern observed does not give meaningful information.

seeing a pattern in shades of a presentation in grey. It can also be a question of interpreting and integrating colors. One of the founders of abstract art, the Russian painter Wassily Kandinsky, is said to have had an epiphany when seeing his easel in half-light and realizing that the remains of paints on it could represent a subject of art by itself. Colors can also be reflected in words. The following citation from James Joyce's *A Portrait of the Artist as a Young Man* gives just one example:

> The phrase and the day and the scene harmonized in a chord. Words. Was it their colors? ... from the reflection of the glowing, sensible world through the prism of a language many colored and richly storied than from the contemplation of an inner world of individual emotions mirrored perfectly in a lucid supple periodic prose?

The sensorial impressions obviously can be influenced by other senses than seeing; like hearing (see Chapter 6), smelling, tasting and/or touching. But let us leave the interpretation of intuition and sensorial processing as a question for further discussion at this point and return to the manners of geniuses.

The pursuits of geniuses are generally intensive and monomaniac and the borderline between genius and madness is fuzzy, as briefly alluded to earlier (Ref. 2, Chapter 8), and the subject of many books. In the world of literature authors like Friedrich Nietzsche, Søren A. Kierkegaard and Fjodor Dostoyevsky, who balanced between genius and madness, have been a particular focus of interest. Many of the potential geniuses may be derailed and forestalled in their activities. Although geniuses are obsessive in their engagements they, like other human beings, are also influenced by the social circumstances under which they live.

A number of geniuses are said to have been left-handed, but this may be one of many myths that surrounds this condition. Left-handed people are also said to be more intelligent and creative, but again there is no evidence giving substance to this statement[6]. There must be some other explanation for the fact that about half of all American Presidents have been left-handed. One could analyze the occurrence of left-handedness in Nobel laureates, but to my knowledge this has not been done. It is possible that previously, when left-handedness was considered a defect to be corrected, children with this condition had to find ways of defending it. They might have been forced to develop both their left and right side capabilities and the resulting adaptability of the brain might have endowed them with what is called *fluctuating asymmetry*. This may in turn have been beneficial to the development of the creativity of the individual.

There is a general agreement that IQ values are not a good indicator of the potential success of the individual as a scientist. There are many qualitative and quantitative aspects to intelligence and only some of these are measured by conventional IQ tests. In order to allow the full use of an advanced receptive capacity it is necessary for the individual to be able to combine this resource with other qualities that allow its full use — perseverance, energy to take initiatives, a heterodox attitude, etc.

It is a truism to note that the environment has a major influence on the development of the personality of an individual. Earlier sociological studies of the prototype successful scientist showed that he — sadly the group is dominated by the one sex — was frequently the oldest in a family with many children, the father of which had died when the children were young. To digress it should be noticed in this context that as long as we do not have a roughly equal proportion of female and male scientists we are not taking full advantage of the total human intellectual resources. As is apparent from the scarcity of female Nobel laureates we still have a long way to go before the development of the minds of both sexes is properly catered for. The taking of major responsibilities at a young age due to circumstantial events might be beneficial for some personalities, but in the end it may be difficult to distinguish what is the cause and what is the effect. There can be many kinds of environmental conditions forcing an independence and accentuated maturity of individuals. For example there are dramatic differences between the scientific outputs of peoples representing different ethnic groups. The remarkable overrepresentation of people of Jewish ethnic background among scientists was discussed earlier (Ref. 2, Chapter 1) and also mentioned in several instances in this book. Their exposure to new and different environments in the Diaspora could be one important factor in this case. In Chapter 5 the importance for the development of scientists of being forced to change homeland was exemplified. In the end it is a question of attempting to understand what conditions may favor the elicitation of Eureka events of discoveries. Because this problem is so many-faceted, it is probably best to illustrate the richness of the individual rocky roads to paradigmatic discoveries by citing examples of individuals, environments and events. This is exactly what this book and my preceding one aim at.

Since the success of the endeavours of a scientist depends both on his innate intellectual capacity and, equally importantly, on his environment, it is worth discussing the importance of choice of life style.

The Importance of Lifestyle

Mens sana in corpore sano — a healthy mind in a healthy body, is a statement that does not need any explanation. Murray, who we met in Chapter 4, seems to have been a very harmonious person. His wife literally brought music into the life of the family, which came to include many children. Two paragraphs in his auto-presentation preceding the Nobel lecture[7] deserve to be cited.

> My life as a surgeon-scientist, combining humanity and science, has been fantastically rewarding. In our daily patients we witness human nature in the raw — fear, despair, courage, understanding, hope, resignation, heroism. If alert, we can detect new problems to solve, new paths to investigate.

It is at the bed-side of hospitalized patients that new problems to be solved for improving human health are identified. The last paragraph read:

> We have been blessed in our lives beyond my wildest dreams. My only wish would be to have 10 more lives to live on this planet. If that were possible, I'd spend one lifetime each in embryology, genetics, physics, astronomy and geology. The other lifetimes would be as a pianist, backwoodsman, tennis player, or writer for the *National Geographic*. If anyone has bothered to read this far, you would note that I still have one future lifetime unaccounted for. That is because I'd like to keep open the option for another lifetime as a surgeon-scientist.

Murray also noted that for recreation he had always been an enthusiast for physical exercise. He clearly believed that a healthy body is conducive to the maintenance of a healthy soul. He was also to have a long life dying at the age of 93 in November of 2012, survived by his wife, six children and 18 grandchildren.

Murray's choice of lifestyle has a particular appeal to me since I myself am an avid jogger and out door person. In 2010, at the age of 73, I accomplished my twenty-fifth 30 kilometres cross-country competition. Jogging is a good catalyst for intellectual work and several books have been written about jogging and writing. It is not a matter of developing a competitive spirit but rather of accentuating your self-discipline and keep in good physical shape. The one you compete with in a race is yourself. Less has been written about jogging and scientific pursuits, but I know from experience that many scientists are joggers. It frequently happens that by chance one gets acquainted with a colleague when jogging in connection with conferences in different corners of the world. Harold Varmus, the 1989 Nobel Prize recipient in physiology or medicine is an active jogger and cyclist and he used the latter unconventional means of transport during his time as Director of the National Institutes of Health (NIH) in Bethesda, Maryland. He has compared his experiences in scientific research to the challenges of a long-distance cyclist:

> Long flat intervals. Steep, sweaty, even competitive climbs, an occasional cresting of a mountain pass, with the triumphal downhill coast. Always work. Sometimes pain. Rare exhilaration. Delicious fatigue and well-earned rests.

The physical exercise can weed out emotional turmoil, clear your thinking and assist in problem-solving and it may even spawn heterodox ideas. The antipodal situation is to have, like Medawar (Chapter 2), during the time he was Director of the Institute for Medical Research at Mill Hill, a private chauffeur to transport you back and forth to work and various social events. This certainly can make the use of time temporarily more effective and allow a more liberal enjoyment of social pleasures, but it definitely is not as helpful as physical exercise to maintaining good health.

There are obviously many human vices and virtues that might be discussed in a search for understanding of the source of exceptional human creativity. It is sometimes said in a shallow way that there are two things that drive people — sex and money; and the one can be bought by the other. Such a vulgar statement does not belong in a book of this kind, which of course does not mean that sex is not as important to scientists as it is to other people. In fact it is possible that scientists, being driven by a considerable life energy, might have even a larger than normal representation of erotomaniac individuals. Examples may easily be found; Schrödinger (shared 1932 Nobel Prize in physics) moved to Ireland because there was a more liberal view there of his *ménage-à-trois* lifestyle; Svedberg (1926 Nobel Prize in chemistry; Chapter 5) was married four times and had 12 children, six boys and six girls; Bernal's liberal view on relations between the sexes was repeatedly cited in Chapter 7, etc. However, I leave to others to discuss the importance of this private matter, which by definition must be very difficult to research. When it comes to money, we have already noted that this is not an important driving force in scientific pursuits. The intellectual satisfaction of managing to establish hybridomas producing monoclonal antibodies was more important than patenting the methodology and making money (Chapter 3). Access to and control over money generally is a good measure of power and influence. This is not the case in the world of science. In fact scientists making a lot of money are sometimes even looked upon with a certain suspicion by their colleagues. Scientists use another currency than the ones used in regular financial transactions. Their currency is knowledge. It is by their capacity to generate new knowledge and hereby transform the landscape of learning that scientists can excite respect among their colleagues. Invitations to be a key lecturer and to write influential reviews are one indicator on the standing of a scientist. For a scientist the jury is always out — his colleagues, and peers, are always monitoring his performance.

Murray also emphasized the importance of a happy family situation. Many Nobel laureates have made references to the importance of their life partners, usually women because of the regrettable overwhelming dominance of men among the prize recipients. Many books could be written on this theme. Sometimes it might be a matter of money, in particular if there has been a divorce. Albert Einstein made an agreement with his wife Mileva Maric when they separated in 1919 that she would receive his Nobel Prize money. Thus in 1922 the prize money was sent to her and she bought three houses in Zürich, which she was able to use to cover the living expenses of herself and their two sons. During my time as permanent secretary at the Royal Swedish Academy of Sciences there was one case where a divorced wife of a laureate received 50% of the prize sum. On this theme a single particular situation might be mentioned. When Abdus Salam, the recipient of a shared physics prize in 1979, trained in Great Britain, but originally from Pakistan, came to Stockholm he brought two wives. One accompanied him to the Nobel Prize ceremony and banquet and the other to the King's dinner the following day. Lack of solid information, as in the cases of choice of life partners and the importance of sexual habits, also makes it of less value to reflect on the importance of the use of stimulants like alcohol, a potentially serious vice in situations of licentious use. Maybe a harmless anecdote would still be in place.

All Nobel Prize recipients are allocated a personal attaché to care for all their wishes and whims during their visit to Stockholm. In 1962 it was time to find an attaché for John Steinbeck, who had been awarded the prize in literature that year (p. 298). The young career diplomat Ramel (p. 101), already referred to in Chapters 3 and 6, was selected. He was introduced to this task by the Executive Director of the Nobel Foundation Envoy Nils K. Ståhle (p. 247), who emphasized that it was a demanding responsibility. The reason was that Steinbeck was well known to have a bohemian nature and also to become somewhat disorderly after intake of alcohol. Ramel had a very intense week together with Steinbeck, but it all worked out well[8]. It was possible to keep him sober by substituting the whisky by a weaker vermouth drink. After Steinbeck had left Stockholm it did not take long before Ramel received a greeting of thanks from him. It was in the form of a personally delivered case containing 12 bottles of whiskey. On an attached letter Steinbeck had written "This is all the whiskey I did not drink in Stockholm thanks to you." But this episode had one more important consequence. In 1972 when Ståhle was leaving his responsibility for the Nobel Foundation he came to think of the attaché who had been so successful in managing Steinbeck during the Nobel Prize week of 1962. He called Ramel and asked if he might be interested in the position of Executive Director of the Foundation. This turned out to be the case and eventually Ramel was selected to become the new Executive Director, a task he managed effectively from 1972 to 1992 (Ref. 2, Chapter 1).

Many other aspects on the interplay of personality traits and the environment could be given in this context. Maybe the major omission is a discussion of the great value of having a good sense of humor providing some perspective on the challenges of being a scientist. The RNA tie club presented in Chapter 8 is a good example of how to mix serious intellectual exchanges and play. Having fun together obviously furthers social cohesion and it may also carry the individuals engaged through periods when the work is stalling and the opportunities for further advance appear very bleak.

In his book *The Act of Creation* Arthur Koestler compared the conscious and unconscious underpinnings of scientific discoveries, artistic creations and jokes. He argued that they have a basic pattern in common, which he referred to as "bisociative" thinking. The comparison departs from the analysis of how two independent matrices of perception or reasoning interact with each other. He outlines three different outcomes. The first one is the exploratory scientific fusion of the matrices into a new intellectual synthesis. The second is the participatory artistic management of the situation of confrontation resulting in an aesthetic experience. Finally there may be a situation of incongruence resulting in an irreconcilable collision of the matrices. This situation of tension is conjectured to potentially be resolved by laughter. Although many successful scientists have a qualified sense of humor and are good at telling jokes this does not apply in any general sense. The presence of a sense of humor among scientists appears to me to be distributed just as in people in general. The strength of a successful scientist is to exaggerate the relevant and simplify or ignore the irrelevant aspects of reality as mentioned above. It is probably also helpful to keep some distance from the present situation and even look at it from a somewhat humorous perspective when experimental conditions are persistently uphill.

The Driving Force in the Pursuit of Science

Both Burnet and Medawar, the central figures in Chapters 1 and 2, were exceptionally productive scientists and it would be appropriate to reflect on what drove them in their professional pursuits. They were energetic polymaths and to use a neologism introduced by Medawar — they were obsessionalists. They put in a massive amount of work, but it is worth emphasizing that, as in any challenge in life, only a minor part of these efforts had a positive outcome. It was not a long march of triumphs, but mostly setbacks and reaching of points of no return. Without a belief in a mission it would have been hard to prevail. But it is not enough to do hard work to make important discoveries in science. It is also important to choose the right problem — i.e. a very important and fundamental one. It is only attacks on large problems that allow the making of major new discoveries as mentioned in Chapter 8.

The substrate for the fertile scientific intellect is ignorance and in particular the absence of insights into phenomena of general significance. Perutz (Chapter 7) has formulated this in the following way "the unknown is more invigorating than the known. Once the fertile mind of a creative scientist has become hooked on a problem there is no way out". It is an expression of our "restless endeavor to make sense of things" to use an expression from Kant. What comes first is the scientist's obsession of the call of the wild from the unsolved problem. On this issue it was remarked by Robert Musil in his book *The Man Without Qualities* that "It is not true that a scientist goes after the truth. The truth goes after him." And in a review of Jim Watson's book *The Double Helix* Ernest Chargaff noted "One can almost say that, with very few exceptions, it is not the men that make the science, it is science that makes men." These are different ways of highlighting the emphasis in the intercourse between the scientist and the problem he has chosen to pursue.

When describing impressive scientific personalities like Burnet and Medawar it is easy to be lured into believing that things came easily to them and that they had almost superhuman qualities. This impression most likely is wrong because for each and every human being there are periods when things come more easily and bring joy and euphoria, but most of the time it is a dull, dogged work. The professor of positive development psychology Mihaly Csikszentmihalyi — a spelling challenge — previously at the University of Chicago and presently at the Claremont Graduate University in California, has referred to the former state as *flow*, which is also the name of one of his many books[9]. However, according to him this is a rare state of positive emotions, in precious instances epitomized by an experience of Eureka, from Greek heúréka, meaning "I have found (it)" (see Chapter 8). Most of the time there is the everyday toil and struggle, even for a scientist who may have a very stimulating professional post with a high degree of freedom to choose the direction of his work. Like anyone else the scientist has to manage the rhythm of the day and fundamental bodily needs, like food and sex as was briefly alluded to earlier in this chapter. It should also be added that the pursuit of science is a very, sometimes even fiercely competitive business. Many scientists have pronounced competitive personalities. Priority issues are always central in discussion of candidates for Nobel Prizes. Being humans, scientists sometimes may be so intensively driven by competitiveness that it pushes them overboard. This has been well described in the recent book *Prize Fight* by Morton A. Meyers[10].

In the US the post Second World War period led to a democratization of scientific environments which markedly improved the creative environments and made this country the leading one in spawning Nobel Prize recipients in the natural sciences (Ref. 2, Chapter 1). In other countries the scientific environments have remained more hierarchical holding back the blooming of young and dynamic minds. Many comparisons of the role of national traits and scientific creativity can be made[11]. Let us take Sweden and Japan as an example. There are many similarities between the cultures of these two countries. Originally they were relatively isolated peninsula/island cultures with homogenous populations. During the last 50 years the Swedish population has become somewhat more heterogeneous because of a liberal immigration policy. Also the general atmosphere has become much less authoritarian. By way of contrast immigration to Japan is still negligible and the culture of the country remains authoritarian. Both countries are highly organized and patterns of life are reasonably well structured and safe. Still there are differences partly also due to distinctive geographical conditions. In Sweden there is a lot of room for the nine million people to enjoy in their large country and hence natural romanticism is widely shared in the appreciation of life. In Japan too there is a pronounced veneration of nature but because of the much larger population and the restricted space available for each individual different considerations apply. Moreover, the impact of religions differs with Sweden, because of its history, markedly influenced by its Lutheran heritage, doing away with a State church as late as 2000, and Japan instead applying a much wider tolerance reflecting the diversity of polytheistic religions defining its culture for a long time. The differences between the cultures of the two countries are also apparent from their national flags. The Japanese flag has the red sun on a white background where the Swedish flag has a yellow cross — a Christian symbol — against a medium blue background. Whereas the Japanese celebrate the rising sun — *ex oriente lux*; light come from the east — the Swedes enjoy the end of a working day, with Luther sitting on their shoulder, and therefore enjoy more the nostalgic moment of the setting sun — *ex occidente flux*; the deed comes from the west. The discipline and ambitions of both Japan and Sweden when it comes to the development of science are very high. The future will tell if the results obtained will be mostly high quality predictable findings or if they will also include occasional paradigmatic discoveries recognized by Nobel Prizes. At the beginning of the 21st century Japan with its 14 times larger population than Sweden has had its shares of Nobel laureates, whereas Sweden is still waiting for its next recipient.

In my own endeavors I have appreciated both the sunsets and sunrises. During the third through fifth decades of my life I did all my writing at night starting at about 10 p.m. when the house was quiet. There was always the challenge of reaching the goal set. The traditional scientific article was divided into a summary, introduction, material and methods, experimental (results), discussion, acknowledgments and a reference list. The goal could be to finish one or more of these parts of a manuscript. If the proper degree of concentration developed it was easy to lose all sense of the passing of time. In this state of flow the goal might have been reached four to five hours later. If it happened to be a May spring morning it was a precious feeling to take a few minutes in the hammock in the garden, enjoying the light of the rising sun in this northern part of the world before going to bed for a short and intense sleep. After a night shift a Swede too can appreciate the rising sun.

We will now return to the issue of whether it is the scientist himself who drives his creative environment or if there are external forces that push the accumulation of knowledge in human civilizations. What is the role of curiosity of the individual?

Internalism and Externalism

The natural sciences have a proud history of being accumulative. The situation is not the same for humanistic sciences, although branches of them may pass through major transformative transitions. The already introduced concept of paradigmatic shift, like the Copernican, Newtonian, Darwinian and the DNA revolution, cannot be applied in a strictly comparative way to these kinds of sciences. Still there is a need for communication between these qualitatively different categories of sciences as emphasized by C. P. Snow in 1959 in a lecture on *The Two Cultures*. Bernal (Chapter 7) was a good friend of Snow and they had many opportunities to discuss the driving force behind natural sciences. One possibility was that developments of science were driven solely from within the researcher by curiosity, perseverance, skill and heterodox thinking. The alternative was that science was driven by the surrounding societal and economical environment. As separate entities these two schools, or rather models, are referred to as *internalism* and *externalism*. The extreme form of externalism included dogmatic Marxism, for which Bernal may have argued — see his four books on *Science in history*, which include subtitles like *The Emergence of Science*, *The Scientific and Industrial Revolution*, *The Natural Sciences in Our Time* and *The Social Sciences: Conclusion*. The worst form of externalism is the proposal that scientific data represent social constructs lacking the requirement of proven causation or objective validation. Of course if one thinks that the belief in gravity is a social construct one can always test this by jumping out of the window. One consequence of the prevailing Marxist dogmatic attitude in the former Soviet Union was the Lysenko affair, as discussed briefly in the context of Hašek in Chapter 2.

The truth obviously must be that none of the extreme attitudes can provide a full explanation. In fact the situation is much more complex and needs to be discussed in relation to both the character of the scientific endeavor and also to the source of money for the research. The character of science ranges from a fundamental basic science, developed by discoveries of different order of magnitudes to highly applied science. The latter form of science shares a border with developmental work, which, because its outcome can be foretold, should not be listed under science. It needs to be repeated emphatically that science *is not* a predictable venture. Basic science is irrevocably dependent on the qualities that characterize curiosity-driven endeavors, already cited above. A great discovery, like the identification of the periodic system by Dmitri Mendeleev discussed in Chapter 5, provided a unique opportunity to make predictions. The complete table of 92 naturally occurring elements was not finished until in the 1940s, 70 years after it was originally proposed.

The relative importance of externalism versus internalism increases the more of an applied character a certain science has. This is also reflected in the source of financial resources that allows a particular kind of research to be pursued. There are three sources; governmental taxation-derived money; private means deposited in a foundation and industrial financial resources. Together they support the wide-ranging scale of different forms of science extending from very fundamental to highly applied developmental work. The relations are not defined by a rigid matrix, since, for example fundamental research may sometimes be pursued within an industrial setting, as exemplified by the Bell Laboratories in the mid-20th century[12]. The Bell Labs for short were previously a division of the American Telephone and Telegraph Company. Researchers at Bell Labs developed radio astronomy, the transistor, the laser, information theory etc. Their achievements were recognized by seven Nobel Prizes.

Another way of shunting industry money into basic science work is to use industrial returns for the establishment of a foundation. A shining example is the Rockefeller Foundation[13] and its establishment of the Rockefeller Institute, later called University. A more recent example is the private research establishment that supports the J. Craig Venter Institute (JCVI), which I know well since it is my responsibility to be the vice-chairman of its Board of Trustees. The money that Venter received when he stepped down as President of the company Celera, which he had developed as a vehicle to sequence the fruit fly and the human genome, was used to establish a foundation which has formed the basis for the partial management of JCVI. This private money allowed investment into research projects which might not be granted support by governmental or by other private foundation sources. When Venter and his collaborators published the first full genome of a prokaryote, *Haemophilus influenza*, in 1995, they had just been informed about the rejection of their grant application to the National Institutes of Health in Bethesda, MD. It had been judged that the project was not possible to realize. There are two major eyes of needles to pass through in the sciencific endeavors. One is to get grant money to pursue the selected science and the other is to get heterodox data published. The problems related to the latter were briefly referred to in Chapter 5 (p. 212).

A discussion of the character of research is important also in the context of Nobel Prizes in the natural sciences. The reason is that the prizes prioritize *discoveries* made by basic research studies, but in some cases they may also recognize more applied science, since an *invention* may form the basis for an award in physics and an *improvement* may be recognized by a prize in chemistry.

One may ask in this context if a discovery may rank qualitatively higher than the other two possible motivations for a prize. Intuitively this might be so but there is no formal motivation for such an attitude. This is a kind of discussion which might have had relevance for the deliberations of a prize either to Perutz and Kendrew or to Watson, Crick and Wilkins. As was discussed in Chapter 7, Perutz's and Kendrew's contributions were not considered to represent a discovery, but rather an improvement, and in spite of this it was prioritized *before* the discovery of the DNA double-helix structure by the chemistry committee in 1962.

As already indicated it is not a straightforward issue to judge the relative role of the two principal models developed by historians, internalism and externalism in scientific endeavors. The balance of importance is dependent on the nature of the research pursued. A generalizing example of a more poised position can be found in publications by one of the authorities on social sciences Robert K. Merton, mentioned in my previous book[2]. Merton referred to Marxist presentations of history as vulgar and presented himself a special model of relations anchored in social sciences, called the Science-Technology-Society model. The unique contributions of selected individuals and certain environmental and societal conditions have allowed the advance of science by leaps. It is a truism to conclude that Science and Technology are the prime movers in modern society and that we ought to try to understand the essence of their nature.

Science and Politics

The organizational structure of research departments to a large extent depends on how they are embedded in institutional environments. In most countries research is mainly supported by tax revenues. This generally leads to the development of highly institutional organizations with a relatively rigid structure. By way of contrast some of the private elite universities and research institutes in the United States have a weaker institutional environment, which sometimes correlates with a relatively higher production of major discoveries[13]. Powerful private research institutions are also found in other countries, like the Max Planck Institutes in Germany. Disregarding the institutional organization one can say that scientists often have a uniquely privileged situation. They can satisfy their curiosity and independently build new knowledge and at the same time receive a salary for their efforts. It behooves the scientist to acknowledge this favored situation and be grateful to those ultimately responsible for this —

politicians in the case of tax revenues and managers of trusts and foundations in other cases. It is the unconventional and often high-risk research that may give the best return, but, as has been repeatedly stressed, the emergence of major discoveries, by definition, is not predictable.

A relationship of trust must be established between scientists and politicians so that inappropriate dependences do not develop. It is not an uncommon situation when politicians feel that they should direct the orientation of a certain sector of research. Thus for example they may want, not unsurprisingly in our present times, to prioritize special sectors like environmental or energy research. This may be accepted provided that the criteria on quality and originality remain unaltered. However, not infrequently, the criteria applied are less rigorous with the result that opportunistic and mediocre research will be pursued. It is ideas and not money that should guide research.

In Chapter 2 we discussed how Hašek adjusted his approach to science to satisfy the political wish that Lysenkoism should prevail. In this case it was the scientist who erred and his opportunism temporarily gave him privileged conditions for his research. In the end he was at loss when he was rejected by the political establishment. A detestable particular situation of expression of political power is when scientists of a certain ethnic background are excluded from the scientific community. The situation which applied to people of Jewish ethnic background in Nazi Germany was an obvious and unforgettable example. This kind of situation is referred to in a number of cases in this book, in particular in Chapter 5. It has taken a long time for Germany to recover its once very dominant influence on the development of the sciences[11].

Discussions of priority and rivalry between research groups are recurrent themes in this book and they represent a challenge that Nobel committees have to manage. When Gallo and collaborators had developed a test that could be used to screen blood for the presence of antibodies against HIV (Chapter 3) it was advised by the NIH that the test should be patented. This was the first time that Gallo's group had experience of such a procedure. The patent was used for non-exclusive licensing. It was then learnt that Montagnier's group at the Pasteur Institute in Paris had also submitted a patent, in fact a few months earlier than the NIH group. The test was of a different kind and of less practical value. The first attempts at reconciliation between the two groups aiming at a sharing of revenues failed. Never-ending lawsuits as it seemed were pursued until the matter was settled in 1987. Prior to that Jonas Salk, the polio vaccine pioneer (Ref. 2, Chapter 5) had been involved in shuttle diplomacy of a Kissinger mode. Gallo and Montagnier managed to agree on formulating a joint historical description of the discovery of the virus, which was published in the journal *Nature*. This resolved the rivalry situation and offered a resolution to the conflict. The top politicians of the two countries at the time, the French premier Jacques Chirac and President Reagan, sealed the agreement when Chirac was visiting the White House. In the end only a minor fraction of the revenues were collected by the two institutions and the scientists involved. The main part was used to build up the World Aids Foundation. This foundation is associated with the NIH and provides support for research and education relating to AIDS in the developing world. The Nobel Prize in physiology or medicine in 2008 for the discovery of HIV was a challenge to the truce established between Gallo's and Montagnier's laboratories. Diverging opinions on the scientists to be included in the prize were expressed by a number of scientists, including also some influential Swedish researchers and published in *Science*. In this case the committee decided to use a narrow definition of the discovery, not considering its consequences. The proper delimitation of a discovery is an eternally recurring theme of relevance to Nobel committees[2], as discussed repeatedly.

Seeds and Deeds

There are only two forms of immortality of an individual. If one is fortunate enough to have offspring (see picture on p. 402) shows my wife's and my three children, to whom this book is dedicated) the genes will continue to dance in a potentially unlimited number of consecutive generations. The information carried by DNA may survive through time eternal. The second way to immortality is to contribute knowledge that survives for the future. This is an area where the contributions by Nobel laureates are particularly apparent and important. Their deeds can make them immortal. Watson and Crick represent a shining example. Their revelation of the structure of DNA became a central part of the *cultural* inheritance that has been so uniquely developed and expressed by modern man and his civilization.

The position of an individual in relation to preceding and posterior generations can be imagined as located to the narrow neck connecting the two globular parts of the traditional hour-glass. The numbers of genes that transitorily represent the individual derive from a huge number of genomes of previous ancestors. As can be appreciated from the story about the requested reward to the inventor of the game chess — one seed for the first square, two for the next, four for the third, eight for the fourth, etc. — the power of two results in a rapid expansion towards huge numbers. All the grains in the world would be required to fill just a fraction of all the 64 squares of the chessboard. Thus, in the case of genes, for a single individual there are more than thousand individuals living some 300 years back in time who contribute to the DNA of his genome. And as a mirror image the genes of the individual potentially may spread among the same number of individuals some three hundred years hence. Of course reproduction strategies can influence the relative representation of genes from a single individual among the population at large. It has been estimated that genes from Genghis Khan are represented in one of 200 modern men.

Sand as a metaphor for life took on a special meaning for me on a beach at the lonely Ascension Island on the Southern mid-Atlantic ridge. This island, visited in 2005, was the second to last harbor for Craig Venter's sailing yacht Sorcerer II in her global circumnavigation to sample all microscopic life in oceans using the metagenomic DNA technology. When stretching out on one of the beaches of the island to view the elegant and equilibristic flights of frigate birds I noticed that the sand in contrast to normal quartz sand stuck much more firmly to my skin. It turned out to be composed of finely ground organic material, such as corals and shellfish. This DNA-containing kind of sand readily stimulated an association to the well-known poem by William Blake (1757–1827):

> To see a World in a Grain of Sand
> And a Heaven in a Wild Flower,
> Hold Infinity in the palm of your hand
> And Eternity in an hour.

Sand as a metaphor in the discussion of existential problems has also been used by Ronald Dworkin, a professor of law and philosophy in New York. He finished his book *Justice for Hedgehogs*[14] in the following way:

> Without dignity our lives are only blinks of duration. But if we manage to lead a good life well, we create something more. We write a subscript to our mortality. We make our lives tiny diamonds in the cosmic sand.

The reading of the books of life by use of the rapidly advancing techniques of sequencing of DNA is dramatically changing our insights into biology and also our daily life. We accumulate new understandings of the diversity of species and their relationships to each other. However, determining the order of bases in a certain DNA also has many other important uses; paternity issues can now be categorically settled, perpetrators and victims in criminal cases can be revealed and not the least this kind of analysis can be used in archeological contexts to trace our history. Recently it has been demonstrated that humans, *homo sapiens*, who had moved out of Africa some 60,000 years ago, have had sexual contacts with their relative, the now extinct species of hominids, the Neanderthal people. Our genome contains some 1–4% Neanderthal DNA. Our relatives who remained in Africa have no such DNA.

A special aspect of the immortality of an individual is the case when cells from a person have been allowed to replicate in the laboratory. Normally the cells subjected to such artificial cultivation outside the body show a trait of senescence. They eventually stop dividing after a number of consecutive transfers between cultivation vessels, as if they had an inbuilt clock. However, under particular conditions they may take on immortality. A particular case was the so called HeLa cells from a cancer of the African–American woman Henrietta Lacks, discussed in a recent book[15]. These HeLa cells have an unlimited capacity to divide. They have therefore become a convenient object of study by cell biologists. lt has been estimated that scientists have grown as much as 20 tons of her cells, although this must be a wild guess, and there are 11,000 patents involving HeLa cells. Another aspect of immortality is the technique of cloning, first applied to sheep, the famous Dolly. The technique of cloning which in principle can be used for mammals in general by definition also could be developed for use in humans. Obvious ethical barriers prevent such an application, but what about the favorite pet dog?

In his Nobel lecture on December 8 in 2012 at the Karolinska Institute Shinya Yamanaka described his work on reversing a cell to a stem cell stage by activation of a few genes. On one of the slides the word "immortality" by a Freudian slip had become "immorality". Having a healthy sense of humor Yamanaka took this in his stride. Although fortunately physical immortality of the life of an individual cannot be achieved, it is possible to influence longevity by choice of lifestyle. Thus moral issues are of importance. It has turned out that the best stepping stone to a long life is wide reaching knowledge that implicitly also allows choices of life style. Just to finish a PhD has been documented to add an average of three months to the average life span of an individual. Hence not surprisingly Nobel laureates have a long life. One *grande dame* among female Nobelists, Rita Levi-Montalcini died in 2012 at the age of 103. The Nobel laureates are people privileged with possibilities to search for new knowledge under conditions which they to a large extent have under their own control. Knowledge gives happiness and happiness contributes to a long life. So what about candidates for a Nobel Prize who never received one? There is in fact some evidence that their life span may be somewhat shorter than those who did receive the prize. Nevertheless this effect should be marginal and hence not detract from the possibility of a rich life as a scientist, also in the case when the results of the work have not become recognized by a Nobel Prize.

Since choice of lifestyle is very important for the life span of an individual one may ask to what extent characterization of our genome might provide valuable information guiding us in this endeavor. The most extensively analyzed genome is that of Craig Venter. In his biography *A Life Decoded*[16] one can find examples of insights that can be of value in selecting a style of life. However, as discussed at the end of Chapter 8, the expanded understanding of the complexity of the genome with its structural and regulatory genes focusing either on protein and RNA products makes it difficult to draw any simplified and general conclusions. We need more knowledge before we can extract validated information of practical use from the analysis of our genomes. Because of the rapidly improving possibilities for sequencing genomes at high speed and at a low cost we can anticipate having a lot of new critical information in the near future. When a number of scientists actively participating in the Nobel Week Dialogue in December 2012 (p. 387) were asked if they would like to have their genome sequenced, most of them said no. This attitude may change as the field advances. However, to repeat, the search for new knowledge by itself provides for a stimulating life and hence also one of a longer duration. As Thomas Jefferson said "knowledge indeed is a desirable, a lovely possession". And so life will go on — towards new discoveries allowing us to improve our care for the temporary existence that is fortuitously given to us.

References

Chapter 1

1. Burnet, M. (1969) *Changing Patterns. An Atypical Autobiography.* American Elsevier Publishing, New York.
2. Sexton, C. (1999) *Burnet. A Life, 2nd ed.* Oxford University Press.
3. Norrby, E. (2010) *Nobel Prizes and Life Sciences.* World Scientific, Singapore.
4. Lewis, S. (1925) *Arrowsmith.* Buccaneer Books, New York.
5. Burnet, F. M. (1945) *Virus as Organism: Evolutionary and Ecological Aspects of Some Human Diseases.* Harvard University Press.
6. Burnet, F. M. (1955) *Viruses and Man, 2nd ed.* Penguin Books, Harmondworth, Middlesex.
7. Burnet, F. M. (1934) The Bacteriophages. *Biol. Rev.* 6:332–350.
8. Stent, G. S. (1963) *Molecular Biology of Bacterial Viruses.* W. H. Freeman, San Francisco.
9. Brock, T. D. (1990) *The Emergence of Bacterial Genetics.* Cold Spring Harbor Press, New York.
10. Schlesinger, M. (1934) Zur frage der chemischen zusammensetzung des bakteriophagen. *Biochemische Zeitschrift* 273:306–311.
11. Fenner, F. and Ratcliffe, F. N. (1965) *Myxomatosis.* Cambridge University Press, Cambridge.
12. Stolt, C.-M. (2002) Moniz, lobotomy, and the 1949 Nobel Prize. In *Historical Studies in the Nobel Archives. The Prizes in Science and Medicine* (Ed. Crawford, E.) Universal Academy Press, Tokyo.
13. Burnet, F. M. (1959) *The Clonal Selection Theory of Acquired Immunity.* Vanderbilt University Press, Nashville.
14. Klein, G. (1984) … *i stället för hemland* (in Swedish). Bonniers, Stockholm.
15. Medawar, P. (1982) *Pluto's Republic.* Incorporating *The Art of the Soluble* and *Induction and Intuition in Scientific Thought.* Oxford University Press, USA.
16. Murphy, F. A. (2012) *The Foundations of Virology.* Infinity Publishing, West Conshohocken, PA.

Chapter 2

1. Lagerkvist, U. (2003) *Pioneers of Microbiology and the Nobel Prize.* World Scientific, Singapore.
2. Norrby, E. (2010) *Nobel Prizes and Life Sciences.* World Scientific, Singapore.
3. Burnet, F. M. and Fenner, F. (1949) *The Production of Antibodies, 2nd ed.* Walter and Eliza Hall Institute for Medical Research in Pathology and Medicine. Monograph No. 1, Macmillan, Melbourne.
4. Burnet, M. (1969) *Changing Patterns. An Atypical Autobiography.* American Elsevier Publishing, New York.
5. Huxley, A. (2006) *Brave New World.* Harper Perennial Modern Classics; reprint edition.
6. Burnet, F. M. (1957) A modification of Jerne's theory of antibody production using the concept of clonal selection. *Aust. J. Sci.* 20:67–72.
7. Medawar, P. B. (1986) *Memoirs of a Thinking Radish: An Autobiography.* Oxford University Press, Oxford.
8. Medawar, J. (1991) *A Very Decided Preference. Life with Peter Medawar.* Oxford University Press, Oxford.
9. Gibson, T. and Medawar, P. B. (1943) The fate of skin homografts in man. *J. Anat.* 77:299–310.
10. Anderson, D., Billingham, R. E., Lampkin, G. H., and Medawar P. B. (1951) The use of skin grafting to distinguish between monozygotic and dizygotic twins in cattle. *Heredity* 5:379–397.
11. Snell, G. D., Winn, H. J., Stimpfling, J. H., and Parker, S. J. (1957) The homograft reaction. *Ann. Rev. Microbiol.* 11:439–458.
12. Medawar, P. B. (1990) *The Threat and the Glory. Reflections on Science and Scientists.* Oxford University Press, Oxford.
13. Billingham, R. E., Brent, L., and Medawar, P. B. (1953) Actively induced tolerance of foreign cells. *Nature* 172:603-606.
14. Ivanyi, J. (2003) Milan Hašek and the discovery of immunological tolerance. *Nature Reviews* 3:591-597.
15. Billingham, R. E., Brent, L., and Medawar, P. B. (1956) The antigenic stimulus in transplantation immunity. *Nature* 178:514–519.
16. Doherty, P. (2006) *The Beginner's Guide to Winning the Nobel Prize. A Life in Science.* Columbia University Press, New York.
17. Burnet, F. M. (1959) *The Clonal Selection Theory of Acquired Immunity.* Vanderbilt University Press, Nashville.
18. Burnet, F. M. (1945) *Virus as Organism: Evolutionary and Ecological Aspects of Some Human Virus Diseases.* Harvard University Press.
19. Burnet, F. M. (1961) Immunological recognition of self. In *Les Prix Nobel en 1960.* Imprimerie Royale, P. A. Norstedt & Söner, pp. 113–124.
20. Medawar, P. B. (1961) Immunological tolerance. In *Les Prix Nobel en 1960.* Imprimerie Royal, P. A. Norstedt & Söner, pp. 125–134.
21. Sexton, C. (1999) *Burnet. A Life., 2nd ed.* Oxford University Press.
22. Burnet, F. M. (1955) *Viruses and Man, 2nd ed.* Penguin Books, Harmondworth, Middlesex.

23. Burnet, F. M. (1978) *Endurance of Life. The Implications of Genetics for Human Life.* Cambridge University Press, London.
24. Burnet, F. M. (1979) *Credo and Comment: A Scientist Reflects.* Melbourne University Press, Melbourne.
25. Medawar, P. B. (1957) *The Uniqueness of the Individual.* Dover Publications.
26. Medawar, P. B. (1982) *Pluto's Republic.* Incorporating *The Art of the Soluble* and *Induction and Intuition in Scientific Thought.* Oxford University Press, USA.
27. Medawar, P. B. (1988) *The Limits of Science. Paperback.* Oxford University Press, USA.
28. Medawar, P. B. (1981) *Advice to a Young Scientist* (Alfred P. Sloan Foundation Series). Basic Books, New York.
29. Medawar, P. B. and Medawar, J. (1983) *Aristotle to Zoos: A Philosophical Dictionary of Biology.* Harvard University Press, Cambridge, Mass.
30. Thomas, L. (1984) *Late Night Thoughts on Listening to Mahler's Ninth Symphony.* Bantam Books, New York.
31. Ohlmarks, Åke (1969) *Nobelpristagarna* (in Swedish). (Ed. Forssell, G. B.) F. Beck & Son, Stockholm.

Chapter 3

1. Miller, J. F. A. P. (2011) The golden anniversary of the thymus. *Nature Reviews Immunology* 11:489–495.
2. Martinez, C., Kersey, J., Papermaster, B. W., and Good, R. A. (1962) Skin homograft survival in thymectomized mice. *Proc. Soc. Exp. Biol. Med.* 109:193–196.
3. Arnason, B. G., Jankovic, B. D., and Waksman, B. H. (1962) Effect of thymetomy on "delayed" hypersensitivity reactions. *Nature* 194:99–100.
4. Möller, G. (1961) Demonstration of mouse isoantigens at the cellular level by the fluorescent antibody technique. *J. Exp. Med.* 121:415–434.
5. Medawar, P. B. (1986) *Memoirs of a Thinking Radish: An Autobiography.* American Elsevier Publishing, New York.
6. Medawar, P. B. (1990) *The Threat and the Glory. Reflections on Science and Scientists.* Oxford University Press, Oxford.
7. Zuckerman, H. (1996) *Scientific Elite. Nobel Laureates in the United States. New Edition with a New Introduction.* Transaction Publishers, New Brunswick.
8. Hollingsworth, J. R. and Hollingsworth, E. J. (2011) *Major Discoveries, Creativity, and the Dynamics of Science.* Complexity Design Society, Vol. 15. Remaprint, Vienna.
9. Norrby, E. (2010) *Nobel Prizes and Life Sciences.* World Scientific, Singapore.
10. Gardner, H., Czikszentmihalyi, M. and Damon, W. (2001) *Good Work: When Excellence and Ethics Meet.* New York, Basic Books.
11. Porter, R. R. (1973) Structural studies of immunoglobulins. In *Les Prix Nobel en 1972.* Imprimerie Royal, P. A. Norstedt & Söner, pp. 174–183.
12. Landsteiner, K. (1946) *The Specificity of Serological Reaction.* Harvard University Press, Cambridge.
13. Edelman, G. M. (1973) Antibody structure and molecular immunology. In *Les Prix Nobel en 1972*, Imprimerie Royal, P. A. Norstedt & Söner, pp. 147–170.

14. Ramel, S. (1994) *Pojken i Dörren. Minnen* (in Swedish). Atlantis, Stockholm, p. 247.
15. Vandvik, B. and Norrby, E. (1973) Oligoclonal IgG antibody response in the central nervous system to different measles virus antigens in subacute sclerosing panencephalitis. *Proc. Nat. Acad. Sci., USA* 70:1060–1063.
16. Köhler, G. and Milstein, C. (1975) Continuous culture of fused cells secreting antibody of predefined specificity. *Nature* 256:495–497.
17. Köhler, G. (1985) Derivation and diversification of monoclonal antibodies. In *Les Prix Nobel en 1984.* Almquist & Wiksell International, Stockholm, pp. 174–189.
18. Milstein, C. (1985) From the structure of antibodies to the diversification of the immune response. In *Les Prix Nobel en 1984.* Almquist & Wiksell International, Stockholm, pp. 194–216.
19. Norrby, E., Biberfeld, G., Chiodi, F., von Gegerfeldt, A., Nauclér, A., Parks, E., and Lerner, R. (1987) Discrimination between antibodies to HIV and to related retroviruses using site-directed serology. *Nature* 329:248–250.
20. Tonegawa, S. (1988) Somatic generation of immune diversity. In *Les Prix Nobel en 1987,* Almqvist & Wiksell International, Stockholm, pp. 203–227.
21. Dausset, J. (1981) Concepts passés, presents et futures sur le complexe majeur d'histocompatibilite de l'homme (HLA). In *Les Prix Nobel en 1980,* Almquist & Wiksell International, Stockholm, pp. 196–211.
22. Benacerraf, B. (1981) The role of MHC gene products in immune regulation and its relevance to alloreactivity. In *Les Prix Nobel en 1980,* Almquist & Wiksell International, Stockholm, pp. 165–191.
23. Doherty, P. (2006) *The Beginner's Guide to Winning the Nobel Prize. A Life in Science.* Columbia University Press, New York.
24. Klareskog, L. (1997) The Nobel Prize in Physiology or Medicine. In *Les Prix Nobel en 1996,* Almquist & Wiksell International, Stockholm, pp. 25–26.
25. Murphy, F. A. (2012) *The Foundations of Virology.* Infinity Publishing, West Conshohocken, PA.

Chapter 4

1. Olson, S. (2002) *Mapping Human History. Genes, Race, and our Common Origin.* Houghton Mifflin Company, Boston.
2. Oppenheimer, S. (2003) *Out of Africa's Eden. The Peopling of the World.* Jonathan Ball Publishers, Johannesburg.
3. Diamond, J. (1997) *Guns, Germs and Steel.* W. W. Norton, New York.
4. McNeill, W. H. (1976) *Plagues and Peoples.* Anchor Books, New York.
5. Boorstin, D. J. (1985) *The Discoverers. A History of Man's Search to Know His World and Himself.* Vintage Books, New York.
6. Mann, C. C. (2011) 1493. *Uncovering the New World Columbus Created.* Alfred A. Knopf, New York.
7. Norrby, E. (2010) *Nobel Prizes and Life Sciences.* World Scientific, Singapore.
8. Gibson, D. G., Glass, J. I., Lartigue, C. *et al.* (2010) Creation of a bacterial cell controlled only by a chemically synthesized genome. *Science* 329:52–56.
9. Murray, J. E. (1991) The first successful organ transplants in man. In *Les Prix Nobel 1990,* Almqvist & Wiksell International, Stockholm, pp. 204–216.

10. Murray, J. E. (1991) Autobiography. In *Les Prix Nobel en 1990*, Almquist & Wiksell International, Stockholm, pp. 201–203.
11. Thomas, E. D. (1991) Bone marrow transplantation — past, present and future. In *Les Prix Nobel en 1990*. Almqvist & Wiksell International, Stockholm, pp. 222–230.
12. Hargittai, I. (2011) *Drive and Curiosity. What Fuels the Passion for Science*. P. B. Prometeus Books, New York.
13. Elion, G. B. (1989) The purine path to chemotherapy. In *Les Prix Nobel en 1988*, Almquist & Wiksell International, Stockholm, pp. 267–288.
14. Elion, G. B. (1989) Autobiography. In *Les Prix Nobel en 1988*. Almquist & Wiksell International, Stockholm, pp. 263–266.
15. zur Hausen, H. (2009) The search for infectious causes of human cancers: Where and why. In *Les Prix Nobel en 2008*, Edita Norstedts tryckeri, Stockholm, pp. 223–243.
16. Murphy, F. A. (2012) *The Foundations of Virology*. Infinity Publishing, West Conshohocken, PA.

Chapter 5

1. Levi, H. (1985) *George de Hevesy. Life and Work*. Rhodos, Copenhagen.
2. Niese, S. (2009) *Georg von Hevesy*. Wissenschaftler ohne Grenzen (in German). Principal Verlag, Münster, Westfahlen.
3. Marx, G. (2001) *The Voice of the Martians. Hungarian Scientists Who Shaped the 20th Century in the West.*, 3rd ed. Akadémiai Kiadó, Budapest.
4. McCagg, W. O. (1972) *Jewish Nobles and Geniuses in Modern Hungary*. Columbia University Press, New York.
5. Klein, G. (2011) *Jag återvänder aldrig. Essäer i förintelsens skugga* (in Swedish). Albert Bonnier, Stockholm.
6. Hevesy, G. (1962) *Adventures in Radioisotope Research*. 2 vols. Pergamon Press, London.
7. Hevesy, G. (1946) Some applications of isotope indicators. In *Les Prix Nobel en 1940–1946*. Imprimerie Royale, P. A. Norstedt & Söner, Stockholm, pp. 95–127.
8. Soddy, F. (1923) The origins of the conception of isotopes. In *Les Prix Nobel en 1921–1922*. Imprimerie Royal, P. A. Norstedt & Söner, Stockholm, pp. 1–29.
9. Pais, A. (1991) *Niels Bohr's Times, in Physics, Philosophy and Polity*. Clarendon Press, Oxford, p. 154.
10. Hevesy, G. and Paneth, F. (1913) RaD als "Indikator" des Bleis. *Z anorg. Chem.* 82:323.
11. Hevesy, G. and Paneth, F. (1923) *Lehrbuch der Radioaktivität*. Joh. Ambr. Barth, Leipzig.
12. Lagerkvist, U. (2012) *The Periodic Table and a Missed Nobel Prize in Chemistry*. World Scientific, Singapore.
13. Hevesy, G. (1923) On the new element hafnium. *Chemy. Ind.* 42:258.
14. Coster, D. and Hevesy, G. (1923) On the missing element of atomic number 72. *Nature* 111:79.
15. Bohr, N. (1923) Om atomers bygning (in Danish). *Les Prix Nobel en 1921–1922*. Imprimerie Royale, P. A. Norstedt & Söner, Stockholm, pp. 1–37.

16. Friedman, R. M. (2001) *The Politics of Excellence: Behind the Nobel Prize in Science.* Henry Holt & Co., New York.
17. Arrhenius, G. and Levi, H. (1988) *The Era of Cosmochemistry and Geochemistry. George de Hevesy 1885–1966.* Festschrift (ed. Marx, G.) Akademiai Kiado, Budapest, pp. 11–36.
18. Hevesy, G. (1923) Jordens alder (in Danish) Medd. *Fra Dansk Geol. Forening*, p. 13.
19. Hevesy, G. (1929) Das Alter der Grundstoffe. Vortrag in der Freiburger Wissensch. *Ges. Heft* 17.
20. Hevesy, G. (1930) The Age of the Earth. *Science* 77:509.
21. Hevesy, G., Hofer, E., and Krogh, A. (1935) The permeability of skin of frogs to water, as determined by D_2O and H_2O. *Scand. Arch. Physiol.* 72:199.
22. Norrby, E. (2010) *Nobel Prizes and Life Sciences.* World Scientific, pp. 155–157.
23. Chievitz, O. and de Hevesy, G. (1935) Radioactive indicators in the study of phosphorous metabolism in rats. *Nature* 136:754.
24. Hevesy, G. (1958) A scientific career. *Perspec. Biol. Med.* I:345.
25. Westgren, A. (1946) Det kemiska Nobelpriset för år 1943 (in Swedish and also in French). *Les Prix Nobel en 1940–1944.* Imprimerie Royale, P. A. Norstedt & Söner, Stockholm, pp. 15–22.
26. Hevesy, P. (1965) *The Unification of the World: Proposals of a Diplomatist.* Pergamon Press, Oxford.
27. Kovács, L. and Kovács, L., Jr. *George de Hevesy 1885–1966.* Berzsenyi College, Szombathely/Hungary.
28. Norrby, E., Magnusson, P., Falksveden, L-G., and Grönberg, M. (1964) Separation of measles virus components by equilibrium centrifugation in CsCl gradients. II. Studies of the large and small hemagglutinin. *Arch. Ges. Virusforsch.* 14:462-473.
29. Yalow, R. S. (1977) Radioimmunoassay. A probe for the fine structure of biological systems. *Les Prix Nobel en 1977.* Almqvist & Wiksell International, Stockholm, pp. 447–468.
30. Norrby, E., Chen, S.-N., Togashi, T., Sheshberadaran, H., and Johnson, K. P. (1982) Five measles virus antigens demonstrated by use of mouse hybridoma antibodies in productively infected tissue culture cells. *Arch. Virol.* 71:1-11.
31. Libby, W. F. (1961) Radiocarbon dating. In *Les Prix Nobel en 1960.* Imprimerie Royale. P. A. Norstedt & Söner. Stockholm, pp. 95–112.
32. Bergmann, O., Bhardwaj, R. D., Bernard, S., *et al.* (2009) Evidence for cardiomyocyte renewal in humans. *Science* 324:98-102.

Chapter 6

1. Ratliff, F. (1976) *Georg von Békésy 1899–1972.* Biographical Memoir. National Academy of Sciences, Washington, D.C.
2. Ratliff, F. (1974) *Georg von Békésy. His Life, His Work, and His "Friends".* Preface to the catalogue of the exhibition at the East Asiatic Museum in Stockholm of T*he Georg von Békésy Collection — Selected Objects from the Collection of Georg Von Békésy Bequeathed to the Nobel Foundation.* Ed. Jan Wirgin. Allhems Förlag, Malmö, pp. 9–26.

3. Marx, G. (2001) *The Voice of the Martians. Hungarian Scientists Who Shaped the 20th Century in the West, 3rd ed.* Akadémiai Kiadó, Budapest, pp. 341–355.
4. Von Bekesy, G. (1962) Concerning the pleasures of observing, and the mechanics of the inner ear. In *Les Prix Nobel en 1961*, Imprimerie Royale, P. A. Norstedt & Söner, Stockholm, pp. 184–208.
5. Von Békésy, G. (1928). Zur theorie des Hörens. Die Schwingungsform der Basilarmembran. *Physikalische Zeitschrift* 29:793–810.
6. Norrby, E. (2010) *Nobel Prizes and Life Sciences.* World Scientific, p. 23.
7. Hargittai, I. (2000). George A. Olah. Chapter 21 in *Candid Science: Conversations with Famous chemists.* World Scientific. Singapore, pp. 271–283.
8. Von Békésy, G. (1956) Current status of theories of hearing. *Science* 123:779–783.
9. Von Békésy, G. (1957) The ear. *Scientific American* 197:66–78.
10. Bernhard, C. G. (2000) *Huset på höjden. Självbiografiska Anteckningar* (in Swedish). Atlantis, Stockholm, pp. 335–340.
11. Bernhard, C. G. (1962). Presentation speech for the Nobel Prize for physiology or medicine 1961. In *Les Prix Nobel en 1961*, Imprimerie Royale, P. A. Norstedt & Söner, Stockholm, pp. 34–36.
12. Von Békésy, G. (1962) Speech at the Nobel banquet 1961. In *Les Prix Nobel en 1961*, Imprimerie Royale, P. A. Norstedt & Söner, Stockholm, pp. 50–51.
13. Söderlind, U. (2010) *The Nobel Banquets. A Century of Culinary History (1901-2001).* World Scientific, Singapore.
14. Friedman, R. M. (2001) *The Politics of Excellence.* Henry Holt, New York.
15. Ramel S. (1994) *Pojken I dörren. Minnen.* (in Swedish). Atlantis, Stockholm, pp. 260–263.
16. Wirgin J. (1974). *The Georg von Békésy Collection.* Allhems Förlag, Malmö. copyright The Nobel Foundation, Stockholm.
17. Ohlmarks, Å. (1969) *Nobelpristagarna* (in Swedish; ed. Forssell, G. B.) F. Beck & Son, Stockholm.

Chapter 7

1. Liljas, A. (2012) Background to the Nobel Prizes to the Braggs. *Acta Cryst.* A69:10–15.
2. Hunter, G. K. (2004) *Light Is a Messenger: The Life and Science of William Lawrence Bragg.* Oxford University Press.
3. Brown, A. (2005) *J. D. Bernal: The Sage of Science.* Oxford University Press.
4. Perutz, M. F. (1963). X-ray analysis of haemoglobin. In *Les Prix Nobel en 1962.* Imprimerie Royale, P. A. Norstedt & Söner, Stockholm, pp. 82–102.
5. Norrby, E. (2010) *Nobel Prizes and Life Sciences.* World Scientific, Singapore.
6. Crowfoot Hodgkin, D. (1965) The X-ray analysis of complicated molecules. In *Les Prix Nobel en 1964.* Imprimerie Royale, P. A. Norstedt & Söner, Stockholm, pp. 157–178.
7. Ferry, G. (1998) *Dorothy Hodgkin: A Life.* Granta Books, London
8. Ferry, G. (2007) *Max Perutz and the Secret of Life.* Chatto & Windus, London.
9. Pauling, L. (1960) *The Nature of the Chemical Bond and the Structure of Molecules,* new edition, Cornell University Press.

10. Hargittai, I. (2002) *Candid Science II. Conversations with Famous Biomedical Scientists*. Imperial College Press, London.
11. Hager, T. (1995) *Force of Nature. The Life of Linus Pauling*. Simon and Schuster, New York.
12. Hägg, G. (1955) In *Les Prix Nobel en 1954*. Imprimerie Royale, P. A. Norstedt & Söner, Stockholm, pp. 29–32.
13. Pauling, L. (1955) Modern structural chemistry. In *Les Prix Nobel en 1954*. Imprimerie Royale, P. A. Norstedt & Söner, Stockholm, pp. 91–99
14. Perutz, M. (2003) *I wish I'd Made You Angry Earlier: Essays on Science, Scientists and Humanity*, expanded edition, Cold Spring Harbor Laboratory Press.
15. Kendrew, J. C. (1963) Myoglobin and the structure of proteins. In *Les Prix Nobel en 1962*. Imprimerie Royale, P. A. Norstedt & Söner, Stockholm, pp. 103–125.
16. Westgren, A. (1972) *The Prize in Chemistry*. In *Nobel, the Man and His Prizes*, 3rd ed. Odelberg, W. Elsevier, New York, pp. 119–133.
17. Hargittai, I. (2007) *The DNA Doctor. Candid Conversations with James D. Watson*. World Scientific, p. 61.
18. Hägg, G. (1965) The introductory speech to the 1964 Nobel Prize in chemistry. In *Les Prix Nobel en 1964*. Imprimerie Royale, P. A. Norstedt & Söner, pp. 30–33.
19. Hägg, G. (1963) The introductory speech to the 1962 Nobel Prize in chemistry. In *Les Prix Nobel en 1962*. Imprimerie Royale, P. A. Norstedt & Söner, pp. 30–33.
20. Finch, J. (2008) *A Nobel Fellow on Every Floor. A History of the Medical Research Council Laboratory of Molecular Biology*. Icon Books, Cambridge.
21. Perutz, M. (1991) *Is Science Necessary? Essays on Science and Scientists*. Oxford University Press.
22. Ohlmarks, Å. (1969) *Nobelpristagarna* (in Swedish; ed. Forssell, G. B.) F. Beck & Son, Stockholm.

Chapter 8

1. Crick, F. H. C. (1988) *What Mad Pursuit: A Personal View of Scientific Discovery*. Basic Books, New York.
2. Watson, J. D. and Crick, F. H. C. (1953) Molecular structure of nucleic acids. A structure for deoxyribose nucleic acid. *Nature* 171:737–738.
3. Olby, R. (1974) *The Path to the Double Helix: The Discovery of DNA*. Macmillan, London; revised edition (1994), Dover, New York.
4. Judson, H. (1996) *The Eighth Day of Creation: Makers of the Revolution in Biology*, expanded edition. Cold Spring Harbor laboratory Press, New York.
5. Watson, J. D. (1968) *The Double Helix. A Personal Account of the Discovery of the Structure of DNA*. Weidenfeld and Nicolson, London.
6. Wilkins, M. (2003) *The Third Man and the Double Helix: The Autobiography of Maurice Wilkins*. Oxford University Press, Oxford.
7. Schrödinger, E. (1944) *What Is Life? The Physical Aspect of the Living Cell*. Cambridge University Press, Cambridge.
8. Olby, R. (2009) *Francis Crick. Hunter of Life's Secrets*. Cold Spring Harbor Laboratory Press, New York.

9. Cochran, W., Crick, R. H. C., and Vand, V. (1952) Structure of synthetic polypeptides I. The transform of atoms on a helix. *Acta Crystallogr.* 5:581–586.
10. Hager, T. (1995) *Force of Nature. The Life of Linus Pauling.* Simon & Schuster, New York.
11. Roberts, R. M. (1989) *Serendipity. Accidental Discoveries in Science.* John Wiley & Sons, New York.
12. Wilkins, M. H. F., Stokes, A. R., and Wilson, H. R. (1953) Molecular structure of deoxypentose nucleic acids. *Nature* 171:738–740.
13. Franklin, R. E. and Gosling, R. G. (1953) Molecular configuration in sodium thymonucleate. *Nature* 171:740–741.
14. Watson, J. D. and Crick, F. H. C. (1953) Genetic implications of the structure of deoxyribonucleic acid. *Nature* 171:964–967.
15. Crick, F. H. C. and Watson, J. D. (1954) The complementary structure of deoxyribonucleic acid. *Proc. Royal Society* 223:80–96.
16. Norrby, E. (2010) *Nobel Prizes and Life Sciences.* World Scientific, Singapore.
17. Tatum, E. L. (1959) A case history in biological research. In *Les Prix Nobel en 1958.* Imprimerie Royale, P. A. Norstedt & Söner, Stockholm, pp. 160–169.
18. Lederberg, J. (1959) A view of genetics. In *Les Prix Nobel en 1958.* Imprimerie Royale, P. A. Norstedt & Söner, Stockholm, pp. 170–189.
19. Norrby, E. and Albertsson, P.-Å. (1960) Concentration of poliovirus by an aqueous polymer two-phase system. *Nature* 188:1047–1048.
20. Franklin, R. E. and Gosling, R. G. (1953) The structure of sodium thymonucleate fibres. I. The influence of the water content. *Acta Crystallogr.* 6:673–677.
21. Franklin, R. E. and Gosling, R. G. (1953) The structure of sodium thymonucleate fibres. II. The cylindrically symmetrical Patterson Function. *Acta Crystallogr.* 678–685.
22. Meselson, M. and Stahl, F. W. (1958) The replication of DNA in *Escherichia coli. Proc. Natl. Acad. Sci.*, 44:671–682.
23. Franklin, R. E. (1955) Structure of tobacco mosaic virus. *Nature* 175:379–382.
24. Crick, F. H. C. and Watson, J. D. (1956) The structure of small viruses. *Nature* 177:473–475.
25. Maddox, B. (2002) *Rosalind Franklin. The Dark Lady of DNA.* HarperCollins New York.
26. Sayre, A. (1975) *Rosalind Franklin and DNA.* W. W. Norton, New York.
27. Klug, A. (1968) Rosalind Franklin and the discovery of the structure of DNA. *Nature* 219:808–810 and 843–844.
28. Klug, A. (1974) Rosalind Franklin and the double helix. *Nature* 248:787–788.
29. Franklin, R. E. and Gosling, R. G. (1953) Evidence for a two-chain helix in crystalline structure of sodium deoxyribonucleate. *Nature* 172:156–157.
30. Franklin, R. E. and Gosling, R. G. (1955) The structure of sodium thymonucleate fibres. III. The three-dimensional Patterson function. *Acta Crystallogr.* 8:151–156.
31. Klug, A. (1983) Curriculum vitae. In *Les Prix Nobel en 1982.* Imprimerie Royale, P. A. Norstedt & Söner, Stockholm, pp. 89–92.
32. Finch, J. T. A. and Klug, A. (1959) Structure of poliomyelitis virus. *Nature* 183:476–477.
33. Hogle, J. M., Chow, M., and Filman, D. J. (1985) Three-dimensional structure of poliovirus at 2.9 Å resolution. *Science* 229:1358–1366.

34. Caspar, D. L. D. and Klug, A. (1962) Physical principles in the construction of regular viruses. *Cold Spring Harbor Symp.* 27:1–24.
35. Norrby, E. (1966) The relationship between the soluble antigens and the virion of adenovirus type 3. I. Morphological characteristics. *Virology* 28:236–248.
36. Virus taxonomy. *Ninth Report of the International Committee on Taxonomy of viruses.* (Eds. King, A. M. Q., Adams, M. J., Carstens, E. B., and Lefkowitz, M. J.) (2011) Academic Press, London.
37. Hunter, G. K. (2004) *Light Is a Messenger. The Life and Science of William Lawrence Bragg.* Oxford University Press, Oxford.
38. Wilkins, M. H. F. (1963) The molecular configuration of nucleic acids. In *Les Prix Nobel en 1962.* Imprimerie Royale, P. A. Norstedt & Söner, Stockholm, pp. 126–154.
39. Klug, A. (1983) From macromolecules to biological assemblies. In *Les Prix Nobel en 1982.* Imprimerie Royale, Norstedt & Söner, Stockholm, pp. 93–125.
40. Engström, A. V. (1963) Introductory speech to the Nobel Prize in physiology or medicine 1962. In *Les Prix Nobel en 1962.* Imprimerie Royale, P. A. Norstedt & Söner, Stockholm, pp. 38–40.
41. Crick, F. (1979) How to live with a golden helix. A DNA pioneer takes another look at his seminal discovery. *The Sciences.* Sep. pp. 6–9.
42. Watson, J. D. (2007) *Avoid Boring People. Lessons from a Life in Science.* Alfred A. Knopf, New York.
43. Crick, F. C. H. (1963) On the genetic code. In *Les Prix Nobel en 1962.* Imprimerie Royale, P. A. Norstedt & Söner, Stockholm, pp. 179–187.
44. Watson, J. D. (1963) The involvement of RNA in the synthesis of proteins. In *Les Prix Nobel en 1962.* Imprimerie Royale, P. A. Norstedt & Söner, Stockholm, pp. 155–178.
45. Watson, J. D. (2000) *A Passion for DNA: Genes, Genomes, and Society.* Cold Spring Harbor Laboratory Press, New York.
46. Watson, J. D. (2002) *Genes, Girls, and Gamow: After the Double Helix.* Oxford University Press, Oxford.
47. Watson, J. D. (with Andrew Berry) (2004) *DNA. The Secret of Life.* Arrow Books, London.
48. Hargittai, I. (2007) *The DNA Doctor. Candid Conversations with James D. Watson.* World Scientific, Singapore.
49. The ENCODE Project Consortium (2012) An integrated encyclopedia of DNA elements in the human genome. *Nature* 489:57–64.
50. Scherrer, K. and Jost, J. (2007) The gene and the genon concept: A functional and information-theory analysis. *Molecular Systems Biology* 3:87–98.
51. Darnell, J. (2011) *RNA. Life's Indispensible Molecule.* Cold Spring Harbor Laboratory Press, New York.
52. Murphy, F. A. (2012) *The Foundations of Virology.* Infinity Publishing, West Conshohocken, PA.
53. Ohlmarks, Å. (1969) *Nobelpristagarna* (in Swedish; Ed. Forssell, G. B.). F. Beck & Son, Stockholm.

Chapter 9

1. Kuhn, S. K. (1996) *Structure of Scientific Revolutions.* Chicago University Press, Chicago, Ill.
2. Norrby, E. (2010) *Nobel Prizes and Life Sciences.* World Scientific, Singapore.
3. Gleick, J. (1992) *Genius. The Life and Science of Richard Feynman.* Pantheon Books, New York.
4. Feynman, R. P. (1997) *Surely You're Joking, Mr Feynman.* W. W. Norton & Co., New York.
5. Miller, A. J. (1996) *Insight of Genius. Imaginary and Creativity in Science and Art.* Springer-Verlag, New York.
6. McManus, C. (2002) *Right Hand, Left Hand. The Origins of Asymmetry in Brains, Bodies, Atoms and Cultures.* Harvard University Press, Mass.
7. Murray, J. E. (1991) Autobiography. In *Les Prix Nobel en 1990.* Norstedts Tryckeri AB, Stockholm, pp. 201–203
8. Ramel, S. (1994) *Pojken i dörren. Minnen.* (in Swedish). Atlantis, Stockholm.
9. Csikszentmihalyi, M. (1990) *Flow: The Psychology of Optimal Experience.* Harper and Row, New York.
10. Meyers, M. A. (2012) *Prize Fight. The Race and the Rivalry to be the First in Science.* Palgrave Macmillan, New York.
11. Hollingsworth, J. R. and Gear, D. M. (2013) The rise and decline of hegemonic systems of scientific creativity in *Exceptional Creativity in Science and Technology. Individuals, Institutions and Innovations* (Ed. Robinson, A.). Templeton Press, West Conshohocken, PA, pp. 25–52.
12. Anderson, P. W. (2011) *More and Different: Notes from a Thoughtful Curmudgeon.* World Scientific, Singapore.
13. Hollingsworth, J. R. and Hollingsworth, E. J. (2011) *Major Discoveries, Creativity and the Dynamics of Science.* Remaprint, Wien.
14. Dworkin, R. (2011) *Justice for Hedgehogs.* Harvard University Press, Mass.
15. Skloot, R. (2011) *The Immortal Life of Henrietta Lacks.* Broadway, New York
16. Venter, J. C. (2007) *A Life Decoded. My Genome. My Life.* Penguin Group, New York.

Index

A

B

C

D

E

H

I

J

K

L

M

N

O

P

Q

R

S

W

X

Y

Z